A Textbook of Social Work

D0153654

Where did professional social work originate from? How effective are social work interpretations in the lives of vulnerable people?

A Textbook of Social Work provides a comprehensive discussion of social work practice and its evidence base. It strikes a balance between the need for social workers to understand the social, economic, cultural, psychological and interpersonal factors which give rise to clients' problems, and the need for them to know how best to respond with practical measures.

Divided into three parts, the text covers the history and development of social work as a movement and profession in the first part, and social work methods and approaches in the second. The final part looks at the major specialisms, including, among others, chapters on:

- Children and families;
- Youth offenders and substance misusers;
- Social work and mental health;
- Disabled people;
- Older people.

Providing a comprehensive guide to conceptual and methodological issues in social work and containing numerous case studies and examples, this book is an essential read for social work students, as well as a valuable resource for practitioners and academics.

Brian Sheldon is Emeritus Professor of Applied Social Research at the University of Exeter, UK. He was previously Director of the Centre for Evidence-Based Social Services in its medical school.

Geraldine Macdonald is Professor of Social Work and Director of the Institute of Child Care Research at Queen's University Belfast, UK. Previously, she was Director of Information and Knowledge Management at the Commission for Social Care Inspection.

A Textbook of Social Work

Brian Sheldon and
Geraldine Macdonald

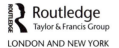

Routledge
Taylor & Francis Group

LONDON AND NEW YORK

First published 2009
by Routledge
2 Park Square, Milton Park, Abingdon, Oxon OX14 4RN

Simultaneously published in the USA and Canada
by Routledge
270 Madison Avenue, New York, NY 10016

Routledge is an imprint of the Taylor & Francis Group, an informa business

Typeset in Galliard by
Keystroke, 28 High Street, Tettenhall, Wolverhampton
Printed and bound in Great Britain by
The Cromwell Press, Trowbridge, Wiltshire

British Library Cataloguing in Publication Data
A catalogue record for this book is available from the British Library

Library of Congress Cataloging in Publication Data
Sheldon, Brian.
Rethinking social work / Brian Sheldon and Geraldine Macdonald.
p. cm.
1. Social service–Great Britain. 2. Social service–Great Britain–History.
3. Social service–Great Britain–Evaluation. I. Macdonald, Geraldine M. II. Title.
HV245.S477 2009
361.30941–dc22
2008019813

ISBN 10: 0–415–34720–3 (hbk)
ISBN 10: 0–415–34721–1 (pbk)
ISBN 10: 0–203–64010–1 (ebk)

ISBN 13: 978–0–415–34720–4 (hbk)
ISBN 13: 978–0–415–34721–1 (pbk)
ISBN 13: 978–0–203–64010–4 (ebk)

For Rita Malpas Sheldon and
Kenneth Iain Macdonald

What if I knew thy speeches word by word?
And if thou knew'st I knew them wouldst thou speak
What if I knew thy speeches word by word. . . .
(Ezra Pound, Satiemus)

Contents

Illustrations

Figures

Plates

Tables

About the authors

Brian Sheldon is Emeritus Professor of Applied Social Research at the University of Exeter and was previously Director of the Centre for Evidence-based Social Services in the medical school there. Before that he was Director of Applied Social Studies at Royal Holloway College, University of London, where he and G.M. worked together for eleven years.

Geraldine Macdonald is Professor of Social Work and Director of the Institute of Child Care Research at Queen's University Belfast. Before this appointment she was Professor of Social Work at the University of Bristol, and then Director of Information and Knowledge Management in the Commission for Social Care Inspection. She is Coordinating Editor of the Cochrane Developmental, Psychosocial and Learning Problems Review Group, which is jointly registered with the Campbell Collaboration.

Both authors are qualified social workers with considerable practice experience. Both have written and researched extensively on questions regarding the effectiveness of professional social work and on ways to improve services in the light of current best evidence.

disciplinary climate seems better disposed to the idea of evidence-based practice, we offer this book as an attempt at a consolidation of what we know about (a) the origins of these problems, and the insider views of those who face them; and (b) about what interventions enjoy the best scientific support regarding their amelioration.

2   We train our students in a strange way. Different courses have their own, embedded, 'these truths we hold to be self-evident' assumptions, and strong antibody reactions to foreign material which might threaten them. It should not be so because first CCETSW and now the Social Care Councils have published yards of guidelines regarding what every social work student needs to know and to be able to do. The problem with these is that, in the effort to avoid jargon (they fail miserably at this) and to be inclusive, they say very little. Thus 'problems' don't occur, only 'challenges', and the resultant pronouncements amount to a politically correct Rorschach test, within which any approach, either to curriculum content or teaching methods, can be vindicated. But imagine a medical school where diseases of the gut was the main specialty because Professor A had researched these, or a course which never discussed brain disorders because Professor B left two years ago and the new Director, Dr C, is mainly interested in public health. There are many examples where the equivalent of this occurs in our field, and this is *not* creative diversity.

3   All the above problems (sorry, challenges) stem from three sources: (a) the tendency for staff in our discipline to become emotionally attached to concordant priorities, explanations and methods; (b) a tendency to favour pleasing research outcomes independently of the means by which these were produced; (c) a culture in which changing one's mind and dealing with critical comments from students is seen as threatening, rather than as a sign of intellectual maturity.

Now we do not assume ourselves to be (Pharisaically) immune to these temptations, but we long ago signed up to the self-denying ordinance that is evidence-based practice (see Chapter 4). This somewhat more obsessive-compulsive approach to recipes from research seems to us the only rational answer to the difficulties described above.

Here then are the precepts which have influenced us while writing this book:

1   Textbooks *need not* be boring. They need *not* be devoid of political content or controversy for 'not in front of the children' reasons. In our experience students often suppress their more critical questions under corporate pressures from their universities and their placement agencies, but of course, still have them in their heads. However, whatever the highs and lows of your course or placement (now a 'practice learning opportunity'), you can be advised by the very best experts in the field by going to the library (likely to have a selected range – but then there are always inter-library loans – half-price at your local library), and then there is the internet.

2   This book is avowedly evidence-based but the name does not appear in the title because we do not see such a stance as specialist or partisan. Surely any textbook in any of the helping professions can, for both ethical and technical reasons, on good grounds, now assume this?

3   Textbooks cannot cover everything. In Part I we discuss the history of social work as a movement and a profession. In Part II we review the evidence for different intervention methods. Then in Part III we include chapters which review the best research available to us about the origins and nature of the problems which typically come the way of social services staff, pointing to sources of more specialist knowledge along the way. Nor is this a guide to the large legal framework which influences practice across the different legal systems even of the UK. However, where there are key legal implications we have included them and point the reader to texts which cover them in more detail.

4   We have tried to exercise as much 'cultural competence' as is available to us, but obviously our main experience is with UK institutions. This said, we have taught and conducted research in China, Hong Kong, Scandinavia, Australia, South Africa, Tajikistan and the USA, and our impression is that the problems facing social welfare services in these countries are surprisingly similar. In addition, the discipline is increasingly international – we need to read their outputs and they need to read ours.

5   Some themes crop up in different forms in different branches of the discipline (e.g. substance misuse, prejudice, racism). Substance misuse ruins the lives of youngsters and of the mentally ill or troubled in subtly different ways; the prejudice that older people experience is subtly different to that experienced by people with learning disabilities, and so on. Therefore, rather than devoting a chapter each to these forms of social oppression, we have included discussions of them in each relevant chapter.

6   We see no contradiction between our avowed aim to establish a scientific basis for social work practice, and our use of literary sources. If anything, social work is much too cut off from general cultural discourse, to our detriment.

7   Our academic position is best summed up by the following quotation from our best-ever cultural historian:

> Our intellectual history is a succession of periods of inflation and deflation; when the imagination grows too luxuriant at the expense of careful observation and detail there is a salutary reaction towards austerity and the unadorned facts; where the accounts of these grow so colourless, bleak and pessimistic that the public begins to wonder why so dreary an activity, so little connected with any human interest, is worth pursuing at all.
>
> (Berlin, 1996: 27)

    In conclusion, this book is intended for social work students, their (all-important) practice teachers, and for academics in our field. It is our hope that it might help to engender a sense of intellectually justified optimism within this somewhat beleaguered profession and could help social work develop a better sense of itself and its contribution to society. It is an attempt at a distillation of past and current evidence. In the end though: 'If you like not this, then get you to another inn' (Richard Burton, *The Anatomy of Melancholy* (1621)). If you can find one, that is.

Part I

The history of social work as a discipline and the intellectual sources on which it has drawn

1   A brief history of social work

Those who know no history are often condemned to re-live it.
Karl Marx, paraphrasing Hegel

This chapter aims to give the reader (particularly if a student) a sense of the town plan equivalent of 'you are here'. Because, contrary to common opinion, or what Larkin (1974) observed in another context, social work did not begin 'in 1963 between the end of the Chatterley ban and the Beatles' first LP'. This was just the period when the legislature began to take an interest. We go back much further in fact. We bubbled up from a thick, nineteenth-century, socio-political soup and shall need to give this a quick stir if we are to get a better look at the main ingredients. However, before we do, let us address the a priori question of what social work is for.

The scope of professional social work

Social work's disciplinary territory is the poor, troubled, abused or discriminated against, neglected, frail and elderly, mentally ill, learning-disabled, addicted, delinquent, or otherwise socially marginalized up-against-it citizen in his or her social circumstances. This is a dauntingly broad remit, particularly since some of these circumstances line up together on the fruit machine of life. Thus, as we write, we have students on placement trying to help psychiatric patients to survive in a community which does not always 'care'; helping to rehabilitate frail elderly people following discharge from hospital when once they would have found themselves on a conveyor belt from medical treatment to nursing home, premature dependency, and eventually death (see Royal Commission on Ageing; Godfrey et al., 2000; Lomax and Ellis, 2002). We have students working to prevent, or to arrange the admission of troubled and troubling children to the public care system – which, research tells us, is not exactly a side-effect-free disposal (see Bullock and Little, 1998; DfES, 2006). They support families with autistic children, sit out the uncertainties of kidney transplant vs. continued dialysis roulette with physically ill clients, and are engaged in projects to reduce the effects of juvenile crime on those who commit it and on those who are its victims. They assist with community projects which seek to help people to reclaim their local environments from the depredations of poverty, infrastructure decay, drug dealing and endemic truancy (see Holman, 1999; Jordan, 1995; Pritchard,

2001). The point is that they are all doing social work. Indeed, a full treatment of the scope of this profession, and of this movement, would fill at least a further 500 pages. So much so that it sometimes seems that unless problems fall exclusively under the duties of the army or the fire service, then social workers are expected to do *something* – whatever that might be.

We have chosen to use the term 'client' throughout this book since we think it better defines the ethical relationship which should exist between would-be helpers and might-be helped. Therefore, respectively, it confers more rights and requires more obligations than 'customer' or 'service user'. While the latter terms might just serve for recipients of practical support, social work has a broader scope and so we must be careful with our choice of words. For example, are people who have to be compulsorily admitted to psychiatric units 'using a service'? Are parents whose children have to be removed from them for reasons of safety in any meaningful sense 'service users' or 'carers'?

Social work as a field of study

The sheer range of social and personal problems for which we have acquired some responsibility has led to the development of a discipline which has always been forced to borrow heavily, and, it must be admitted, on occasion recklessly, from adjacent fields. Thus, in addition to courses on social work methods and client groups, most training courses now contain contributions from psychology (in its developmental, social, abnormal and community forms); from law, sociology, political science, philosophy, social history, gender studies, social administration, social policy, research methodology, and so forth. Indeed, a long-standing challenge for social work students has been to go to the university library and to try to find there books on something *not* plausibly relevant to their future tasks.

Such an embarrassment of intellectual riches, though often celebrated as a deserved benefit of admirable openness to all ideas and experience, does have its burdens (see Macdonald and Sheldon, 1998; Sheldon, 1978). This said, there *is* growing support from scientific commentators (e.g. Dennett, 1991; Wilson, 1998) for the idea of *considered* eclecticism, i.e. 'borrowing freely from various sources' (*Oxford English Dictionary*) and collaboration – 'the rub' is in the italicized word. These proponents hold that many of the best breakthroughs in understanding now come from groups of researchers willing to hop over disciplinary fences in order to meet the neighbours. All very admirable, but one must also consider the tendency it encourages in less-than-settled disciplines such as ours, to flit between and to take up or drop ideas according to current fashion or the congeniality of propositions or findings, rather than taking the longer but safer route of checking out the robustness of ideas before committing to them and, remember, using their prescriptions on vulnerable people:

> Social scientists, like medical scientists, have a vast store of factual information and an arsenal of sophisticated statistical techniques for its analysis. They are intellectually capable. Many of their leading thinkers will tell you, if asked, that all is well, that the disciplines are on track – sort of, more or less. Still, it is obvious to even casual inspection that the efforts of social scientists are snarled by disunity

and a failure of vision. And the reasons for the confusion are becoming increasingly clear. Social scientists by and large spurn the idea of the hierarchical ordering of knowledge that unites and drives the natural sciences. Split into independent cadres, they stress precision in words within their speciality, but seldom speak the same technical language from one speciality to the next. A great many even enjoy the resulting overall atmosphere of chaos, mistaking it for creative ferment.

(Wilson, 1998: 201)

Francis Bacon (1605), the good stepfather of science, addressed the epistemological difficulties alluded to above rather accurately when he declared that: *'What is known depends upon how it is known'*. Here are the complementary views of Thomas Kuhn (an eminent philosopher of science), who takes an example from eighteenth-century physical optics to examine how ideas and propositions are either strengthened or become mired. His conclusions, though from another field and from a long time ago, may yet seem uncomfortably familiar:

Being able to take no common body of belief for granted, each writer on physical optics felt forced to build his field anew from its foundations. In doing so, his choice of supporting observation and experiment was relatively free, for there was no standard set of methods or of phenomena that every optical writer felt forced to employ or explain. Under these circumstances, the dialogue of the resulting books was often directed as much to the members of other schools at it was to nature.

(Kuhn, 1970: 13)

This issue of 'what shall count as evidence?' remains the largest single obstacle to the *cumulative* development (distinct from mere change or fashion) in our discipline.

The point we are trying to make is that, given their remit, social workers need to be quite clever if they are to be good at their jobs. They need to be knowledgeable about studies of the nature and causes of personal and social problems and conversant with the growing body of research on what appears to ameliorate these – research being simply the screened, codified and organized experience of those doing similar work elsewhere, 'recipes' if you like. However, in three large-scale studies of what UK social workers think about their training, and what they know as a result of it (see Marsh and Tresiliotis, 1996; Sheldon and Chilvers, 2000; Sheldon *et al.*, 2005), two themes stand out: (1) the near-complete mental compartmentalization of research, theory and practice; (2) a dire lack of knowledge about the findings of studies of social work effectiveness and of how such research should be appraised (see Chapter 3). The introduction of degree-level entry to social work might provide an opportunity to remedy these matters, but as yet 'the jury is out' on this.

The impulse to help

Let us concentrate now on the strange, apparently Darwinism-defying phenomenon of the widespread human tendency to try to help others less fortunate, and to do so in an organized, socially cooperative way. Here is a good early answer to the conundrum:

cruel use of boy chimney sweeps at another – had this to say about religious influences on welfare:

> We have used the Bible as if it was a constable's handbook. As an opium dose for keeping beasts of burden patient while they are being overloaded.
>
> (Kingsley, 1863: 3)

Thus, to a late eighteenth- or early nineteenth-century gentleman of means, the idea that he had a personal or party-political responsibility to alleviate the suffering of his tenants beyond what was required by 'good husbandry' and homilies from the pulpit on Sundays (its occupant was usually paid by him) would have seemed an impertinent or even a dangerous idea. The prevailing political doctrine was that of *laissez-faire* (literally, 'let do'). This policy of settled, indifferent neglect in the cause of individual freedom stayed in place until the mid-nineteenth century, when even Chadwick's modest public health reforms were resisted by many as 'an intolerable intrusion upon private life'.

The political effects of industrialization

Lying across this established doctrine of *laissez-faire* and its companion comfort that limply organized religious benevolence would continue to mollify the poor and the dispossessed, was the shadow of the French Revolution of 1789. Remember that in the early/mid-nineteenth century the unprecedented social upheaval of the Revolution was only one generation behind. Rudyard Kipling's later poem 'If' – 'If you can keep your head while all about you are losing theirs' (1885) – is perhaps an over-literal interpretation of the motives of the 'haves' grudgingly to follow the advice of a few good men and women (the Earl of Shaftesbury and Elizabeth Fry spring immediately to mind) who urged, citing the principle of 'enlightened self-interest', the moral duty to bring the 'have-nots' a little way into the fold and to weigh the consequences of an oppression too far.

There had been some protests about the forced enclosure of common land during another revolution taking place at about the same time, namely the agrarian revolution, during which improved farming techniques created the scope for larger estates, changing the British countryside forever. Consequently there was less need for the intensive manual labour of old, and so ancient grazing rights on common land, which had hitherto held out the possibility of basic subsistence in the years of bad harvests, were first curtailed and then abolished by large landowners. Open dissidence against this thievery did occur, but more usually opposition was put in coded form, i.e. safely into the mouths of children and singers; for example:

> The fault is great in a man or woman, who steals a goose from off a common, but who can plead that man's excuse, who steals a common from a goose?
>
> (Anon.)

Conditions in Britain were particularly harsh during the Napoleonic wars (1793–1815). The running conflict with France disrupted imports of staples, and so prices rose and agricultural wages fell. Food riots followed, and the breaking by 'Luddites' of the new farm machinery. The storming of a flour mill at Downham Market in East

Anglia, opposed by the local militia, led (note) by the local *vicar* on horseback, gave rise to this moving testimony before sentence at Ely assizes by one of the insurgents:

> Here I stand between earth and sky. So help me God, I would sooner lose my life than live as I am. Bread I want, and bread I will have.
>
> (Mingay, 1976: 95)

Brave, defiant, desperate men; their cry was 'bread or blood', but has this anything to do with us today? We hope to show so. For this is our first historical theme: namely, how far can the state (the ruling class in the present historical case) go in pursuit of its economic goals and its instinct for self-preservation without sparking dissent? We are still not free of these issues, as the increasingly violent, anti-globalization demonstrations and opposition to economic migration reveal – whatever one thinks is the best solution to these issues.

The French Revolution sent a shudder through the privileged classes of Europe. 'The Terror' was only twenty miles across the Channel for the English, not, as in the American revolution (a vicar's tea party by comparison) 3,000 miles away in a colony which, though it would have been nice to have kept, we could still continue to trade with if not milk any more. The continuing reaction of government, landowners, mill owners and the magistracy (virtually interchangeable terms at the time) was repression via military force. Thus the paid poor were set against the unpaid poor; as at St Peter's Fields in Manchester on 16 August 1819 when the mounted Yeomanry charged a crowd of 50,000 peaceful protestors against the unemployment and abject poverty caused by mechanization in the cotton-weaving industry. Men, women and children were cut down with sabres and the massacre became known ironically as 'Peterloo'.

Yet, despite public outrage, further repressive legislation rather than political repentance followed. The hastily passed 'Six Acts' (1819) gave local magistrates fresh powers of summary trial; allowed exemplary punishment for politically motivated offenders; equipped Justices with draconian sanctions to search houses and to confiscate books; to employ spies to infiltrate dissenting groups, and to impose a punitive tax on radical publishers. Thomas Paine's *The Rights of Man* (1791) was a prime target for confiscation since he had written lines such as: 'All delegated power is trust, all assumed power is usurpation.' Paine had also, heretically, proposed the abolition of the Poor Law (see p. 13) and its replacement with a graded tax on estates. This exercise of suppression failed, just as did the attempts to close down the *Samizdat* publishers in the Soviet Union 150 years later.

The mushrooming industrial towns were crucibles of political dissent. The conditions were much worse there than those of the languidly oppressive circumstances of country life. These are the early origins of the idea that governments and municipalities had little time to make up their minds about suppression versus preventative relief. Then there arose another pressing reason for governments to come up with practical schemes to improve social conditions, and to look to the welfare of the citizenry.

The social and public health effects of the Industrial Revolution

It all began in Coalbrookdale in Shropshire in the late eighteenth century, where coal and iron ore were to be found together. The population of Britain was increasing dramatically at this time. The first national census (1801) yields a figure of 9 million, but the figures had risen to 10 million by 1811, and to 12 million by 1821. But the more important data are those for increases in population density per square mile. These doubled in the 100 years between 1721 and 1821, and, over three generations the English, in particular, changed from being largely a nation of country dwellers employed on the land, to a nation of town dwellers engaged in industrial production.

As we have noted, the 'push' for this migration from countryside to town resulted from the fact that jobs in the agricultural economy shrank due to the enclosures and the development of 'more efficient' farming techniques. The 'pull' came from the lure of something close to a living wage in the new manufacturing centres. However, the social consequences of all this were great. How, for example, *was* an agricultural labourer to be transformed in the space of a couple of years into an industrial worker in a very different and more dangerous place, with unfamiliar skills being demanded of him, and oppressive working practices in place?

Here is Trevelyan's (a great historian of this period – but see also Elizabeth Gaskell's novel *Mary Barton*) broader assessment of the social and political consequences of the Industrial Revolution:

> The age of coal and iron had come in earnest. A new order of life was beginning, and the circumstances under which it began led to a new kind of unrest. Immigrants to the mining and industrial districts were leaving an old rural world essentially conservative in its social structure and moral atmosphere, and were dumped down in neglected heaps that soon fermented as neglected heaps will do, becoming highly combustible matter.
>
> (Trevelyan, 1944: 475)

The English in particular have never quite recovered from this rapid change from a predominantly rural to a predominantly urban culture. As in the case of a lost love, the qualities of what once was are idealized, and the heartache forgotten. The writings of Thomas Hardy (1840–1928) capture most honestly both the departed simplicity and the privations of the old life. But still, looking forward, in the pockets of hundreds of soldiers on the Western front in World War I was a slim copy of A.E. Housman's *A Shropshire Lad*, containing lovely lines such as these:

> Into my heart an air that kills
> From yon far country blows:
> What are those blue remembered hills,
> What spires, what farms are those?
> That is the land of lost content,
> I see it shining plain,
> The happy highways where I went
> And cannot come again.
>
> (Housman, 1896: 58)

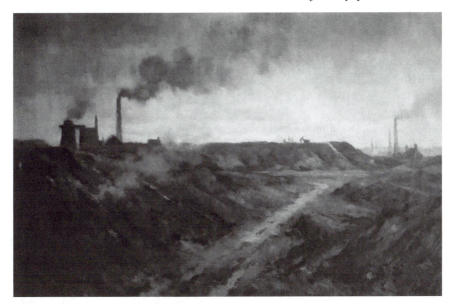

Plate 1.1 Untitled by Edwin Butler Bayliss.
Source: Reprinted courtesy of Wolverhampton Art Gallery

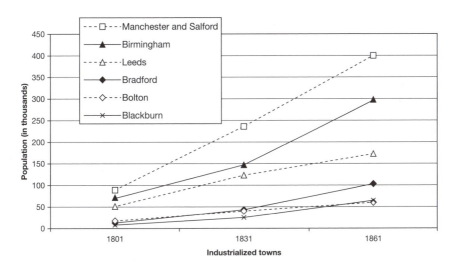

Figure 1.1 Growth of industrial towns during the Industrial Revolution (from Census data)
Note: The figures for London will not fit into the chart above so large are they, i.e. 957,000 for 1801; 2,362 for 1851, and (later) 5,536,000 for 1901.
Source: OPCS

Daily life for working-class people in the new industrial towns of the early to mid-nineteenth century ranged from the abject to the grim. Men and women, and as often as not their children, worked 12-hour days for meagre wages and could be dismissed on the whim of an overseer. Housing conditions were squalid in the extreme. There were few opportunities for education; for leisure; little wholesome food; no access to medical treatment (just as well perhaps); no sanitation to speak of, and no clean water supply. In 1832 alone cholera killed over 5,000 Londoners, and typhoid and smallpox combined, thousands more. In the middle of the century 25,000 lives per annum were claimed by these diseases. Charles Dickens addressed the threatening implications of all this in *Bleak House:*

> There is not an atom of Tom's slime, not a cubic inch of any pestilential gas in which he lives, not one obscenity or degradation about him, not an ignorance, not a wickedness, not a brutality of his committing, but shall work its retribution through every order of society up to the proudest of the proud and to the highest of the high.
>
> (Dickens, 1852: 141)

The need for reform, or what was called by opponents 'interference', became compelling to those in power by reason of the *force majeure* of mortality statistics and the daily evidence of their own noses. The Thames had by then become a different kind of 'liquid history' as Burns (1943) later described it. It was in fact an open sewer; the common description of effects being 'The Great Stink', which miasma led to the suspension of many parliamentary sittings. When Queen Victoria's beloved husband Prince Albert died of typhoid in 1861, the question 'who then is safe?' was on everyone's lips.

We still have trouble today with the idea that poverty, poor housing and class position are major correlates of ill-health. Proving that this connection remains somewhat in place, and that many causes of illness lie outwith the scope of the NHS, the Black Report (Black *et al.*, 1980) on inequalities in health was quietly released on a Bank Holiday weekend.

Sanitary and social conditions which once could have been safely ignored in the open, breezy countryside were now a major threat to life, property and to political stability. Legislation, organization, inspection, municipal intervention and, above all, public money were required, as the link between the social conditions of the poor and public health were established by early epidemiological studies such as Chadwick's (1842) *Report into the Sanitary Conditions of the Labouring Population of Great Britain* (see Table 1.1).

The mortality figures in Table 1.1 (based on a population density of 150,000 per square mile), appalling in their own right, are skewed by the effects of poor pre- and postnatal care, and thus by high levels of infant death. Still, note the differences between town and country survival rates in these ledgers of death, and the class bias in the entries.

New powers were given to local authorities and new Public Health Boards set up under the Public Health Act of 1848 (which was followed by strengthening legislation in 1858). *Laissez-faire* was now effectively dead. Death rates from cholera and typhoid slowly fell as a result of substantial investment in public works, culminating in the monumental creations of Sir Joseph Bazalgette, who oversaw the building of an entire drainage and clean water system for London. The problem confronting him was no less than that the effluent from 2.5 million people was being dumped into the Thames and then siphoned back out as drinking water. He

Table 1.1 Life expectancy by class and location in 1842

Place	Professional/gentry	Tradesmen	Labourers
Bethnal Green	45	26	16
Bolton	34	23	18
Derby	49	38	21
Kendal	45	39	34
Leeds	44	27	19
Liverpool	35	22	15
Manchester	38	20	17
Wiltshire	50	48	33

Source: Chadwick (1842)

oversaw the building of 500 miles of main trunk sewers and 13,000 miles of tributary conduits – the largest engineering project of the nineteenth century – involving 22,000 labourers over a period of eighteen years. This then is our second historical theme: that public health, and political and social conditions cannot sensibly be separated in welfare policy.

Dire necessity was thus the mother of rapid invention, and this was the beginning of organized and expert (by the standards of the time) social intervention, and is part of the answer to the question of where the idea of social welfare came from. The other great example of this new-fangled principle of state interference was the Poor Law, which was redesigned to attack the causes of poverty and degradation through increasingly strategic policies of 'relief', but mainly via a policy of dissuading people from daring to seek it in the first place.

The English Poor Law

Prior to 1834 when the Poor Law Amendment Act was passed, relief for the destitute had from Elizabethan times been based upon grudgingly paid parish rates and church philanthropy. A system of aid, modelled on the practices in what was once a village near Newbury in Berkshire called Speenhamland, was seen as what we would now call a 'best practice model'. Under this scheme, when harvests were bad and prices high, a little cash and a little local work might be offered. However it looks to us now, this was the first example of the state taking direct responsibility for the poor. All interventions have unintended consequences, and Speenhamland relief practices effectively became a subsidy on agricultural labour provided by the tradespeople of boroughs and townships. Rich country landowners were required to stump up next to nothing.

Most of all it was the spiralling costs of the poor rate (eightfold increases in 20 years or so in some parishes) that triggered change. There was much political dispute regarding how to solve this problem. A Royal Commission was set up to concern itself with the economic and moral consequences (a dangerous combination then as now) of existing policies of relief and to produce recommendations for 'improvement'. Here is what they came up with:

from the Liberals and their earlier bequests, certainly no National Health Service – the 'moral glory' of British public policy' – as Aneurin Bevan, its chief architect, rightly described it. We, as the inheritors and beneficiaries of these policies, are currently engaged in a fierce controversy about their future. For some, the Welfare State and the NHS have a sort of listed building status; they are somewhat impractical; they leak and creak; they are expensive to maintain, but they are beautiful. For others, they require urgent rebuilding from the ground up in the modern European style, or at the very least the addition of a couple of privately funded wings. We tend towards the steady repair and maintenance view of these matters, and would wish a similar policy to be applied to social services, which have been subject to constant digging up to see how well they are growing.

Public health concerns intrude once again at the end of the nineteenth century. At the time of the Boer War there was a large-scale recruitment campaign by the army. Applicants – there were thousands who sought to escape poverty and unemployment in this way – had first to be medically examined for physical fitness. Between a half and two-thirds were turned down on grounds of ill-health and incapacity; rickets and TB were the predominant diseases. News of this caused a public scandal. Malnutrition was the overriding cause, and the British Public Health Service owes its origins to this belated, essentially self-interested concern.

The contrast between imperial pomp and the conditions for ordinary people at home had been made clear by the first attempts at what we would now call social-scientific enquiry (by Engels (1844 – but translated from the German only in 1892), and the Rowntree (1901) surveys into the living circumstances of the working class in Manchester and York). 'Dire' was the answer to the question about the effects of social conditions in both cases, but this time the evidence was empirical, large-scale, and less easy to dismiss.

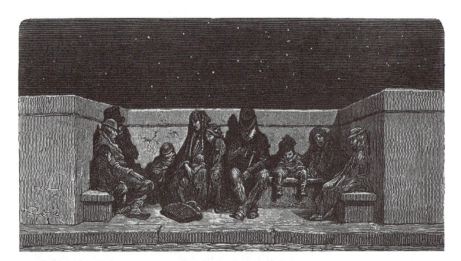

Plate 1.3 The Embankment, London (1868). Gustav Doré *Asleep Under the Stars.*

Note the contrast between the new imperial architecture and the condition of the human beings inhabiting it.

Source: Reprinted by kind permission of Dover Publications Inc.

The Poor Law (the 'black sheep' ancestor of modern Social Services) remained a hated policy among those it set out to 'improve'. The calls for reform from organized labour were strident. This pressure led to the establishment of a Royal Commission on the Poor Law in 1905, which reported in 1909. It was strongly influenced by the work of Sydney and Beatrice Webb, politically inspired social reformers who were campaigning for national insurance and something called *welfare* to replace policies of deterrence. The following passage is from the *majority* report. The minority report by the Webbs and their followers was even more radical in tone, and eventually became the set of arguments that we remember:

> 'Land of Hope and Glory' is a popular and patriotic lyric sung each year by thousands of voices. . . . To certain classes of the community into whose moral and condition it has been our duty to explore, these words are a mockery and a falsehood.
>
> (Report of the Poor Law Commission, 1909)

Labour was, by then, increasingly organized, and trades union representatives wielded a growing influence on the municipalities – for they could no longer be safely ignored. At the same time concerted attempts took place to form a new political party – seeking first to lobby, then to enter Parliament (this in the face of a very limited, indeed, rigged suffrage). The Social Democratic Federation (1884) and the Labour Representation Committee led eventually to the foundation by Kier Hardy, John Burns and Ben Tillett of the Independent Labour Party, which led in 1906 to the formation of the Labour Party, and in 1924 to the first Labour government.

The rise of organized social welfare

This period (the turn of the nineteenth century and immediately after) sees the development of *organized* attempts to improve social conditions for individuals, and this is our third historical theme. The example of university settlements stands out in this regard. These were based upon an extension of the foreign missionary principle to our own country – whereby university undergraduates from Oxford, Cambridge and London set up and staffed welfare centres, clubs and educational groups in the poorer parts of the land, for example, at Toynbee Hall in London, established in 1884 by Canon Samuel Barnett and his wife Henrietta. It was named after Arnold Toynbee (1852–1881), a historian from Balliol, who was a passionate campaigner for free education. It set up community groups, literacy classes, and arranged free country and seaside holidays for city children: early practical social work in action (see Briggs and Maccartney, 1984).

The principle of organized voluntary action assumes increasing prominence at this time. This loose collection of bodies and interest groups was aimed mainly at preventing claimants from exploiting charitable bodies by making multiple applications for aid. It formed itself into the Charity Organisation Society (COS) in 1869 and introduced the idea of 'rational planning' for, and the evaluation of, the practical effectiveness of charitable assistance. Here is what would now be called its 'mission statement':

Saying, Lay not thy hand upon the lad,
Neither do anything to him.
Behold, A ram, caught in a thicket by its horns;
Offer the ram of Pride instead of him.
But the old man would not so, but slew his son,
And half the seed of Europe, one by one.

(Owen, 1916)

Among the combatants on the Western front an increasingly common condition began to arise, that of 'shell-shock'. Later, under the influence of Sigmund Freud's work, this was termed 'war neurosis', although Ivan Pavlov has provided the obvious explanation for this malady (Pavlov, 1927). Despite attempts by the generals

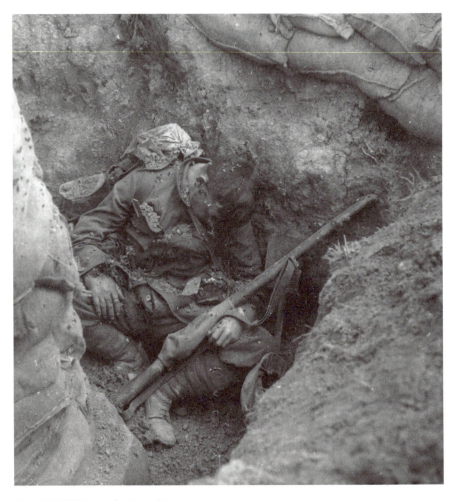

Plate 1.5 WWI battlefield conditions.

The soldier in the pictue is not dead, just totally exhausted.

Source: Reprinted courtesy of the BBC/Imperial War Museum

(quartered comfortably in chateaux behind the lines) to claim that there was no such medical condition, and that the term was simply an excuse for cowardice, the sheer number of troops so afflicted and the fact that brave officers such as Wilfred Owen and Siegfried Sassoon were also sufferers, gradually changed minds. The psychology of post-traumatic stress disorder is now quite well understood (see DSM IVTR; ICD 10; also Ginzburg *et al.*, 2002). Put simply, if human beings are placed in conditions of constant and unavoidable danger with little prospect of tactical action to avoid it, and no scope for the natural instinct of 'flight', and sometimes not even for 'fight', then they descend into a state of 'helplessness', i.e. conditioned, generalized fearfulness and depression (see Seligman, 1975).

Psychiatrists and people whom we would now recognize as social workers were deployed in the new treatment centres (as at Cariglockhart, at Oxford, and in Birmingham). W. H. Rivers (1864–1922), a Major in the Royal Army Medical Corps, pioneered the treatment of these shattered people and played an important part in changing social attitudes to their plight (see Rivers, 1922; Stallworthy, 1974: ch. 8). Abject sympathy aside, this period is important to the development of a profession of social work for the following reasons: (1) psychiatrists (a new discipline themselves then) were asked to treat cases of serious mental illness which were clearly not the result of either 'bad blood' or lunar phases, but clearly of atrocious *environmental* experiences; (2) to assist them in the task of care and resettlement, they needed welfare workers to bridge the gap between treatment and rehabilitation. The psychiatric social worker was thus born, first in the USA, then over here; hospital almoners (already in existence by this time) found a new role in the rehabilitation of soldiers; (3) psychiatrists and their allies turned to psychology for answers to these extreme reactions to trauma, particularly to the then highly risqué work of Sigmund Freud (1856–1939). These ideas influenced both medical and welfare staff (whether they sensibly should have is a different question, and for later); (4) the idea that *knowledge* rather than moral sentiment should inform treatment and other interventions to promote future well-being was loosely established at this time. Thus psychiatry, and on its coat-tails the emerging profession of social work, began tentatively to look for an evidential, head-over-heart basis for attempted remedies.

The 'psychiatric deluge' and the role of knowledge in social work

In respect of our fifth theme – the use of knowledge in social work – it is still possible to tease conference audiences gathered to address the implications of evidence-based practice (see Chapter 4) by reading out the following quotation and attributing it to a recent speech by some adjacent Director of Social Services, and then letting them in on the fact that it was written on the eve of the Russian Revolution:

> With other practitioners – with physicians and lawyers, for example – there was always a basis of knowledge held in common. If a neurologist had occasion to confer with a surgeon, each could assume in the other a mastery of the elements of a whole group of basic sciences and of the formulated and transmitted experience of his own guild besides. But what common knowledge could social workers assume in like case?
>
> (Richmond, 1917: 5)

Richard Cabot, President of the National Association of Social Workers in the USA, went on to direct the first large-scale controlled trial in the field of delinquency prevention (see Powers and Witmer, 1951). Its publication was delayed by World War II, but retained most of its methodological integrity. Unfortunately, this comparison of extensive, psychoanalytically flavoured counselling, conducted over three years, with very high contact levels, produced no significant differences between the experimental (i.e. well-exposed) group and a matched control group which had received no such 'help'.

At the time, where it was known about at all, this study and others with similarly disappointing results were seen as flukes; the results attributable to a naive attempt to apply 'inappropriate' scientific principles to something beyond their capacity to investigate. We return to this issue in Chapters 3, 4 and 5, since it is these very research methods that underpin the idea of evidence-based practice, and which are increasingly recognized as essential in evaluating the effectiveness of professional good intentions (see Sheldon, 1986; Sheldon and Macdonald, 1999). For your comfort, the robust evidence that we now have is very much more extensive and positive.

World War II and the creation of the Welfare State

World War II cost 55 million lives among combatants and civilians. This was 'total war' on all sides, including the British. Few distinctions were made between 'legitimate' and 'illegitimate' targets. If we look at the figures for the military and civilian casualties in any country invaded by Germany and the Axis powers we find that, except in the USSR, where just about all remotely able civilians were conscripted, civilian casualties surpass military deaths. Thus a sense of raw survival, and of the vital need for central planning, if necessary at the expense of civil liberties (as we now see in 'the war on terror'), was ubiquitous.

In the face of this, in September 1939, the largest childcare experiment in history began: the evacuation (see Holman, 1995). One has, when looking at the documents, to feel admiration for the logistical skills of those in charge of it. Three million children were removed from the cities, particularly London, and sent to live in the countryside. The entire railway system was commandeered for this purpose. Invasion was regarded as imminent after Dunkirk and our state of military and civil preparation for it was lamentable.

Studies tell us that the experience of evacuation was as mixed as one would have expected. Genuine grief at separation was countered by a brief but at least understandable explanation as to why they had to endure it.

Thus the scheme amounted to emotional fasting in a just cause. There were limited allowances in place, and there was little choice for country dwellers with even a little space to spare but to leave aside any doubts and to do their duty. This was an obligation briskly enforced by an emerging generation of child welfare workers.

It has taken a long time to bring the experiences of evacuated children together (see Parsons and Starns, 1999) but personal testimonies reveal a wide range of effects. Thus we would see *some* children on the left of the distribution suffering serious abuse – definitely not 'Goodnight Mr Tom' experiences. Some never wanted to return home. Many did all right.

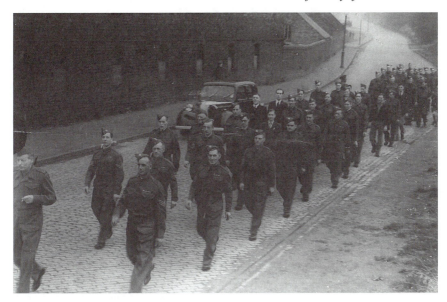

Plate 1.6 The Lye Home Guard, Worcestershire, 1940

Note: The officer in front, smoking a cigarette, is the local dentist; Brian Sheldon's grandfather is third from the left and was the only member of the brigade with any military experience. Note the complete absence of weaponry – they had none until six months later. The dark satanic mill in the backdrop is where he worked. It has now been replaced by a bright satanic mall.

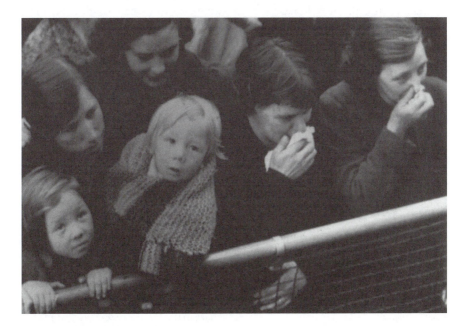

Plate 1.7 Mothers, some with children at an evacuation station, watching evacuees leave for the reception area.

Source: Reprinted courtesy of Parsons and Starns (1999) and the Imperial War Museum

Studies of the experiences of evacuees have, even allowing for the customs of the time, regularly revealed savage experiences such as the above. BS once took a social history from a middle-aged woman who had been an evacuee. She had approached a child guidance clinic over concerns about passing on her own obsessions for cleanliness, constant hand washing and severe fearfulness to her children, having been locked in a hen coop for a day and emerged covered in fleas. 'I've never felt clean since', she observed.

The post-war settlement

The coalition government in the early days of a war which then, it seemed, we could easily lose, set up a comprehensive review of social legislation (recently released German documents show that they were scared stiff of entering '*Die Fleischhak Maschine*' (the mincing machine) of the English Channel. This was an extraordinary act of optimism. It resulted in the 1944 Education Act, promising free education to secondary level for all; a reconstruction plan from the Ministry of Works to rebuild towns ravaged by bombing, but most tellingly, a report (commissioned from Sir William Beveridge) for a design for a post-war Welfare State. This comprehensive set of social security, welfare and health policies set out to attack, in his words, 'the "Five Giants" of *Want, Disease, Ignorance, Squalor and Idleness*' (see Timmins, 2001).

Beveridge's proposals were rapidly translated into practical action over the next five years. Central to the report was the idea that the state should be the main provider of welfare, though the voluntary societies were also to be harnessed. A National Health Service, 'free to all at the point of use', was to be set up. A less stigmatizing National Assistance scheme was to replace the Poor Law. There was to be a new system for childcare, with specialist departments set up to ensure child welfare. There was to be a new scheme for mass housing provision. In addition, existing pension schemes were to be extended so as to encompass all retired people and a comprehensive scheme for unemployment benefit brought in. This was, after all, the sacrifice and hardship of the war years, 'a time for revolutions and not for patching', as Beveridge said in the Preface to his monumental report.

The historical theme with which we began this chapter, i.e. the compact (or once the lack of one) between the state and the citizen, comes powerfully into play again at this point. Winston Churchill, who had inspired the British people by promising only 'blood, sweat and tears', who was loved and admired, both during and at the end of the war, was nevertheless ejected from office by an electoral landslide in 1945 in favour of politicians who supported the idea of a welfare state (see Titmuss, 1951). The privations of the war followed closely on the heels of the economic depression in the 1930s, yet the people had seen that determined work, stoicism, organization and planning had defeated a formidable enemy, so why could not the same strategic principles be applied to long-standing problems at home? It was for this reason that the people voted overwhelmingly for the less charismatic but more socially committed Clement Attlee, and on 'enough is enough' principles, ushered in the most reformist government in our history. Nothing today compares with its progressive and practical accomplishments. All this was achieved on austerity budgets, and through tax rises

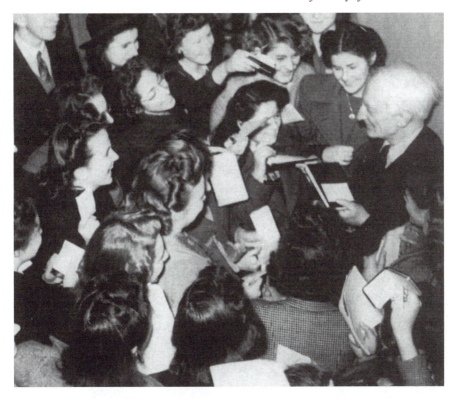

Plate 1.8 The 'People's William', 1944.

Beveridge signing authographs after the publication of *Full Employment in a Free Society*.

Source: Reprinted courtesy of Oxford University Press

from the pre-war 19 per cent to 40 per cent – which were swallowed because the cause was seen as just.

Another political hero of ours, Aneurin Bevan (Minister for Health), travelled the country arguing, persuading and cajoling a reluctant medical profession into signing up for the new NHS (see Foot, 1962: vols 1 and 2). We cannot resist this account: at a public meeting in mid-Wales he met the local Head of Obstetric and Gynaecology services who asked if Bevan was aware that he was 'personally responsible for all the births in a fifty-mile radius'. Bevan asked him (imagine the accent) if he was 'bragging or complaining'. Much laughter, some signing up.

The coming of the Welfare State could either have seen the end of any aspirations for a profession of social work – for what need for individual assistance when the right *policies* were already in place? Pragmatism prevailed again however, and an updated version of Eileen Younghusband's report on the employment of social workers was commissioned in 1951. In Part I she comments on the contribution made by social workers during the war:

> The social worker who was doubtfully regarded as a doer of good works in voluntary organizations is now an accepted part of the machinery of the State

social services, and the term 'caseworker' so far from being a matter of scorn, has even crept into official publications. Almoners and psychiatric social workers have become part of the National Health Service, and Boarding Out and Children's Officers part of the orderly and improved service for homeless children which has succeeded the chaos described in the earlier report.

(Younghusband, 1951: 2)

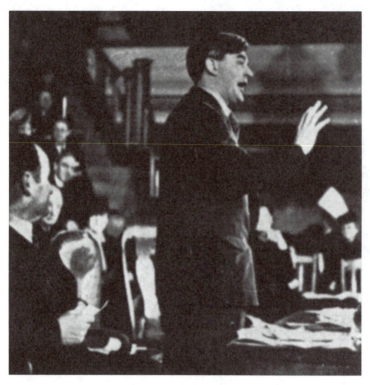

Plate 1.9 Aneurin Bevan, father of the National Health Service in Britain.

Source: By permission of Four Square Books

Training courses for social workers (which began at the University of Birmingham in 1895 and shortly afterwards at the London School of Economics) turned out very small numbers of qualified staff. Even with expansion, awards only in the low hundreds were made between 1945 and 1949, with numbers climbing only gently upward for the next 15 years. Younghusband recommended an expansion of university courses, and gave sensible advice on the need for a thorough grounding in the applied social sciences.

This issue of professional status versus membership of a movement eschewing any such elitist aspirations (and favouring George Bernard Shaw's definition of the word 'profession' as 'a conspiracy against the laity') has caused us much trouble over the years. We see no contradiction in belonging to both camps, but let us pause to consider what membership of a profession entails. The usual candidate rules are as follows:

1   That there exists a distinctive body of knowledge to inform decision-making. We have such without doubt in the theoretical writing and in the empirical studies investigating both the nature of social and personal problems and studies of what might sensibly be done about them (Macdonald and Sheldon, 1992; Davies, 2000; Macdonald, 2001).

2   That staff claiming such status should exercise influence over important matters, i.e. life and death and life chances. It was once held that only law and medicine fulfilled these categories. But do not social workers also hold such matters in their hands? Failure in child protection services has led regularly to the deaths of children (see Sheldon, 1987b; Howitt, 1992; Laming, 2003); failures in mental health care sometimes leads to the deaths of clients or members of the public (see Reed, 1997) or, much more frequently, to the suicides of clients themselves. The point is that social care staff deal with a multitude of demanding, difficult and sometimes dangerous problems.

3   The next requirement is that there should be an ethical code in place. We have long had one, not perfect, but good enough (BASW, 1975, plus revisions). Moreover, all Social Services departments have their own exacting policies regarding the conduct of employees, and now there are Social Councils with disciplinary powers. Where we may perhaps fall short is that such pledges give only limited mention of the requirement for staff to make use of current best evidence as an ethical obligation.

4   In case the reader is thinking that we have left something out (i.e. self-regulation), then this matter can be quickly disposed of, for no professions, not law, not medicine, are really self-governing these days. Policing has now quite properly been placed largely in the hands of independent bodies. QED.

Later attempts at a reform of social work

If we have seen one thing in our historical tour, it is that socio-political and cultural factors powerfully affect definitions of what social work should be for. Imagine for a moment the conditions in the 1960s. Radical left-wing movements abounded; R. D. Laing (1960) was writing his (mistaken) anti-psychiatry tracts (see Sheldon, 1994), and sociologists were producing treatises on youth justice which seemed to suggest that misguided attempts at help by social workers and probation officers were responsible for the cruel 'labelling' of youngsters. This verse from Bernstein's *West Side Story* captures the spirit of the times:

> Officer Krupke, you're really a slob.
> This boy don't need a doctor, just a good honest job.
> Society's played him a terrible trick,
> And sociologic'ly he's sick.
> (Bernstein and Sondheim, 1961)

The 'Radical Social Work' movement reached its apogée in the late 1970s and then, as a result of the following factors, its influence faded: (1) Community development programmes, some of them state-funded, were never able to show that they had

art or an applied social science. Brewer and Lait's amusingly tart conclusion was: 'If social work is an art, then let it be funded by the Arts Council.'

Fast forward: Sir Roy Griffiths (Financial Director of the Sainsbury supermarket chain) was charged in the early 1980s with the production of a plan for the overhaul of Social Services in general and proposals for the development of community care in particular (he had already had a go at the NHS). We pause here, with that due sense of humility rarely extended to our profession, to ask the question: what would a supermarket organized by social workers be like to shop in? (We imagine long queues while variable pricing regulations are assessed against individual need and national standards indicators, and a largely empty aisle for people with 'three problems or fewer'.)

Most of the more extreme versions of purchaser–provider splits and the associated bureaucracy which came in with the NHS and Community Care Act 1990 are now fading, since they are increasingly realized to be less cost-effective ways of delivering services – the concurrent 'Best Value' initiative came in at a modest £15 million in the red, for example. We are left with a partial legacy of better, more strategic management, more detailed service planning, but with increasingly burdensome 'targets' for everything, which distract staff from their face-to-face work, and threaten the inception of 'virtual reality social work' – an activity carried out largely on computers rather than in homes – visiting rates now accounting for less than 20 per cent of the working week.

Recent achievements and future prospects

Obviously, '7,000 planes land safely at Heathrow last week' is no news at all. The same is true in our own field wherein quiet successes are ignored and occasional failures trumpeted. But what could we claim as a cost-effective contribution to the society that picks up the bill for what we do?

1   First, there is the community care project in mental health, whereby thousands of people, once unnecessarily incarcerated, now live better lives in the community. It was always difficult to tell whether any eccentricities of behaviour were due to residues of illness or to the institutional conditions in which they were confined. This is not to detract from the good intentions of previous policies, nor from the many humane reforms and improvements in treatment that had taken place in the 1960s and 1970s (see Chapter 11). Nevertheless, it is close to a psychological fact that the human spirit, especially if weakened by illness, does not thrive in over-regimented, choice-denying conditions.
2   Right next door to the old mental hospitals were the 'mental subnormality hospitals'. Conditions there were even worse, which meant they were dire indeed. The social inclusion of people with learning disabilities is another major social change to which social workers contributed, and continue to advance (see Chapter 14).
3   There is a similar story to tell regarding support for frail, elderly people. Once physical and mental decline were seen as inexorable and irreversible concomitants of old age, this being the predominant 'good innings' view of ageing in our culture. In many areas we now have in place well-organized though logistically

demanding systems of multidisciplinary services designed to support older people in the community. There is much still to do to improve these (and other) services, not least of all to ensure that they are individually tailored to people's needs and aspirations, but social work has made a significant contribution.

4 Childcare and child protection services are altogether more complicated. Failures in this area lead to political knee-jerk reactions, which eventually come to influence virtually all service provision. The public, politicians and journalists have simply failed to grasp the fact that we probably have the safest child protection services in the world, but that a completely accident-proof system, even if remotely achievable, would involve draconian procedures which would freeze virtually all useful preventative work and threaten civil liberties. In addition, below the visible iceberg tip of desperately sad, media-preoccupying child deaths and physical injuries is a mass of less newsworthy misery, emotional damage, neglect and lack of opportunity.

Certain other developments have taken place, not directly regarding social work's primary concern for people in need, but affecting our own ability to get our professional act together and to deliver effective services. Two are compelling; first, increasing governmental concern that social work should be an uncontroversially professional activity. As we have seen, we have been at this issue for over a hundred years, but recent changes in institutional arrangements give cause for optimism. There is now a General Social Care Council to oversee standards in England and Wales, and similar organizations in Scotland and Northern Ireland; there is a requirement that social workers be registered, and for the profession to have a protected title as have doctors and nurses. There is now a mainstream Honours degree route to qualification (in line with many European countries and the USA), and post-qualification courses will continue to be funded. The Social Care Institute for Excellence (SCIE) has been set up to synthesize evidence and to help improve practice (http:// www.scie. org.uk/), one of a number of indicators that an old idea – that of evidence-based practice (see Chapter 4) – has found its time. Various centres exist to encourage this development, for example, *Research in Practice* (aimed at children's social care) and *Research in Practice for Adults* (its predecessor being the *Centre for Evidence-Based Social Services* at the University of Exeter – see CEBSS, 1998–2002), and *Making Research Count*. These schemes are designed to help disseminate research and facilitate its implementation. Use them or lose them is our advice.

Conclusions

1 Social work has its origins in the centuries-old idea of charity, but in its organized forms it is a product of the political, social and public health effects of the Industrial Revolution. Benign intentions were always there, but also the urgent need for state-organized action, well against the political conventions of the time, was forced upon government and the better-off by the threatening consequences of sheer dissent, political necessity, and eventually by enlightened self-interest. Social work and politics were thus never far apart, nor are they now (see Parton, 1998).

2   History teaches us that welfare is here to stay and that social policy, however well framed, will always require its interpreters – since most government proposals come 'flat-packed' and need expert people to put them together. In this regard we agree with the views of the Barclay Report (1982) that if professional social work were to be abolished tomorrow, it would only have to be reinvented under another name later.

3   The history of social work tells us that the problems we face lie along a broad continuum and that therefore, if we are sensible, we should act in concert with allies. This view was forced upon the early public health movement, an under-estimated influence in the few previous histories of social work. Social conditions and health conditions intertwine and require joint action. The remit of public health has now broadened substantially and the overlap with social work is increasingly well recognized.

4   Another of our themes was the purposeful use of knowledge in practice: knowledge about the nature, origins and development of social and personal problems, and about what we know about what might help to ameliorate them. We now have a considerable stack of both types, and the challenge is that of integrating it into the day-to-day decisions of policy-makers and practitioners, i.e. evidence-based practice. This endeavour – to construct a valid and reliable body of knowledge, as free as possible from ideological bewitchment, that informs decision-making in the context of other influences, such as the views of clients, public opinion, and available resources, is an idea long and deeply rooted in the aims of this profession.

You are here.

2 Theory and practice in social work

> There is probably nothing more practical in puzzling circumstances than a good theory.
>
> Karl Popper

Theories and theorizing

The ability to 'integrate theory and practice' appears on all practice assessment schedules and guidelines for essays leading to the award of the professional qualification. It is thus a powerfully sanctioned, if somewhat vaguely defined, expectation of student social workers everywhere. This belief in the superiority of theoretically informed practice and the amendment of theory at the point of use to accommodate individual circumstances has long been an important test of the professional faith. However, general principles (be they ever so wholesome-sounding) which go unanalysed for any length of time tend to degenerate into clichés, and this is what has happened with this idea; the logical implications of the words have been drowned out by the congenial noise they make. We have many words and phrases in modern life which seem to have this effect of switching off the cerebral cortex, from 'organic', 'natural' and 'fresh' in supermarkets, to 'community', 'needs-led', 'strategic' and 'excellence'. The argument is not that these words do not have specific meanings, rather that they should be used with discrimination and due humility if they are not to be quickly worn out, namely:

> 'When *I* use a word', Humpty Dumpty said in a rather scornful tone, 'it means just what I choose it to mean – neither more nor less'.
>
> 'The question is' said Alice, 'whether you *can* make words mean different things.'
>
> 'The question is', said Humpty Dumpty, 'which is to be master – that's all.'
>
> (Carroll, 1872: 197)

Probably because of our long-standing empirical tradition (see Porter, 2000) the British, closely followed by the Americans, but hardly at all by continental Europeans, attach rather dismissive connotations to the word 'theory'. For the British, it implies probable impracticality, 'airy-fairyness' and proper scientific work not yet done. The *Oxford English Dictionary* picks up on both the scientific and vernacular usages thus:

Theory: a plausible or scientifically acceptable general principle or body of knowledge offered to explain phenomena. The analysis of a set of facts in their relation to one another. *Theory*: abstract thought: speculation.

However, whether one tends towards the technical definition – emphasizing the collecting together of separate observations and combining them into something more coherent – or towards the more speculative, hypothetical, vernacular one, the most important point to make about theories and theorizing is that human beings simply cannot not have them or do it. A completely inductive, empirical, non-speculative life would be impossible to live. Only severely neurotic people come close to the precautionary checking out of every prospect or event, thus making themselves miserable and ineffective. Indeed, we seem to have a 'wired-in' tendency to 'join up the dots' of observations and form them into something more explanatory, so as to answer the questions, vital in evolution: 'What will happen next? 'What should I do next?' Theorizing is thus 'future producing' (see Dennett, 1991, 2003) and, through conditioning, leads to learning about what probably goes with what in our danger-avoiding, satisfaction-seeking lives (see Chapter 7).

Over the aeons, we developed raw reflexes which helped us to win out over the ice and the bear, but which subsequently generalized to less physically threatening social circumstances such as those where we need to make a good impression; what the news from a client that 'Dave is being released early' implies for the safety of the children; what 'people have started following me again' implies for future stability in a mental health case, and so forth. In other words, human beings in general, and we in our professional roles, have theories on the brain, only some of which are derived from textbooks. We propose (i.e. we have a theory) that these fall into four main categories.

Perceptual reflex-based theories

Under the influence of Déscartes (1637, 1667/1985) we have been influenced to think – particularly of visual perception – as a two-stage, 'camera-like' activity, as a result of which we first observe and mentally record information about objects and events and then 'develop' more elaborate pictures and thoughts about them in the mind. However, scores of studies challenge such assumptions (see Gregory, 1970, 1988). These show that we see, hear, taste and touch with our *brains*, and that past experiences, emotions and expectations powerfully influence what we perceive or are oblivious to. This is an important topic, since all theories, from the little semi-automatic ones we use to guide us safely through the environment (chairs are usually safe to sit on; people who smile at us and don't have sinister-looking white cats on their laps probably have good intentions) to the more elaborate and formulaic, begin with perceptions.

If we look further into this branch of experimental psychology, the implications for social work should be clear. Let us undertake a few little experiments of our own to illustrate the point that perception is constructive in its nature. If you look at Figure 2.1 you will see that a bright, white triangle dominates the foreground between the black shapes, shining out from the background with a hint of defining lines. Obvious; but the problem is that it has no material existence. The illusion is a

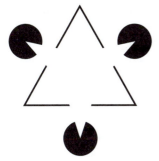

Figure 2.1 Kanizsa Triangle

product of our brains, which when scanning this unlikely array of shapes reflexively determine that the best explanation for its oddness is that a white triangle is between us and some more likely figures. One can even alter the shape of the triangle by narrowing or widening the gaps cut out of the black circles.

Here is another, more complicated example of mental construction at work. Figure 2.2 challenges the *just observe and calculate* abilities with which we are supposed to be equipped. If you look at it, it is obvious that the table on the left is longer and narrower than the one on the right. But if you get out a ruler and check, they are of identical proportions; it is just that we have observational theories about them based on the usual rules of perspective. The point being that we have to take extraordinary cognitive precautions against such 'wired-in' reflex reactions – which is all that science is observational and epistemological paranoia in a good cause.

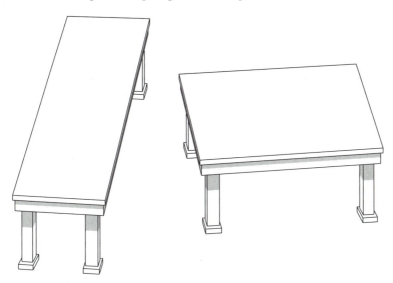

Figure 2.2 Turning the tables

Expectation reflexes also predominate in the next experiment. Try this on your colleagues. Invite them to respond out loud and as spontaneously as possible to a short series of questions; hold up a sheet of white paper and ask: 'What colour is this?' Then repeat the exercise with another, and then another. Then quickly ask: 'What do cows drink?' About 90 per cent will say 'milk'.

Selective perception also influences memory, as Bartlett (1950) showed in his classic experiments at Cambridge. He presented research participants with a short Inuit folktale entitled 'The War of the Ghosts'. This story is (for us) constructed in a haphazard-seeming way and contains many unusual references to the spirit world. The idea in these studies was to produce a test sequence low on cultural cues as to what was or ought to be going on. Here is an extract:

> And the warriors went on up the river to a town on the other side of Kalma. The people came down to the water, and they began to fight, and many were killed. But presently the young man heard one of the warriors say: 'Quick let us go home: that Indian has been hit'. Now he thought: 'Oh! They are ghosts'. He did not feel sick, but they said he had been shot.
>
> (Bartlett, 1950: 97)

Participants were then asked to recall such passages at carefully spaced intervals, and, as might be expected, the longer the interval, the greater the failure of memory – but also the more *invention* took over. The orderliness of the results across respondents suggests that Bartlett and his colleagues were mapping an internal predisposition to subtract from, and add to, weak or ambiguous stimuli until concordant sense could be made of them, involving polar bears and seals not mentioned in the text. The following quotation gives an idea of typical results:

> There was a strong tendency to rationalize, common to all subjects. Whenever anything appeared unusual, incomprehensible, or queer it was either omitted or explained. Rather rarely this rationalization was the effect of conscious effort.
>
> (Bartlett 1950: 201)

This and similar exercises easily replicated in the psychology class have implications for the way social workers make assessments and record data in their cases (issues revisited later in Chapter 5). Indeed, if one examines inquiry reports into failed risk assessments in childcare or mental health cases one can usually detect the implicit theories, sometimes promising but sometimes wrong, at work.

Such routine distortions are based on the fact that, despite our prodigious information-processing capacities, human beings could never, over evolutionary time, afford to respond anew to every sequence of stimuli. Any edible creature which had stood still and pondered whether large dun-coloured animals with manes had the same negative attributes as the smaller spotted ones, would have been unlikely to pass on its genes.

Theories, however elaborate, are only as good as the initial data on which they are based. For example, Sigmund Freud's analyses of the 'neuroses' of six middle-class Viennese women, one of whom was definitely *not* fantasizing and *had* been sexually abused as a child, and another who was *indeed* very physically ill (see Masson, 1985; Eysenck, 1991), led to the development of a large body of influential writings and thousands of clinical and social interventions.

So theories matter, and the validity and reliability of empirical observations on which they are based also matter, as does research on the extent to which they survive selective-perception-squeezing tests, comparisons with other theories, and empirical checks on their practical utility (see Chapter 4). Thus, the fact that we are not natural, unbiased observers means – not what the postmodernists propose, namely, that we should give up on the hopeless pursuit of as much objectivity as we can manage – rather that vigilant precautions against inbuilt subjectivity are all the more necessary.

Implicit theories

These are less automatic and more cognitively based than perceptual reflexes, but nevertheless are often surprisingly unconsidered. They have the intellectual status of 'most favoured concepts'. Here are two examples. The first is the theory that adverse early childhood experiences virtually always result in irreversible damage (e.g. following child sexual abuse, or as a result of being in a caring role where parents have a disability). The evidence suggests that (1) effects differ greatly; (2) that compensatory experiences can strongly counter initially negative ones; (3) that some people have sufficient inbuilt resilience to overcome them and can accurately attribute the causes of distress not to failings in themselves but to those who held the power at the time, or to the 'no-fault' circumstances of the time (see Rutter and Hersov, 1987; Macdonald, 2001). Second is the 'It always helps to talk' theory. Here, the implicit presumption is that a better understanding or greater insight into past problems will yield gains in the present, and that these 'unblockings' can be achieved by sympathetic verbal interchange alone. Yet modern research evidence suggests that the gap between understanding and purposeful action is probably the most under-estimated obstacle to recovery in cases known to all of us in the helping professions (see Bandura, 1969; Rachman and Wilson, 1980; Sheldon, 1995). After all, are not we ourselves full of insight into habitual sequences of less than constructive thinking, untoward emotional reactions and self-defeating behaviour? But then do not we (the much less up against it) often tend to continue in the same patterns?

In other words, just because a theory has a harmonious resonance, supports preferred ways of working and/or is flattering of a given professional role or, as in the case of psychoanalysis, has dramatic 'Wagnerian' features, by no means makes it the best theme to follow. Here is a quote (from one of our best philosophers of science) which sums up the problem:

> We are still so deeply steeped in the tradition of which Blake was one of the founders that we find it difficult to realize that the intensity of the conviction with which we believe a theory to be true has no bearing upon its validity except in so far as it produces a proportionately strong inducement to find out whether it is true or not. Some theories have enjoyed an unduly long lease of life because of a certain, dark visceral appeal.
>
> (Medawar, 1982: 1)

Embedded theories

The organizations to which we belong are also likely to reinforce preferred explanations and ways of evaluating disparate evidence. In other words, corporate cultures favour certain theories about what they are for and how those employed in them should go about their work, and they punish heresies.

Let us consider a historical example of authority-driven theorizing from another rather more certain field than our own. There was once much controversy about the precise number of human chromosome pairs per cell in the human body. Some 12-year-olds can now tell you that it is 23, but in the 1920s staining and microscope slide preparation techniques left the matter in some doubt. In 1923, the eminent American zoologist Theophilus Painter pronounced that there were 24 pairs. This authoritative conclusion was repeated in textbooks over the next 30 years alongside photographs clearly showing (had anyone bothered to count) only 23 pairs. The power of argument from authority, the power of routine 'givens', and the influence of peer-group pressure are all revealed in this case and we have many equivalent examples in our own field.

Such theory-driven observational errors have occurred at both ends of the optical scale. The Dutch astronomer Christian Huygens (1629–1695) first identified pale patches at the poles of Mars using a primitive telescope. Ice? The nineteenth-century Italian astronomer Giovanni Schiaparelli built on this work and in 1877 reported a network of *Canali* criss-crossing from the poles. Waterways? The word *Canali*, which in Italian means 'channels' or 'rifts', was mistranslated into English as 'canals', implying constructed waterways. Under this misapprehension, the American astronomer Percival Lowell wrote three books on what Martian irrigation systems and waterside life might look like (think Canary Wharf). Then H.G. Wells derived a theory that the red planet was red due to water shortages (hence the irrigation scheme) and that 'they' might be coming here to exploit our surplus. Then Orson Wells read *The War of the Worlds* story on radio as if it were an official broadcast, and thousands fled to the hills. What has this to do with social work? Well, the 'wired-in' tendency to join up the dots of separate observations and to theorize about them still influences what we see and believe today. Thus, the 'theory' that people with clean carpets and quiet children are unlikely to be guilty of abuse, or that poor families under stress are more likely to have committed such crimes, is clearly present in the inquiry literature (see Sheldon, 1987a). Later reports then reinterpret such patterns.

Social psychological experiments have long confirmed this tendency to accept ideas and proposals from apparent consensus and from authority, and to ignore disconcerting, even commonsense, evidence (see Asch, 1951; Milgram, 1974). Illustrations of this tendency at work will be found below. The Milgram experiment employed an actor who pretended to receive electric shocks for failing a test (no electricity was involved). An astonishing number (64 per cent) of volunteers moved the lever to the 'Danger 350 volts, dangerous shock' level just because they had been told to by a technician. The implicit theory in these circumstances, and the ones shown in Plates 2.1 and 2.2, is that it is best to think and report what the majority think, or to do what those 'in charge' want.

In the Asch experiments subjects were asked to judge the length of obviously longer or shorter lines shown on a screen. The room was packed with confederates of the experimenters who consistently gave wrong answers. Naive subjects went along with the majority even though the distinctions were obvious. Interestingly, you can see the psychological pressures at work just by looking at the demeanour and gestures of the person who is obviously the naive subject.

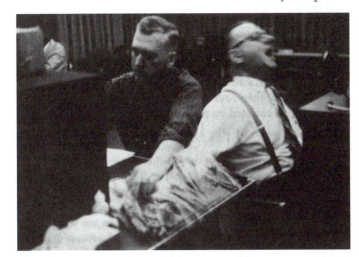

Plate 2.1
The Milgram
experiments
(1974).

Obedient
subject in
touch-proximity
condition.

Source: Reprinted
courtesy of Yale
University Press

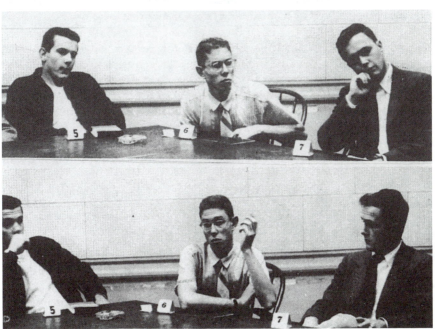

Plate 2.2 The Asch experiments (1951)

Source: Reprinted courtesy of Yale University Press, *The Scientific American*

The catastrophic events of 11 September 2001 in New York provide another example of what happens when members of organizations do what they have always done. The FBI receives hundreds of briefings per day, most of which, thankfully, led to nothing. So how are individual risk assessors to isolate the genuine signals of danger from the (on the face of it) equally threatening background noise? After the attack, disinterred memoranda took on the look of tailor-made predictions which should definitely have been acted upon (for more on this, see Dixon's riveting book *On the Psychology of Military Incompetence* (1976)).

The foregoing is not just an interesting excursion into another field, because exactly the same problems of vigilance and interpretation operate in child abuse and mental health cases. Examining the records of children who have been abused, a range of factors have been identified as being associated with increased risk of child abuse (e.g. a baby in the care of a young, inexperienced single parent whose own childhood had been troubled, who has a visiting partner with social services or police 'form', who lives in relative isolation from the extended family, who is welfare benefit dependant and in poor-quality housing, with a substance misuse problem in the background, perhaps). But these are not reliable predictors of abuse, and to act as if they were would be to bring very large numbers of children into protective care – which disposal itself carries noteworthy risks (see Chapter 10).

We have long known that tensions exist between professional decision-making and organizational rules designed to ensure accountability. Probably we have swung from too much reliance on unaided professional judgement to too much reliance on corporate plans and service frameworks. Here is an awkward idea:

> Only if somewhat immune from ordinary social pressures and free to innovate, to experiment, to take risks without the usual social repercussions of failure, can a professional carry out his work effectively. It is this highly individualized principle which is diametrically opposed to the very essence of the organizational principle of control and co-ordination by superiors – i.e., the principle of administrative authority. In other words the ultimate justification for a professional act is that it is, to the best of the professional's knowledge the right act. The ultimate justification of an administrative act, however, is that it is in line with the organization's rules and regulations.
>
> (Etzioni, 1964: 117)

This tension has not eased over the years; if anything, it has worsened, making the topic worthy of an entire series of Reith lectures in 2002 entitled *A Question of Trust* (O'Neill, 2002 – do read this if you can, it is full of good sense).

Let us conclude this sequence on the critical faculty-bending power of embedded theories and dangerous-to-challenge organizational policies with a further example from the child protection field. The first comes from a tape recording of an interview with one of the children caught up in troubling events on the Orkney Islands in the 1990s. There was then a growing concern in childcare circles regarding the possibility that members of satanic cults were abusing children. This derived mainly from American Christian fundamentalist tracts and from the testimony of allegedly abused children under so-called 'disclosure-interview' questioning. The Orkney raid (what else are we to call it?) was an ideological commitment too far and did great damage to the standing of social work (the police and the judiciary, though main players, were little criticized). Later investigations by the Department of Health indicated that there were indeed children being brought up in less than ideal circumstances, but no evidence of widespread 'satanic abuse', rather more of moral panic (see Clyde, 1992). Here is a section of a transcript from an interview with one of the children. As you read it just think what, if anything, would ever have been considered as counter-evidence against the theory? The questions come in 'coo-ing whispers' to the child whom we will call Gwennie.

Adult:	Where are the dickies and the fannies?
Gwennie:	Don't know.
Adult:	Can you write the word?
Gwennie:	No.
Adult:	. . . a word for when a dickie goes into a fanny?
Gwennie:	Don't know.
Adult:	Would you like to whisper?
Gwennie:	No.
Adult:	Is it yuckie inside and outside . . . is there any other word?
Gwennie:	[anxious to please] Gooey?
Adult:	[amidst childish laughter] Oh, that's a good word . . . what does gooey feel like?
Gwennie:	Here, this . . . (puts finger in mouth and pops).
Adult:	Don't know.
Adult:	Has it got a colour?
Gwennie:	[begins to count slowly up to four]
Adult:	I wonder what this gooey is. Can you tell me?
Gwennie:	No.
Adult:	When you put the dickie into the fanny . . .
Gwennie:	No. [angry] Now can I play? I am going to get my red car. This is boring [gets the car and begins to play]. Go and get me some toys.
Adult:	When you put the dickie into the fanny it's yuckie and gooey and disgusting. Who hurt you most?
Gwennie:	No one did it to me . . .
Adult:	We won't write it down.
Gwennie:	No one has been doing it to me [breaks into a scream]. Nobody has been doing it to me!
Adult:	You can play with the red car. We won't write it down if you want to whisper it . . .
Gwennie:	[shouting even louder] I AM NOT . . . I AM NOT GOING TO WRITE IT DOWN!
Adult:	If it's a name you can see written down you can point to it [shows the child a list of names of people on South Ronaldsay]. Is it a name you see written down?

(Dalrymple, 1994)

Elaborated theories

These are explicated, printed theories about purported causes and effects. Examples are Piaget's theories of intellectual development (Piaget, 1929); Freud's theories on unconscious motivation and repression (Freud, 1940, 1949); feminist theories on the unconscious absorption by women and girls of the embedded assumptions of patriarchy (Greer, 1970); Marx's theory on the 'contradictions' of capitalism and its power to dominate thinking and culture as well as economics (Marx, 1887);

attachment theories which attempt to explain adult mental health problems or failures in social relationships in terms of childhood disconnections (Bowlby and Salter-Ainsworth, 1963); Durkheim's theory of *anomie* (1893, 1933) which seeks to explain suicide rates in terms of social dislocation; conditioning theories by Pavlov (1897), Skinner (1953) and others which seek to explain how we acquire behavioural, cognitive and emotional reflexes and predispositions; systemic theories on how family tensions create self-scapegoating expressions of pain and trouble by children (see Chapter 8); theories of personality development attempting to explain tendencies to think, feel and behave in particular ways semi-independently of environmental circumstances (see Pervin, 1989; Sheldon, 1995); and theories of bereavement purporting to explain the predictable stages of recovery and also why and how some people fail in the attempt to rebalance their lives (Parkes, 1994).

These theories have one thing in common: they are extended attempts to fill in the gaps between experiental, professional or clinical observations. They aim to produce a panoramic view of causes and effects, and so of attendant implications for useful interventions. However, the inescapable question is: Are all such theories created equal? Or do certain explanations have superior qualities which should induce us to prefer them and sideline others? Or is it simply a matter of selecting plausible, experience-confirming proposals and integrating them into our practice, and then just glancing backwards at what happens? The problem with this route seems to be that routine evaluations are generally so subjective as to provide no reliable feedback loop in such a process (see Sheldon, 1995). We recommend, therefore, that 'respectful scepticism' is the right stance with which to begin this process of weighing up different strategies.

The integration of theory and practice

The combined challenges to the idea of a straightforward, reciprocal relationship between theory and practice are that we have (1) a very wide range of potentially useful theories from our own and nearby disciplines, and (2) a wide range of demanding functions in which we might apply such knowledge. These two factors have led to a serious problem in our discipline, i.e. we have ended up with something closer to a knowledge pile than a knowledge base. We propose therefore that the creation of a more orderly relationship between practice and theory has been a neglected priority.

Let us consider next the obstacles to such a shift in our thinking and in our educational arrangements. Here is what we believe the over-lightly used term 'integration' actually implies:

1   It assumes that social work has a distinctive bank of knowledge on which it can draw in trying to come up with plans and schemes to help needy people. We have such a store of intellectual capital as never before, though in research terms the chaff/wheat ratio is still unacceptably high (see Sheldon, 2001; Macdonald, 2003). However, the idea also implies that some kinds of 'drawing and depositing arrangements' have been agreed among the producers and the users of this bank of information, beyond the ad hoc, 'salad bar', 'choose what you fancy and leave the rest' approach redolent of most training courses.

2   The concept further assumes that social workers have been taught how to make other than convenient, comfortable, consonant, or otherwise subjective selections from the theoretical literature.

Two cultures?

It is arguable that two different subcultures, *à la* C. P. Snow (1933), have long existed within social work. In universities and colleges there is a 'theory and research sub-culture' understandably preoccupied with the *discipline* of social work and associated questions of evidence and outcome, occasionally in danger of forgetting its *raison d'être* in its quest for academic respectability. Next there is the much larger 'practice subculture', forced to hang on to its individualistic principles in unpropitious circumstances; somewhat anti-intellectual in its approach to questions of theory and research; a little suspicious of academics, and preferring still to rely largely on 'practice wisdom' as a way of monitoring progress. However, while some practice decisions are indeed wise, some, as we have seen, are foolhardy: telling the two apart prospectively (retrospectively it is easy) is the challenge.

Notwithstanding the fact that they address the same fundamental problems in the longer term, the solutions put forward by these two groups are quite different in relation to questions of effective practice. The theoretical subculture typically offers as its best product the systematic review of controlled trials. Sometimes these suggest that much of what goes on within practice is less useful than is generally supposed, or that the evidence is less than conclusive (see Littel *et al.*, 2005; Turner *et al.*, 2007). However, this rarely has a chastening effect, simply because few people in the practice subculture set much store by these exercises – particularly if the findings are critical of established habits or seem to contradict what fieldworkers regard as the evidence of their own eyes and ears.

The practice subculture offers a less methodologically demanding and more relevant-seeming product, but consequently a less reliable one. The emphasis here is more on the individuality and uniqueness of the problems under review than on general patterns of what might well be called *social epidemiology*. The favoured approach is the case report or small, local evaluation. Such views are often based on the views of a small number of clients and (mistakenly) are seen as atheoretical state-ments – and all the better for it. Thus the question: 'What shall count as evidence?' produces different answers in this constituency. The investigator's involvement with his or her subject matter, not their detachment from it, is seen as the important test of verisimilitude; evaluations of practice or of service patterns are thus often based on the opinions of the deliverer, and on the uncontrolled verbal reports of the recipi-ents. From this source, and from their immediate reference group of colleagues, such staff, where they bother at all, gain their impressions of effectiveness. However, there is much in the literature to caution us against over-reliance on these kinds of highly negotiable data. It is interesting to note that in a number of the classic evaluation studies (see Jones and Borgatta, 1972; Fischer, 1976; Sheldon, 1986; Fischer, 1993) significant numbers of clients, when first interviewed, recalled the experience of seeing a social worker as useful and reassuring. It is arguable that in certain cases such an outcome might be called a success, but these immediate impressions were not what the researchers were investigating. They were not seeking primarily to evaluate settee-side manner or the congeniality of the helping process, but more tangible impacts in respect of pre-set goals (e.g. lower reconviction rates; improved community tenure; better school attendance). Therefore theory is not readily amended by feedback from practice because by and large practice lacks certain qualities. Equally, practice is not affected as much as it might be by research and theory, because these products too are perceived to lack certain qualities. The development of evidence-based practice in social work has made some inroads into this problem, but it remains a rather endemic and protean one (see Sheldon *et al.*, 2005).

Problems with eclecticism

Social work is, and should remain, an eclectic discipline. Its field of operation – the troubled and/or disadvantaged and/or discriminated against individual in society – ensures that it will depend for theoretical sustenance on concepts and findings drawn from a wide variety of sources. The opportunities presented by this kind of relationship have long been celebrated. There are, for example, built-in disincentives to partial or fixed views of problems, and challenges to unduly fixed perspectives are supposedly waiting around any number of corners. The policy of eclecticism thus, allegedly, ensures a 'balanced' curriculum. The approach also leads us away from the dangers of having too many of our eggs in anyone else's theoretical basket: the failure of our investments in psychodynamic psychology and radical politics provided important lessons in this respect. However, proposals that we should invest more judiciously in the future (see Sheldon, 1978) were recognized as potentially controversial and likely to provoke rows among the shareholders. Therefore, by default, we are left with a policy of just investing more widely than before. 'Never mind the quality, feel the *width*' sums up current attitudes.

Thus the problems of *laissez-faire* curriculum development have been less well documented than have the potential benefits. They stem not so much from the diversity of our sources of explanation as from the way in which we relate to these. Eclecticism assumes that *all* knowledge is potentially useful to us, and from there it is but a small step to the even more comfortable assumption that, in the right hands, it is all of equal status and value. Thus different research methodologies for evaluating the effectiveness of what we do are widely regarded as belonging to a continuum rather than a hierarchy: not better or worse, not more or less bias-minimizing, just 'different'. A fool's paradise.

As practitioners, students and teachers we typically 'select such doctrines as please us in every school' (*OED*), the result passing for a 'broad' approach to our subject. If we have Piaget, Vygotsty and Skinner in the curriculum then we must include Foucault and Laing – it seems only fair somehow. So, in the interests of a spurious academic freedom we give too little thought to what *should* please us, for how *long* we should expect it to remain pleasing, and what we should do with theories which, on the empirical evidence, should no longer please us.

Theoretical conflict

The knowledge base of social work is made up of theories and concepts which seek to explain the same phenomena. We should properly think of these as being in competition for the same intellectual territory. But at present there is little creative tension between propositions, and many instances of completely and logically opposed views co-existing peacefully – either explicitly in the curriculum, or implicitly in chosen forms of practice. Consider a practice example first. As things stand, a child with behavioural problems, who is troubled, troubling or both, whatever the reasons for his or her behaviour, may be subjected either to approaches which encourage him or her to 'act out' their antisocial behaviour, or to regimes which seek to inhibit such expressions and encourage something else. Adherents of the former theory view the latter course of action as merely symptomatic treatment or tinkering with surface phenomena. They would expect the 'real causes' to break out elsewhere (perhaps in a more pernicious form) as a result of vain attempts at tying down the child's 'emotional safety-valve'. The latter group see this as an outdated argument and would accuse the proponents of 'acting out' theory of sustaining the very behaviour they say they want to change; of simply relabelling problematic behaviour with some technical term of doubtful validity (e.g. 'antisocial behaviour disorder'; attention deficit hyperactivity disorder) and tautologically calling this the cause. The worst cases will, however, receive something called 'support' in a building named after a tree, and only a little is known about what goes on in such places and what effects these disposals have.

The typical solution to the inconsistencies discussed above has been to argue for a 'third-way' combination of both contending approaches. Theories are often taught alongside each other, the ultimate choice being left to the student. Here, the failure of an individual to develop an adequately functioning conscience may be discussed on Mondays in terms of his or her early feeding experiences (Klein), or on Tuesdays as resulting from a failure to resolve a competitive relationship with his father at age 4 (Freud); on Wednesdays as a disturbance in the discrete stages of moral and intellectual development which exert influence over the next decade might be indicted (Piaget); and on Thursdays, if you are lucky, as resulting from the lifelong process of operant conditioning (Skinner). Fridays are for placement preparation work, where none of these things, from the silly to the sensible, will get much of a mention (see Macdonald and Sheldon, 1998).

Now we may not be able to say with *complete* certainty which of these recipes is the right one (a main course of Piaget and later researchers, with a drizzle of Skinner, Bandura and Pavlov, in a Halsey and Holman sauce would be our order). However, we must be clear that they cannot *all* be, since the proposed causes and time-scales are at odds. We could, however, attempt to decide on some kind of policy which would take account of the methodological sophistication of certain explanations in comparison with others, whether one view or another gives the more economical description of salient factors, or whether views 'A', 'C' or 'D' predict outcomes readily observable in research studies. If a potential user of these theories still finds any resultant recommendation unconvincing, then in opting for view 'A' he or she should surely feel constrained to register the main points of incompatibility with view 'C' or 'D' and attempt to appraise the findings of their proponents before proceeding. Such habits of mind should be inculcated early on our training courses, but probably won't be.

The current practice of presenting logically incompatible theories alongside each other and leaving the choice to the student is closer to academic licence than to academic freedom. It perpetuates a situation where knowledge is merely stored rather than sifted and refined. If we have no broadly agreed, established criteria against which securely to judge the validity, reliability and practical utility of concepts, then it is difficult to know what it is safe to let go of.

There are of course occasions where it is not possible to formulate any firm views from the welter of material available. Where this is the case then the temptation to make snap judgements must also be resisted. There is nothing wrong with the suspension of judgement, providing that this is an active rather than a passive process. By 'active' we mean that suspension of judgement should be at least a little irksome to us, and should follow, not precede, attempts to evaluate the different contributions in the literature. Here is some useful advice on the matter:

> In studying a philosopher, the right attitude is neither reverence nor contempt, but first a kind of hypothetical sympathy, until it is possible to know what it feels like to believe in his theories, and only then a revival of the critical attitude, which should resemble, as far as possible, the state of mind of a person abandoning opinions which he has hitherto held. Contempt interferes with the first part of this process and reverence with the second.
>
> (Russell, 1946: 58)

However awkward for classroom and office harmony, explanations must be made to compete: in practice, in supervision, at case conferences, in tutorials, seminars and lectures – wherever social workers discuss the ideas behind what they are trying to achieve. The current situation, in which students are encouraged to believe virtually anything they like as if, like religious or political affiliation, it were a matter of individual choice with no vulnerable consumers in the picture, is untenable:

> Alice laughed. 'There's no use trying', she said: 'One can't believe impossible things'.
>
> 'I dare say you haven't had much practice', said the Duchess. 'When I was your age, I always did it for half an hour a day. Why sometimes I've believed as many as six impossible things before breakfast'.
>
> (Carroll, 1865)

The qualities of theories

Pursuing the contention that theories are not created equal, that many are logically incompatible with each other, and that we should *mind* that this is so and try to achieve a more coherent synthesis, we should now consider the means by which such a change might be achieved. Our first piece of advice is that the philosophy of science has already provided some good guidance (see Popper, 1963; Oakley, 2000). Here is a list of what we regard as reasonable tests of beliefs and propositions:

1   First, in order to check up on the status of a theory at all it must be potentially refutable. This is Karl Popper's demarcation between what counts as scientific knowledge and what does not. Some theories contain inbuilt defences against disbelief (e.g. much of Freud's and Marx's work; the literatures on 'recovered

memory' effects in the child sexual abuse field). Although the arguments have great explanatory range (we dearly miss the presence of the occasional 'somewhat' or 'sometimes' in such accounts), they must occupy a lower position in any hierarchy stressing validity and reliability. The personal 'blind spots' of the unanalysed critic on the one hand, or the prejudices of class or gender on the other, withhold 'true understanding'. Daniel Dennett (2006) aptly calls this 'pre-emptive disqualification'. New interpretations arise to cope with each successive attack and the theory is in all cases left intact, or, as in debates about religion, there is a general charge of 'disrespect'. This intellectual sleight of hand is also to be found at the level of practice: if the goals of intervention are loosely defined ('flexible goals' as they are euphemistically called; see Chapter 5), then how are we to know what has been achieved?

Einstein once said of a paper critical of his work that it was 'not even wrong'. Irrefutability, either at the level of theories for practice or practice theory, is not a virtue but a vice. In case you think such comments far-fetched, consider the following quotation from the family therapy field:

> During a session on supervision, many of the participants spoke eloquently about their non-hierarchical relationships with their supervisors, about how they considered all ideas equally valid, and about how there is from a social constructivist perspective, no objective place to stand and judge another therapist's work as either good or bad.
>
> (Flemons *et al.*, 1995: 43)

'Postmodernism' is to blame for the contemporary manifestations of this nonsense, but the origins of such self-serving evasiveness go back much further; for example:

> You can believe me when I tell you that we do not enjoy giving an impression of being members of a secret society and of practicing a mystical science. Yet we have been obliged to recognize and express as our conviction that no one has the right to join in a discussion of psychoanalysis who has not had particular experiences which can only be observed by being analysed oneself.
>
> (Freud, 1949: 26)

But then no one ever completes an analysis successfully who has *any* unresolved doubts about the theory behind it all.

Is this still a relevant concern today? Not in the 'care-management' field it isn't, but it is regarding the hundreds of counsellors now being employed in primary care and the hundreds of private jobbing therapists now bought in by social and health services.

2   Popper's second criterion of worth is that of 'riskiness of prediction'. The preferable theory is, contra-intuitively, the one that *prohibits* the most. Thus we should learn to prefer those explanations which place themselves at the greatest risk of refutation by predicting what ought *not* to occur. Cognitive-behavioural theories are thus preferable to psychodynamic and family therapy theories in this respect since they predict that direct intervention will not produce symptom substitution. If they do (they don't), the theory is endangered. Freudian

concepts and 'Humanistic psychology' run no such risks since, if the right degree or direction of behavioural change does not follow, then clients are deemed, retrospectively, not to have attained 'true insight' but merely to be engaging in 'defensive intellectualization' or to be 'unmotivated'.

3   The next point of evaluation concerns testability. The good theory is that which produces relevant and testable hypotheses. Many quite elaborate social work theories produce very low yields of these operational, 'so, on the best current evidence, what we should consider doing is . . .' statements, contrary to what we expect from our medical advisers and gas fitters.

4   Obviously the next point must concern the history of any attempts which have been made to test a theory or concept. Social workers often respond to ideas because they are attractive in themselves; because they find ready support in an established system of values, or because they have flattering implications. Thus R.D. Laing's proposition that schizophrenia is a product of disturbed family functioning (a dimension familiar to social workers) never had to fight hard for a place in the curriculum, whereas H.J. Eysenck's and Vaughan and Leff's more sophisticated empirical work did. Bowlby's (1951) ideas on maternal deprivation are still in there, but Michael Rutter's work modifying these ideas often is not.

5   The next test is concerned with the degree of simplicity in a given theory. This test is called variously 'Occam's Razor' or the 'law of parsimony'. It proposes that the more economical the explanation of a given set of factors or events, the more preferable. In other words, the fewer red herrings that might be pursued, the better. Thus 'persuasion' or 'selective reinforcement of responses' may be preferable concepts to 'insight' for explaining therapeutically derived changes in clients.

6   Logical consistency comes next: the greater the harmony or internal consistency within a theory, the more preferable. Freud's adaptation of the Oedipus theory to cover little girls, the 'Electra Complex', has been taken up by feminist writers, who have largely ignored the fact that it has problems of internal inconsistency. What Freud predicts should happen is logically at odds with the rest of his theory (see Brown, 1986). In case you think all this a little arcane, consider this glossary definition of The Enlightenment from Margaret Ledwith:

> This is the philosophy that developed in Western Europe in the 17th and 18th Century which rejected previous supernatural ways of making sense of the world in favour of an objective, rational, unemotional, scientific knowledge embedded in masculinity.
>
> (Ledwith, 2003: 26)

Clarity of expression: the less ambiguous the presentation of a theory, the more preferable. This is not simply a reference to style, which can be a problem, but to the quality and clarity of the prescription contained within a statement. Thus if the phrase 'family homeostasis' is used it must be operationally defined, otherwise potential users of the concept are entitled to ask how they will recognize this phenomenon should they come across it or think it absent. Getting the research question and attendant propositions right is a major feature of systematic reviews (see Chapter 4). But what are we to do with this sort of situation?

> We can clearly see that there is no bi-univocal correspondence between linear signifying links or archi-writing, depending on the author, and this multi-referential, multi-dimensional machine catalysis.
>
> (Guttari, in Dawkins, 2003: 47)

This is a quotation from the psychoanalyst Félix Guttari who is also keen to 'remove us from the logic of the excluded middle and reinforce us in our dismissal of ontological binarism' (thank heavens someone has their eye on that). This 'speaking in tongues' is a reaction to the Sokal and Bricmont (1998) spoof, dealt with on p. 54, and though entirely devoid of intelligible content, tells us, if we 'deconstruct' it, three interesting things:

- Psychoanalysis has re-morphed itself in virus-like fashion by combining with post-modernist delusions so as further to defeat our intellectual immune systems.
- This and its like seek to persuade us that the benefits of the Enlightenment and of science are illusions; that all is chaos and flux, and that the best guide to finding out anything with even passable caché is to consult a French or Italian social philosopher.
- If you cannot make sense of such writing then the fault definitely lies with you, and further education might be necessary.

There is no suggestion here that there is a danger that busy social workers will be beguiled by this sort of theorizing, rather that a considerable minority of social work academics are, and they use it to advance preoccupations of their own, to excuse failures, and to distract attention from the project of developing a practical, evidence-based curriculum for professional training.

7   In circumstances where no convincing explanation is available, the best that can be done is to attempt to develop what Karl Popper called 'criteria of relative potential satisfactoriness'. That is, we should try to construct the best 'template' possible as a guide to future investigation.

Whether the reader will wish to add items to, or subtract items from, this list will depend largely on which of the social science traditions he/she has been brought up in. The two rival positions on these questions of evidence are positivism and idealism. The views presented in this chapter favour the former stance, holding that certain aspects of the process of evaluating ideas are interchangeable between the natural and social sciences (Homans, 1967; Sheldon and Macdonald, 1999). A good summary of the positivist position is contained in the following quotation:

> All that we can know of reality is what we can observe or can legitimately deduce from what we observe. That is to say, we can only know phenomena, and the laws of relation and succession of phenomena and it follows that everything we can claim to know must be capable of empirical verification.
>
> (Charlton, 1959: 112)

The key assumption here is that what we believe with any firmness ought to be anchored in verifiable sensory experience. In social work this is the position of the cognitive-behavioural school (see Sheldon, 1995; Cigno and Bourne, 2000) who aim at tangible behavioural change and regard forms of mental adjustment as largely concomitant, problem-maintenance factors rather than as primarily causal.

Here is one example of how causes and effects can easily be confused; it concerns the widely held belief that the negative, self-blaming cognitions frequently reported by clinically depressed people might have led to their illnesses in the first place. Lewinsohn and colleagues simply selected a wide sample of people with no particular clinical history; administered a standardized test of negative self-attribution; waited to see which of them became depressed, and then carried out correlational comparisons between the ill and the well. Here is a summary of the results:

> Prior to becoming depressed, these future depressives did not subscribe to irrational beliefs, they did not have lower expectancies for positive outcomes, or higher expectations for negative outcomes, they did not attribute success experiences to external causes and failure experiences to internal causes, nor did they perceive themselves as having less control over the events in their lives.
>
> (Lewinsohn *et al.*, 1981: 218)

While there is now ample evidence that prior to becoming depressed, and upon remission, the cognitions of depressed patients do not differ from others who do not, it seems that, once activated, such thoughts contribute to *maintaining* depressed mood, and research by Teasdale (1978) suggests that it is the impact that negative automatic thoughts can have in times of mild depression (which many of us experience from time to time) that is to blame for the development of clinical levels of depression in those whose latent schema render them vulnerable. In other words, the history of cognitive-behavioural therapy exemplifies the testing and refining processes outlined in Chapter 7. Thus the advantages of the positivist approach lie in its rigour and in the replicability and transferability of its findings.

The idealist position is in some ways closer to mainstream social work. It states that social reality is not so much discovered as invented, socially constructed, by its residents – which category includes any would-be investigators, namely:

> The exploration of the general principles to which man in daily life organises experiences, and especially those of the social world, is the first task of the methodology of the social sciences.
>
> (Schutz, 1954: 267)

The dilemma of these two positions on evidence is mirrored exactly by the dilemma of how to turn social work into a more rigorous discipline, and yet retain the 'idealist' features of close identification with the experiences of clients and a consequent attempt to understand problems from as close to the 'inside' as we can get. It would be nice to have both, but would an attempt at a synthesis produce yet more philosophical and methodological inconsistencies? Happily, there are writers who think not. Ford (1976) and Oakley (2000) have long put forward the view that we can refuse to accept the stark choices presented by settled proponents of either view and that a combination of the best of both approaches is not inconsistent if we view the possibility in the light of Popper's 'two-stage' model of science described earlier, and regard each as the solution to a different problem. Thus, we can agree that what happens and the sense that people make of it, like it or not at the conjectural and problem-identification level, follows most closely the guiding principles of idealism; whereas future attempts to test and evaluate these ideas, so that one's own interpretation might become acceptable to others, brings one almost inevitably into the positivist camp – like it or not.

In the light of such a merger, we need to add one further awkward item to our list of criteria for evaluating competing theories:

8   For a theory to be useful as a medium for social understanding, or for the promotion of social change, it must take some account of the subjective understanding of relevant problems or phenomena held by those experiencing the effects. The good theory, then, must go some ways towards satisfying taken-for-granted conceptions of the matter being studied.

Our aims in mounting this discussion are threefold. First, to show that modern conceptions of the nature of the scientific process do not necessarily clash (either at a philosophical or a methodological level) with many of the accepted beliefs and practices of social work. Second, that science provides us with the key to the development of a cumulative knowledge base, in that ready-made criteria are available for the competitive evaluation of its different theoretical components. Third, we have implied that there are important similarities between the work of the researcher and the practitioner: both erect hypotheses (know it or not) about possible associations between events. Therefore, both ought to be required to pay attention to phrasing these so that they are placed at risk via subsequent experience.

Attitudes to science

The next troublesome obstacle to coherent theory–practice integration deserves a subheading to itself, so large a problem is it. The idea here is that science should be seen as the tried and tested answer to the problems discussed in this chapter, but this notion has many opponents in our field. They rightly point out that, ethics aside, we in the *applied* social sciences do not have the methodological option of screwing down what we wish to observe to the laboratory bench – but then increasingly, neither do physical scientists. Quantum physics is increasingly theoretical, grabbing a (temporary) empirical verification or refutation where it can. But then, our subject matter looks back at us up the microscope and changes its behaviour in the knowledge that it is being studied. So is the idea of the 'appliance of science' (in some suitably adapted form) a mistaken one? We argue that there are several basic ideas which do have immediate application, notably: the idea of hypotheses which are testable; the need for pre-stating what contrary evidence might look like; the ideas of sample representativeness and of validity and reliability tests; and the notion of taking due precautions against known sources of observational and interpretive bias when designing studies or reviewing cases (see Chapter 4).

Conclusions

1   In this age of the internet, where thousands of potentially relevant studies are available on personal computers, *theories* about how they might combine into something more coherent and usable are now *more* rather than less important.
2   Theories are *not* created equal. Some are more systematically arrived at on the basis of more and better empirical evidence; some are frankly fanciful and based on the too little examined influence of authoritative figures and their disciples.
3   Some grand theories place themselves beyond the influence of attempts at refutation either by pre-explaining why such attempts only go to prove the case, or by re-morphing themselves after each critical prod. For example, in 1996 Sokal published a spoof postmodernist treatise on relativity theory, full of nonsense. It was accepted by *Social Text*, a cultural studies journal, and widely debated there and elsewhere. When the gaff was blown no minds were changed; there was instead considerable personal acrimony, and the common cognitive-dissonance reducing ploy was to the effect that the authors *had* in fact come up with something important, but their destructive motives forbade them (unconsciously of course) to recognize the fact. The lesson here is that mega-explanatory, panacea-promising, protean, irrefutable ideas should be treated with caution by those of us with practical goals in mind. See Sokal and Briemont (1998).
4   If some theories prove more valid and reliable than others that are less testable, then the latter must be relegated. We are not always in a position to say which ideas and findings are clearly convincing, but we must acknowledge that not all can be if the proposed causes, effects and time-scales are different among them. Sometimes a synthesis is possible, sometimes not. The important point here is that comparisons of research of good or less good methodological quality, and attention to logical incompatibilities, should be a routine feature of how our subject is taught. Sadly, this is only sometimes the case, so *caveat emptor* (let the buyer beware).
5   Social workers, like most within the helping professions, have to become closely involved with those whom they try to assist. Therefore, due objectivity at the level of theory and research often seems like an alien idea. Our counter-argument is that soft-heartedness need not imply soft-headedness.
6   The demanding purposes of the job, the emotion-arousing plight of those we seek to help, plus the fact that we have to invest something of ourselves in every intendedly helpful encounter, routinely produce obstacles to rational decision-making. The theoretical principles through which we are (explicitly or implicitly) trying to operate become part of us. Thus, it is understandable that we tend to develop 'crushes' on theories which we find 'helpful', rather than being 'just good friends' with them. It is also understandable that we resent detractors and suspect them of malign intentions; that we forgive evidential lapses; and that we sulk in the face of criticism of ideas to which we are emotionally committed. We should instead save our commitment for our clients, and, as we used to say, 'stay

cool' about what we believe might be the best way to help them. The economist John Maynard Keynes put this argument for considered pragmatism well when, after being berated by a reporter for altering his position on monetary policy, replied: 'When the facts change, I change my mind. Pray Sir, what do you do?'

much material as to make them unmanageable. Thus, later, more specialist collections of studies (e.g. McGuire, 1995; Macdonald, 2001; Sheldon *et al.*, 2005) and the material available on specialist websites are all based on empirical assessments of what helps regarding *particular* problems, with *particular* client groups.

Service patterns

Social workers try to do two sets of things: (1) to prevent a deterioration in functioning and/or circumstances and to maintain a tolerably good status quo for fear of something worse; (2) to try also positively to improve circumstances/social functioning (e.g. through training in non-aggressive, disciplinary skills for parents trying to cope with behavioural problems in their children (whosesover's fault, if anyone's, the problem is). They have to develop self-care skills, coping skills, engagement with supportive aspects of the local community, and so forth. Using social functioning as an example, these twin functions may be modelled along the lines of Figure 3.1.

Figure 3.1a covers what social workers do when they are acting as 'buoyancy aids' for clients and/or carers. That is, following some crisis, chronic difficulties, or in the face of increasing infirmity, their role is to maintain a tolerable set of circumstances, and through small, continuous, maintenance interventions to stabilize the situation and prevent relapse (dotted line). In these circumstances, where needs are roughly predictable, it is the *logistics* of care that are the challenge. One used to see jugglers who could spin a row of 36 plates at once. They managed it by giving special attention only to those showing signs of wobbling dangerously: an analogy close to the daily realities of community care.

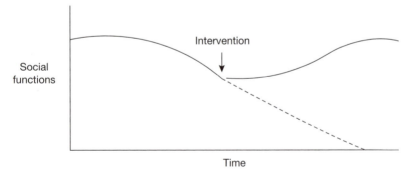

Figure 3.1a Social workers' role as 'buoyancy aids' for clients and/or carers

Then there are other kinds of cases, more acute in nature, which require that urgent changes take place either in behaviour or circumstances (see Figure 3.1b). The point is that if change is required or new skills are pressingly needed – say to control children without hitting them or, in the case of a learning disabled person in danger of becoming a recluse after a bad experience of rejection, then 'drip-feed' stability maintenance regimes are unlikely to be sufficient. No sensible person takes 20-minute driving or computer lessons fortnightly for two years. Let us examine this question further.

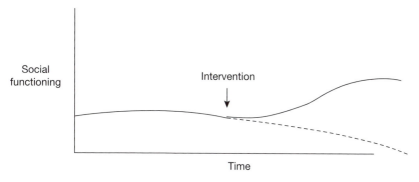

Figure 3.1b Cases requiring urgent changes in either behaviour or circumstances

Thought experiment: supposing the fixed, or close to fixed resources (time, skill, material help) available to a case could be represented by a ball of plasticine of a given size (Figure 3.2, this page and see also page 60).

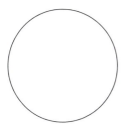

Figure 3.2 Service patterns and their influence on outcomes

Then there are several options open.

1 One could roll the ball out long and thin:

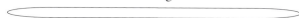

2 Or it could be rolled out short and fat:

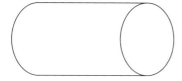

3 Or, since some cases which appear to require only background support flare up in unforeseen ways, it could, to use the technical research term, be rolled out in 'knobbly' fashion:

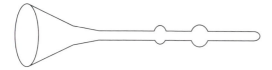

Stitches in time

The next set of findings arises from more recent research on social work effectiveness, and concerns the possibilities of prevention. Social work suffers more than other helping professions from dauntingly high eligibility-for-service thresholds. These are little to do with 'concentrating help on those most in need' – a favourite political mantra when money is short. Instead they are about cost containment and encouraging the not yet desperate to look after themselves. This is quite a sudden change from the original Welfare State principles of 'cradle-to-grave' care as an individual right under the post-war settlement (see Chapter 1), and we in Britain (the fifth largest economy in the world) are not exactly in penury, though we were flat broke when the promises were made and (largely) kept.

These pressures mean that social workers are largely allowed only to engage with clients in a crisis, when many opportunities for therapeutic solutions have evaporated or the chance of anything beyond problem containment is off the agenda. Ex-Prime Minister Blair discovered the importance of prevention regarding very young disturbed/disturbing, poorly brought up children, and proposed a future concentration of resources on such families. He was right that we usually learn in severe cases that there is a long history of disruption and neglect stretching back to early childhoods, but academics have been arguing for preventive approaches for years. It was the previous (Conservative) government's policies that closed down the relatively less stigmatized child and family guidance services and urged that prevention was unaffordable.

The problem we have, in research terms, is that little empirical work is done on these high-threshold, routine services that are currently the norm. Indeed, standard services tend to be in the control groups of experiments as something that we probably need to improve upon. Thus we are in a situation where specialist, preventive projects, which focus their energies on clients' developing problems before they have irreversible consequences, give our most encouraging results. A good example of such programmes is the Cornwall Child and Adolescent Mental Health (CAMHS) project (known popularly as 'Scallywags'; see Lovering *et al.*, 2006). It began life after staff started to debate the fact that many young people excluded from school, received into care, or with escalating patterns of offending, were almost always well known to staff prior to crises, but had received only sporadic help.

The project outlined above had the following features: (1) a specially recruited group of staff; (2) specific training in focused family support and cognitive-behavioural methods; (3) the active involvement of teachers, health personnel and the police, with some of their senior representatives on the steering group; (4) an independent evaluation officer who put standardized, pre-post measures into place and fed back interim information as the project proceeded; (5) intensive, multi-disciplinary involvement with families against contractual guidelines reflecting internal and external concerns; (6) advertisements for the service in 'ordinary' places (e.g. libraries, fish and chip shops, doctors' surgeries, video outlets). You have in that list of factors an example of exactly the recipe which seems to work in this field of community social work.

This point about preventive services is common sense really, because most of us in our daily lives take precautions, never perfectly, but generally speaking we do not visit

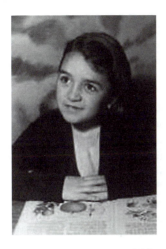

Plate 3.1 Rose West as a child

Source: Reprinted courtesy of
Picture Desk, www.swns.com

the dentist only when our teeth drop out, or disregard the blue smoke emanating from under the bonnet until it becomes really noxious. Look at Plate 3.1. Consider the promise in the expression, but also the malign influences that may be lying in wait for such a child, and when (sooner? later?) might be a good time to address them.

Plate 3.1 is a picture of Rose West as a schoolgirl. As an adult she was implicated in the killings of several people with her husband, with horrific sexual practices as a main feature of these murders. Two generations of the family were vaguely known to Social Services but contacts were intermittent. Her photographed face as an adult convict was widely referred to as 'the face of evil'. Can you spot any of this predetermined evil in the picture?

The problem with prevention is that social workers have to deal both with the emergencies *and* try to do something timely about accelerating need. The triage principle used in health therefore does not really work for us. We do not have the option, because of the costs, of public health-style early interventions; nor the option, even should we ever want it, of assessing clients as 'beyond effective help' and referring them on to some other form of 'palliative care'.

Elected members often ask academics such as ourselves: 'How then would *you* improve services without having any extra money to spend?' This is supposed to be a 'checkmate' question, but there is one move worth considering: Social Services budgets have increased steadily over the decades, and the question is how much of this extra income goes into client care, and how much into the servicing of bureaucratic requirements. Government, national and local, might actually get a better deal for its (our) cash if it backed off a little (see O'Neill, 2002).

Project work

Paul Halmos (drawing on C. Wright Mills' work) criticized social workers in his influencial book for their seeming inability to rise above the experience of a series of individual cases (Halmos, 1965). Pincus and Minahan (1973; see also Chapter 9, this volume) later drew to the profession's attention the need to address problems according to their origins and their prevalence, rather than encasing individual quanta of them in manila folders and treating them singly and symptomatically.

Another feature of project work is that such schemes are usually externally funded and have demanding evaluation requirements. Indeed, it would be possible to collapse a large part of this literature into the conclusion that social workers do better when their minds are concentrated by the existence of a rigorous evaluation programme integrated into the service.

Group work

This is a simple point: earlier reviews containing substantial evidence of positive outcomes contain many studies where therapeutic and supportive services were delivered to groups of clients. This is an efficient use of staff time, but seems to have gone out of fashion, in Britain at least (most of studies now coming from the USA, with the exception of the probation and juvenile justice field in the UK and Canada which have also yielded some good results). Two factors seem to be associated with positive outcomes: (1) that clients should have comparable problems rather than just being lumped together because they have problems per se; (2) that discussions of the probable origins of difficulties, and what clients feel and think about them might well be a necessary clarifying stage in such work, but there must then be a stage within which clients are encouraged to rehearse new behavioural options which might help to ameliorate them. We can find no examples of group work where the reflected-upon dynamics of the group itself are an effective vehicle of measurably useful behavioural or circumstantial change.

Are all intervention methods created equal?

A very strange thing happened recently. The editor of a premier US psychology journal called for *less* research, arguing that we have no further need of more controlled studies of cognitive-behavioural therapy for a wide range of problems. He went on to observe that given the existence of scores of trials with positive outcomes (see Sheldon, 2001; and Chapter 7, this volume) that the key priorities should now be the training of front-line staff in these skills. The government, under the influence of NIHCE reviews, has set aside £177 million for this.

The results of systematic reviews and experiments show that in juvenile justice and probation, in cases of depression, in relapse prevention, in schizophrenia, in the field of child behavioural problems, in helping families to cope with an autistic child, and so forth, cognitive-behavioural approaches never come second to anything. It should therefore be the preferred therapeutic option. Perversely, and unethically, it is probably the approach least likely to be taught on qualifying courses, even though relevant textbooks aimed specifically at social workers have been in print since the mid-1960s.

Individual factors in helping

Clients greatly value the *way* in which help is provided; they like the fact that they are listened to, not judged, not ordered about, and not regarded as 'non-compliant' if they are not always able to carry out the advice they have been given. Outcome research suggests that this is a necessary but not a sufficient set of skills. Most of us have had the experience of kindly, approachable, but in terms of exam-passing track records, hopeless teachers. Conversely, many of us have had the experience of being turned off subjects by knowledgeable but unsympathetic teaching. Both sets of factors are necessary if constructive engagement and change to circumstances or behaviour are to be achieved. We have some theoretical studies (see Rogers, 1951), some empirical studies (Truax and Carkhuff, 1966; Bergin and Garfield, 1986) of what features of personality and interviewing style are important. The three main variables for constructive engagement are *warmth, genuineness and accurate empathy*, and the point is that empirical researchers have refined these concepts so that they are identifiable on videotape and can be scaled for reliability. Let us now look at each of these factors in more detail.

- *Non-possessive warmth.* This consists of (1) getting across to clients feelings of respect, liking, caring, acceptance and concern; (2) managing to do this in a non-threatening way so that there is no question of the client feeling managed or taken over.
- *Genuineness.* Truax and Carkhuff (1966) have given us the best definition of this attribute by telling us what it is not. To be 'genuine' is not to be 'phoney', not to hide behind a professional façade or 'image', not to be defensive in the face of criticism or challenge, and not to be unpredictable in the type of responses made to the client.
- *Accurate empathy* is also a type of *behaviour* required to be *shown* by the would-be helper, because positive feelings they may have inside their heads are of little practical use unless communicated. There are three key elements in this process: (1) accuracy of understanding – letting the client know that you think you have a tentative grasp of his or her problems and dilemmas; (2) showing the client that you are trying to see things from their vantage point; (3) letting clients see that your own mood and feelings are in tune with theirs (see Chapter 6 for more such factors).

Having reviewed general trends from studies of social work effectiveness, we turn next to the evidence-based practice and the challenges it presents to practitioners, policy-makers and researchers.

4 Evidence-based practice

> The enquiry of truth, which is the love-making, or wooing of it, the knowledge of truth, which is the presence of it, is the sovereign good of human nature.
>
> Francis Bacon, 1627

Origins

The concept of evidence-based practice, so long under development, with its regularly changing brand names, seems now to have found its time. There are several reasons for the current level of interest among politicians, managers, front-line staff, and even a few academics. First, the personal social services are labour-intensive and therefore costly; and both state and voluntary funders increasingly require to be assured that their (or, lest we forget, *our*) money is being spent effectively. Unsubstantiated authority-based predictions, self-interested pressure group activity, and cosy evaluations of services from the professionals who provide them, are no longer seen as a tradable currency. Second, social work, more particularly social work academics in the USA, followed by a few in the UK later (see Goldberg, 1970; Rose and Marshall, 1975; Sheldon, 1986) tried to put the matter of service effectiveness beyond the reach of shifting political ideologies long ago, at least as far as studies where a comparison group of clients receives no service, a different service or lesser exposure, and their results are compared over time against outcome indicators, is concerned. The first large-scale controlled trials were begun in the USA in the 1930s, but due to World War II were reported only in the late 1940s and early 1950s (see Lehrman, 1949; Powers and Witmer, 1951). Incidentally, the first medical trials (of Streptomycin for pulmonary tuberculosis) were published at about the same time, just too late for George Orwell and others who continued to die of it (see Daniels and Hill (1952) for a compendium report).

The problem was, as we saw in Chapter 3, that the results of the early social work experiments were almost wholly disappointing. They should therefore have taught us something which the helping professions have only recently begun to acknowledge: namely that it is perfectly possible for good-hearted, well-trained, well-meaning staff, employing the most promising approaches and theories available to them, to make no difference at all to, or even to worsen, the condition of those they are seeking to help.

Thus the fact that there are disappointingly few 'magic bullets' for the social problems in governmental sights was not lost on politicians; indeed, an earlier generation of professionals taught them to expect too much in their claims for legislative and financial backing. Neither did we approach the problem of evidence and cost-effectiveness with due methodological caution. We did not, as would have been sensible, set up a few, tentative, representative, interview-based studies to get clients to tell us what they knew about the practical effects of our good intentions. These came later and out of sequence, and so the first attempt to engage service users in constructive dialogue appeared in 1970 (see Mayer and Timms, 1970). The results were salutary. The respondents seemed, ungratefully, to prefer practical help to the 'in-depth relationships' then in fashion. Nor did we afterwards, encouraged by *some* positive results, then invest in a few 'riskier', pre-post tests of professional influence. Nor did we take much advantage of area or regional differences in service provision, where the same problems existed but were approached differently, and noting differences in outcome. We charged ahead instead with some of the most formidable methodological approaches to evaluation. Politicians therefore heard rumours of the negative results, but not necessarily of more positive later results. Some were, and remain, closet opponents of allegedly initiative-sapping social welfare provision; the more honest aim of others is to ensure that the most vulnerable groups received the most effective help. Virtually *all*, interestingly, are now in favour of evidence-based practice.

The evidence of social work's effectiveness is today of increased volume, based on robustly designed studies. Results regularly point to positive outcomes in difficult fields (see Chapter 3), whereas earlier, negative results often came from less demanding circumstances. Therefore we can surely live now in this environment of higher methodological expectations and higher levels of accountability, and renounce special pleading about social work just being 'different' from all other forms of help and based on will o' the wisp factors too ephemeral to capture.

The health field, again under the influence of a few pioneers (see Cochrane, 1973; Chalmers, 1989, Sackett *et al.*, 1996), introduced the unsettling idea of evidence-based medicine to the world – unsettling because most of the general public thought the matter of the evidential basis of medical treatment a given at about the time that Dr Finlay took up his post at Tannoch Brae (ask your parents). Systematic reviews of randomized controlled trials produced some surprises in the 1990s however (e.g. regarding the efficacy of the widely used drug Lidocaine for heart attack prevention). When all the evidence was in, patients were seen to be statistically better off in the control condition, and the same applies to human albumin in the treatment of serious burns (see www.cochrane.org). Those familiar with evidence-based health care, but concerned with social interventions, brought the issue of evidence-based social care under the spotlight. The President of the Royal Statistical Society, writing in 1995, commented favourably on the work of the Cochrane collaboration in preparing and disseminating systematic reviews of the effects of health care interventions and proposed that its methods be extended to other areas of public activity such as education and the penal system.

Political support for evidence-based social care came, somewhat surprisingly, from the last Conservative government. Here is the announcement from the then Secretary of State for Health and Social Services:

> The commitment to evidence-based medicine pervades modern medical practice. This kind of commitment should be extended to the social services world.
>
> (Dorrell, 1997)

Those of us who had long been arguing for just such a policy were well advised *not* to write the pained letter, but to look out our long spoons instead. The idea was given substantial political backing via the funding of the Centre for Evidence-Based Social Services at the University of Exeter (now merged with Research in Practice at Dartington), bringing the university and 20 Social Services departments into close collaboration. Similar developments (e.g. the Barnardo's 'What Works' project in the childcare field, the 'Making Knowledge Count' initiative administered from Royal Holloway College (University of London), and the ESRC Evidence-Based Policy and Practice Unit) have produced something close to a 'critical mass' of academic and Social Services departments interested in this idea. Staying power versus 'initiative fatigue' is the tension we now have to manage.

Definition and implications

Here is a definition of evidence-based practice (adapted from that of Sackett *et al.*, 1996):

> Evidence-based social care is the conscientious, explicit and judicious use of current best evidence in making decisions regarding the welfare of individuals, groups and communities.
>
> (Macdonald and Sheldon, 1998: 1)

How does this definition translate to our field? *Conscientious* surely reminds us of our ethical obligations to clients, not least among which to try to keep abreast of research which (1) helps us to understand the nature and development of social and personal problems, and (2) provides results on the effectiveness of what has been tried before. There is after all little point in a shared, happy-clappy, non-discriminatory, non-postcode lottery, commitment to equal and speedy access to ineffective services.

Hippocrates (400 BC) counselled his student physicians thus: 'First do no harm.' Can it be said that we in the personal social services do no harm? A glance at the child abuse tragedies discussed in Chapters 5 and 10 should settle the matter. Any intervention with a capacity for good probably carries with it a capacity for ill (you can overdose on vitamin supplements if you try hard enough). Sins of omission and commission are therefore part of our world and need to be guarded against by looking at the evidential back catalogue and then taking stock of what side-effects were revealed.

The next keyword is *explicit*: that is, the need for an open, negotiating, contractual style when working with clients. This emerged as a predictor of positive outcomes in effectiveness research from the mid to late 1970s onwards (see Sheldon, 1980, 1986). Previously, clients tended to be regarded as something close to psychotherapy patients, and Micawberist ('something will definitely turn up one of these days') expectations were the norm. There are two sets of factors associated with the later, much better, results: first, those identified by Reid and Shyne (1969) and Reid and Epstein (1972), whose research and subsequent textbook established the then controversial principles of task-centred social work (see Chapter 6). These results showed that short-term, intensive, focused, pre-planned interventions were at least or more effective as longer term, more expensive ones. This is the phenomenon of

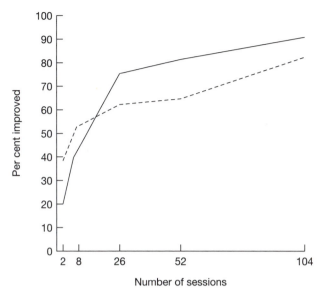

Figure 4.1 Relation of number of sessions and percentage of patients/clients improved

Note: Objective ratings at termination (dotted line); subjective ratings during interventions (broken line).

Source: Reproduced with permission from Howard *et al.* and *American Psychologist* (1986)

'decreasing marginal utility' – the law of diminishing returns, which applies across the helping professions (see Figure 4.1). The solid line represents client-opinion evaluations; the dotted line standardized outcome measures at follow-up (see Howard *et al.*, 1986). One can think of exceptions to this trend (e.g. very emotionally damaged and/or abused children who need longer term help). But then there need be no tension between such help and the need for focus and rigour in the way that we go about providing it – as the work of Michael Rutter (1972; Rutter and Hersov, 1987) illustrates well.

A key figure in the development of evidence-based practice is Eileen Gambrill (University of California, Berkeley). In 1997 she conducted, with her colleague Stein, a randomized controlled study to compare the relative effectiveness of a very explicit, contract-based approach with standard services in reuniting children in foster care with their birth parents. The context was one in which 'decisional drift' was well recognized. The resultant differences in rehabilitation rates and preventions of reception into care were striking. It is strange that this idea of explicit negotiations still gives us such trouble, since research reviews containing positive results have long been clear about its importance; for example:

> In brief, one is struck by the dominance of structured forms of practice in these experiments – that is, of practice that takes the form of well-explicated, well-organised procedures usually carried out in a stepwise manner and designed to achieve relatively specific goals. The influence of the behavioural movement is quite apparent and pervasive.
>
> (Reid and Hanrahan, 1980: 11–12)

Research regularly tells us about the need to avoid over-directive advice-giving which may well be nodded at but not followed. However, tip-toeing up to problems and reflecting back feelings as a way of clarifying them, as is widely taught on courses, can be frustrating for clients who are looking for more straightforward guidance. Most client-opinion studies testify to patterns of miscommunication between workers and clients (see Mayer and Timms, 1970; Fisher *et al.*, 1984). For instance:

> These examples seemed to point to the conclusion that it was not unreasonable for clients to perceive social work as a relatively timeless friendship, in which help was available to weather crises rather than to resolve or avoid them.
>
> (Fisher *et al.*, 1984: 63)

This doesn't happen now of course.

The enemies of the principle of explicitness are methods-led, 'this-is-what-I-usually-do-in-these-circumstances' routines. We tend to dislike the ECT-happy psychiatrist and the Prozac-happy GP, but how often is our own practice similarly Pavlovian? 'The answer's a family centre (whatever goes on there); a group discussion; counselling; or a care plan – now what's the problem?' Reflexive reactions regarding service provision often fly in the face of major findings. For example, there is significant undiagnosed depression amongst older people but as long as they have a roof over their head and perhaps a 'meals on wheels' service, plus a few mobility aids, this feeling of basic safety filters out their other, psychological concerns (loneliness and loss are the predominant problems alongside illness, yet are barely mentioned on most 'comprehensive needs assessment' schedules.

The evidence suggests that 'one-size-fits-all' solutions are unlikely to be useful, by comparison with tailor-made ones. This was the original idea behind the term 'needs-led services' before it became a euphemism for 'cost-led services'. Here is the 2002 Reith lecturer – a philosopher – on these matters:

> A look into the vast database of documents on the Department of Health website arouses a mixture of despair and disbelief. Central planning may have failed in the former Soviet Union but it is alive and well in Britain today.
>
> (O'Neill, 2002: 46)

The principle of explicitness therefore requires the transparent reviewing of problems and their origins with clients, plus a suitably adapted discussion regarding what research of good quality has to say about what has been tried in cases such as theirs and to what effect. What stands in the way of this simple idea is pessimistic assessments of clients' motivation for change. But then motivation is not a commodity that can be dipped like engine oil – 'you seem to be a little low on motivation Mrs Smith'. What it usually means is that clients do not want straight away what we would like them to want. Some of our clients, for example, serial juvenile offenders, are *highly* motivated people, exercising great skill and determination to achieve their ends. Open negotiation, unambiguous discussion of the likely consequences of cooperation and of non-cooperation, even the arrival at, by small steps, 'lowest common denominator' options, have been shown to be influential (see McGuire, 1995; Sheldon, 1995).

Albert Bandura (1977) discerned two central features in these problems of engagement, persuasability, cooperation and motivation: (1) *Outcome expectations* – does
the client think that doing X will achieve the desired outcome; and (2) *Efficacy
expectations* – whether they are, potentially, able to do X. Stein and Gambrill's
work (1976) was based not only on explicit negotiation but also on intensive help
to overcome agreed substantive problems. In other words, there is no point having
'comprehensive assessments' and 'clear goals' if concordant help is not available to
address the problems identified – a common difficulty in modern social work.

The next keyword in our definition is *judicious* – that is, the exercise of considered,
prudent, judgement. Our stock (and that of the policy-makers) is not high in this
matter, and considered pragmatism has been out of fashion for three decades at least.
Social work, in lacking a healthy professional immune system, seems to be particularly
prone to infection by fads and fashions.

This principle of judiciousness presses upon us that not all that *could* be done
should be done, and that some things which appear expensive in the short term may
turn out to be a bargain in the longer term. Potential risks, either in cases or in
policies, should, of course, be assessed, but in the knowledge that not all eventualities
can be predicted – all else is pretence. In the childcare field, for example, the rise
of child protection squads from the 1980s onward (under the influence of a short
series of dramatic, single cases which became the subject of inquiries) brought
thousands of families into a system originally designed for a few seriously dangerous
situations. Only now is the policy of 'refocusing' (who blurred our vision in the first
place is a little discussed question) beginning to make an impact.

Onward in the same vein; 'short sharp shocks' for juvenile offenders, though
appealing to car theft victims and to the *Daily Mail*, do *not* in fact reduce re-offending
(they produce leaner, fitter burglars); nor do any of the 'get tough', 'scare 'em
straight' policies tried out in the USA (see Chapter 12, this volume).

Thus evidence-based practice is about considered action informed by robust
research; i.e. by studies which attempt to cater for, and to reduce, known sources of
bias in interpreting findings. This idea, if it is to be further implemented, requires a
well-educated workforce equipped critically to appraise findings, and free, or partly
free, to make informed judgements regarding the actions they propose to take or
not to take. It requires a workforce with reasonable access to user-friendly reviews
of empirical research, supported by practice supervisors who routinely discuss
case-specific questions of evidence. It requires regular top-up training courses based
on research trends and their implications; a workforce within which managers
routinely make reference to service-effectiveness research when reviewing or evaluating services; a culture of accountability within which elected members sometimes
ask officers to justify new proposals on the basis of international research on the same
issues.

The endless, distracting 'reorganizations' which go on whenever a new Director
of Adult or Children's Services is appointed are a case in point. Indeed, those who
doubt the relevance of scientific principles to social life should consider the
Newtonian predictability of such events – they are as reliable as solar eclipses. In this
regard one cannot but be attracted to the advice of Napoleon's first foreign minister
Tallyrand, who at a passing-out ceremony for the elite *Corps Diplomatiques* advised:
'Above all gentlemen, *please*, no zeal.'

Obstacles to evidence-based practice

There are many such blockages, and some are quite formidable. We begin by looking at general background belief systems prevalent in the professional and disciplinary culture; then at the workplace conditions which either discourage, or encourage, evidence-based practice, confining ourselves as far as possible to the empirical research in these matters. We then look at the current state of social work training, where early habits regarding questions of evidence could be inculcated, but usually are not, before turning to address what is known from evaluations of attempts to remedy the difficulties identified.

Methodological questions

The a priori obstacle to evidence-based practice follows from the fact that a properly calm and considered debate has not taken place among the staff who train social workers regarding questions of *attributive confidence*. This refers to the degree to which a particular set of findings and recommendations can validly and reliably be causally related to intervention that was the focus of a study, and not to other, confounding factors. At many academic and governmental gatherings on how best to improve services, this issue – on which *all* else depends – is usually ruled out of order at the first dangerous signs of dispute. It is thus regarded as an arcane and unanswerable question likely to spoil everyone's day. The discipline prefers, instead, a loose confederation of views on questions of evidence of effectiveness, within which different approaches are held to be equal, and wherein an implicit policy of methodological *détente* is upheld so as to prevent discord. Our experience indicates that it is perfectly possible for questions of evidence to be debated under the Marquis of Queensberry's boxing rules: No hitting below the belt, no biting, no gouging, no spitting (mmm . . .). The present tribal customs, however, assume the following:

1   Different methodological approaches in evaluation research are not seen as potentially better than others, just different. They are held to lie along a *continuum* of options, each band of which could, if sympathetically applied, yield valuable answers (cf. Chapter 2).

2   Researchers are good at different things (true) and so some need to specialize in certain approaches to research questions on grounds of preference, training, 'ethics' and the sorts of scholars they see themselves as being. This view is another example of methods-led, 'this-is-how-I-prefer-to-work' interventions. Our view, regarded as somewhat eccentric, is that there are 'horses for courses' in research methods, and that some approaches are simply incapable of finishing in the service-effectiveness stakes. Pre-race warm-ups are a different matter.

3   Within the academy there are held to be two different types of research: 'qualitative' and 'quantitative'. In a Pavlovian way, the word 'qualitative' seems to trigger in many the warm feelings that the words 'quality' or 'wholemeal' do in everyday life, whereas 'quantitative' is associated with what accountants, pollsters and economists do. This is however, a false polarization. It takes a great deal of self-deception to exclude qualitative findings from quantitative research (see Boyle, 2000). Look at the side-effects of any NHS or social services

'target' evaluation. However, it is equally impossible to exclude quantitative factors from qualitative research (i.e. is it statistically significant in a given sample that N^1 sets of views outnumbers N^2 sets of views by 5 per cent or could these differences be due to chance?). Such questions depend on the clarity of the original questions, the sample frame and its representativeness, on the selection procedures, and on attrition rates. This is not just our opinion; it is a simple, methodological, statistical fact.

4   If positivist methodologies (the term is close to one of abuse in some circles) produce less gratifying results plausibly attributable to professional intervention (they tend to do so in all fields, not just in our own), then they are often deemed 'inappropriate'. Therefore, it is argued, we would do better to snuggle up to the idea that the verbal testimony of service users contains a special kind of truth. Client satisfaction measures are indeed a necessary but not a sufficient measure of the effectiveness of social work. For when we seek to evaluate our impact on the problems to which clients so eloquently testify, more methodologically demanding, bias-reducing precautions are necessary. We urgently need a merger of 'why?' and 'how?' methodologies with 'how much?', 'by when? and 'because of what? approaches. There are some good examples to follow (see Oakley, 2000; Macdonald, 2001; Trappes-Lomax *et al.*, 2003). In trying to make this case, we are not unaware of the possibility that a kind of 'Academic Asperger's Syndrome' might take over systematic reviews, and that methodological rectitude – in horse-riding terms, 'dressage' (hooves and tails up, but going nowhere) as opposed to point-to-point gallops across rough country – might become the favoured intellectual sport. But then methodological horsing around is a far more typical pursuit.

The foregoing arguments imply an argued-out, 'best-we-can-manage-in-the-circumstances' compromise between intellectual rigour and practical reality; something which academics are by training and culture shy of. The philosopher Arthur Schopenhaur's parable of academics cast as porcupines springs to mind. They were portrayed by him as likely to gather together in search of warmth in chilly circumstances but, when spiked by each other's quills, would scuttle around until they found the optimum distance between prickly companionability and comfortable isolation.

   Thus, effectiveness research is not always seen in our field as a special form of enquiry requiring particular methodological safeguards. We disagree. If research is undertaken to gain information on what life is like for children in care, then a qualitative, interview-based approach is the more appropriate, provided that due attention is given to issues of sample representativeness. Children come into care for many different reasons; they have suffered from many different types of abuse and neglect; they come from many different backgrounds, and have many different positive and negative experiences. All these factors need to be represented in our studies of their different plights before we dare to suggest what might be best done to help them. But if we want to determine how best to help prevent them from coming into care, or how best to make the transition to adult life, then something more is needed.

   We are therefore not suggesting that randomized controlled trials are the only fruit (they are, in social work, as rare as pink oranges), but we need more of them to top out more conjectural trends from qualitative and pre-/post-investigations. The presumed ethical objections to them surely do not hold water. We can – apparently – do something to *all* children in care without assessing its effectiveness but not to 'half' in an endeavour to find out whether we are likely to do more harm than good. Most experiments in social work entail comparing the effects of a new intervention with 'management as usual'. In effect, we often do not know whether an intervention will do any good, make no difference, or do harm – the principle of 'equipoise'. Moreover, in many circumstances, high eligibility thresholds mean that there are natural control groups from whom we could learn a great deal. Table 4.1 summarizes our position on questions of attributive confidence in different types of research.

Attributive confidence in different types of research

The contents of Table 4.1 would be regarded as uncontroversial in many fields, yet we seem stuck in a pre-paradigmatic state regarding them (See Kuhn, 1970). This limits the development of a cumulative body of knowledge for our field and leads to the following type of situation:

> The epistemic sequence is initiated by the epistemic purpose, that is the social workers' interest in a given item of data or information as it relates to their practical concerns. The principle of rationality at work is 'If an agent has knowledge that one of its actions will lead to one of its goals, then the agent will select that action' (Newell, 1990, p. 10). This formulation results in the law of behaviour at the knowledge level. Thus, there is a direct connection between goals, knowledge and subsequent actions.
>
> (Webb, 2001: 63)

What on earth does this mean? It is intended as criticism of evidence-based approaches, but in respect of the last sentence one dearly hopes that what is feared is increasingly the case. Apart from the impenetrability of such prose, the research methods the author feels are not being given due respect would simply have no capacity to come up with outcomes likely to convince anyone that something positive (or neutral, or negative) has happened as a result of a given intervention.

To clarify all of this, let us take an example from the work of the founding father of psychoanalysis. This concerns the case of Emma B. who was being treated for 'hysterical nosebleeds'. It later transpired that a ribbon of surgical gauze had been left in her nasal cavities after an operation. What was the reaction to this evidence of misdiagnosis? A letter to Freud's collaborator Fliess contains these views:

> Freud happily tells Fliess of Emma's confession that in the sanatorium, after the incident of the removal of the gauze; 'She began to feel restless out of unconscious longing and the intention of drawing me to her side'. He continues, 'And since I did not come during the night, she renewed the haemorrhage as an unfailing means of reawakening my affection'.
>
> (See Malcolm, 1984: 49)

Table 4.1 Questions of attributive confidence in different types of research

Methodology	Procedure	Attributive confidence
Systematic reviews of randomized controlled trials: These synthesize the evidence from research on the effects of an intervention designed to address an issue for a pre-specified sample population. Where possible, effect sizes from comparisons of one approach with another, or with no intervention, are calculated.	Reviews are conducted in line with a pre-specified protocol, in which reviewers make explicit their working assumptions and proposed methodology. Exhaustive searches for relevant studies, an unvarnished presentation of results and implications, plus regular updating, are other hallmarks.	Well-conducted systematic reviews minimize sources of reviewer bias. If well conducted, they provide our most secure results. Negative conclusions are also valuable.
Randomized controlled trials in which participants are randomly allocated to an experimental intervention or a control group, and the results compared.	One group (the experimental group) receives as consistent as possible an exposure to the intervention under test. The other receives no service, or management as usual, or a non-specific attention or another service (since attention and belief in the expertise of helpers also have strong effects). Rarely, studies have three conditions – no intervention, standard intervention and test intervention – compared. Outcomes are assessed against specific quantitative outcome indicators (e.g. readmission to hospital, recidivism).	Well-conducted trials minimize a number of sources of bias, but each of these needs to be carefully assessed, including confounders such as significant baseline differences across groups (which randomization may not eliminate); biases in allocation concealment, outcome assessment and differential drop-out rates between the two groups.
Quasi-experimental studies.	These are comparison studies in which participants have been matched on variables known to confound results (i.e. influence outcomes, e.g. race, gender, class).	Useful in Social Services where different services are routinely introduced in one area but not in another and a good source of hypotheses for more rigorous tests. The absence of random allocation means we can never be sure that we are comparing like with like, given that 'unknown' factors may also influence outcome.

Table 4.1 (continued)

Methodology	Procedure	Attributive confidence
Single group, pre-post tests. Sometimes known as time-series designs, these procedures compare problems and gains on a before-and-after basis in a single sample.	Baseline (i.e. pre-intervention (preferably standardized)) measures are taken in key problem areas prior to intervention (see Fischer and Corcoran (1994) for an accessible manual). They are then repeated at the end of the programme for comparison purposes.	Most evaluations in Social Services are post-only (see below) and so it is difficult to calculate the value added. This approach takes 'snapshots' of functions on a before-and-after basis. Nevertheless, it cannot determine the extent to which any improvements that occur are due to the mere passage of time (maturational factors) or to other conflicting factors unconnected with the intervention.
Post test-only measures. This approach reviews outcomes only, without benefit of specific pre-intervention (baseline) measures.	A sample is chosen against criteria of need, type and extent of problem(s). The intervention is made, and then measures of outcomes are implemented.	Since most Social Services approaches and projects are still not evaluated at all, this may be better than nothing. It can be improved by standardized referral criteria being in place at the outset.
Client-opinion studies. Largely qualitative studies (occasionally with quantitative elements). Usually post-only, but there is no reason why pre-post qualitative measures should not be taken (there are, however, few examples of this happening).	A sample of clients receiving a particular intervention, or those with a particular set of problems, receiving a range of interventions from Social Services, are interviewed for their opinions on the effects of services and, usually, on the way in which services were provided.	These studies are rich in qualitative detail about what it is like to be on the receiving end of services. However, a common problem is representativeness. Do the respondents in the sample reflect the range of service user and problem characteristics? Random sampling of populations helps here. Should be routine in Social Services as part of the service-planning process.
Single case designs. Largely quantitative measures (though there is no reason why standardized qualitative measures should not be included) (see Fischer and Corcoran (1994), vols 1 and 2) applied to single cases.	Measures are taken on a before-and-after (AB design) or before/after/follow-up basis (ABA designs) or even in experimental forms (ABAB designs) where interventions are baselined, the intervention made, then withdrawn, and then	Should be more widely used by practitioners whatever the intervention method in use. Enable staff and clients to assess progress and adjust accordingly.

Table 4.1 (continued)

Methodology	Procedure	Attributive confidence
	reinstated and differences noted. Mainly used in behaviour therapy, though there is no reason why this should be so, providing that case-specific behavioural change in line with the aims of a given approach are prespecified.	
Narrative reviews: These are not usually as exhaustive as systematic reviews and tend to have less explicit inclusion and exclusion criteria.	Authors draw up a list of topics which they wish to search (e.g. 'social work in general hospitals'; 'supported housing for learning disabled people') and then track down likely sources and look for emergent trends and implications.	They suffer from the problem of 'convenience samples' (i.e. sources readily available to the authors), and from a higher possibility of selective perception than where a very tight, prepublished protocol is in place. Reviewers are more susceptible to privileging evidence that supports their preferred worldviews. Nevertheless, they are a good starting point in the absence of something more rigorous.

Note here the absence of repentance; the preservation of the theory is all – whatever the consequences. The foregoing criticisms of evidence-based approaches are not so much a tenable methodological position, more a fashion statement. But this is where we are stuck, and this kind of material is often taught on qualifying courses instead of critical appraisal skills and research methods.

Stones in the road

We promised an empirical investigation into obstacles to evidence-based approaches. Our searches suggest that we have only two large, representative studies (see Sheldon and Chilvers, 2000; Sheldon *et al.*, 2005). Some demographic comparisons were also possible with the LGMB study of employment trends in social care (1997). A sample of professional-grade staff (e.g. social workers, occupational therapists, care managers, heads of residential facilities and community project leaders) were asked for their views on the prospects for the idea of evidence-based practice (the key ideas having been defined in the questionnaire).

A 42-item instrument was sent out to a random, stratified tranche of professional-grade staff in the south and south-west of England with a comparison with demographic factors elsewhere in the UK. A total of 1,341 replies were received (a

58.7 per cent response rate – good for a postal questionnaire). Let us now concentrate on a few key issues in describing its findings (Figure 4.2). The qualitative results from this questionnaire are overwhelmingly positive, with over half of the sample having 'no misgivings' about evidence-based practice, and a more cautious one-fifth having only 'some misgivings'. This came as a surprise from a group of front-line staff over whom new initiatives flow year in year out. The 'nothing-new' and 'don't-like-the-idea' responses accounted for only 5.5 per cent of reactions. This appears to us as a vote of confidence.

Respondents were invited to explain any doubts or misgivings about the greater emphasis being placed on research evidence in planning and delivering social services. Responses concentrated on organizational issues and complexities, including the need for better critical appraisal skills.

In terms of the conduct of the research, the main themes were: (1) that the right people, with people who use services and carers as an essential part of the equation, are often not properly consulted; (2) that sufficient resources are not allocated to support such activities, and (3) that research does not keep up with the speed at which changes take place within departments – the 'wedding photographer effect' known to all researchers, where the main challenge is to get people to stand still long enough to have their picture taken.

Let us turn next to the views of respondents regarding their opinions on specific obstacles to the idea of evidence-based practice and its implementation. It depends largely upon *reading*, whether on screens, or in books and articles. Gore Vidal made a concordant point in the *New York Review of Books* seven years ago: 'At present, we probably have too many writers and not enough readers.'

It appears from other data in this exercise that if staff read anything at all they are most likely to read *Community Care* (which bits, other than the job adverts, we do not know). This free publication is a large-circulation magazine with topical stories and, commendably, the occasional issue on research, but it too operates the 'equal ops' principle regarding methodology. Nevertheless, here is a real opportunity for academics to put practical ideas and findings into circulation, though the government's star rating system for research would probably punish such eccentricity. Yet in a list of reading options, staff were least likely to look at an academic research article. Their reasons centred on the impenetrability of the prose and lack of understanding of research and how to appraise it.

Respondents were next asked for their views on the obstacles to reading professionally relevant publications (Figure 4.3). Qualitative data from this study, and discussions of these findings with staff at conferences, suggest two things. First, that this general reaction breaks down according to respondents' main areas of responsibility. Typically, childcare staff have moderate caseloads but these are made up of very demanding clients, and so they are preoccupied with questions of risk (see Chapter 5). Second, as in health and education, bureaucratic requirements are high, preoccupying and rising inexorably. Those working with older people most often mentioned the sheer size of their caseload and the logistics of servicing a wide range of needs with severely restricted resources. They have 'time to do for, but not with' was the conclusion of one research review (Godfrey *et al.*, 2000). Those working in the statutory mental health field also appear to be increasingly preoccupied with (not always evidentially based) risks (see Chapter 15).

Perceived relevance of research to practice (%)

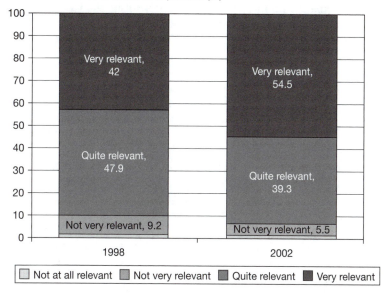

Figure 4.2 A pre-post-empirical study of perceptions of evidence-based practice in social care
Source: from Sheldon *et al.* (2005)

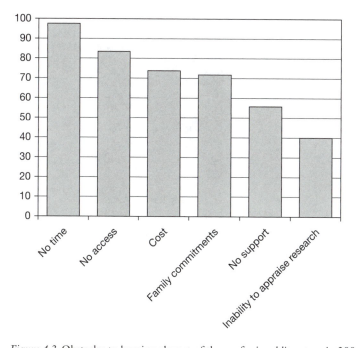

Figure 4.3 Obstacles to keeping abreast of the professional literature in 2002 (%)
Source: from Sheldon *et al.* (2005)

The issue of *access* to literature is seen as a significant obstacle by 83.6 per cent of respondents, justifying the priority being given to this within the CEBSS project, despite the development of library, internet and information services. The associated item on whether staff felt limited in their reading, due to lack of knowledge of what to read and how to interpret it, produced a divided response. Forty-two per cent saw this as an important obstacle.

This study however, went beyond the attitudinal measures associated with questionnaires; it also included tests of actual knowledge. Respondents were first asked a general question about their knowledge of evaluative research; that is, a study designed to establish the impact on the measurable difference made to the lives of clients by given interventions. Forty per cent of staff reported acquaintance with such material – a disturbingly low figure since this is a representative sample of qualified staff. Respondents were then asked to give a few basic details of their knowledge. They were first invited to identify a client-opinion study. General descriptions, author(s) or subject matter were accepted (Figure 4.4).

The first thing to note is that 792 (of 1,341) respondents did not answer this question. Many of the remaining contributors produced answers too vague to analyse (70 per cent of replies); others tried, but nominated either research which came nowhere near the criteria, or were plainly mistaken about what constitutes client-opinion research. Thus, only 145 respondents could identify a study of client reactions to services, the majority of these selecting a historically interesting study from 1970 based on working practices which no longer pertain (Mayer and Timms,

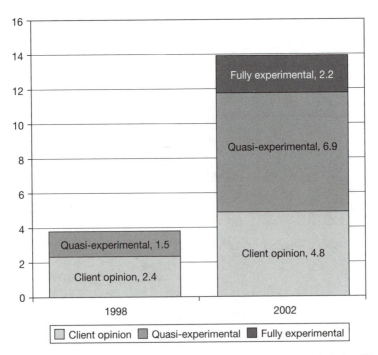

Figure 4.4 Ability correctly to identify an evaluative study by research design (%)

Source: from Sheldon *et al.* (2005)

1970). This is not very reassuring about current teaching on this issue, given that 'user involvement' is allegedly at the top of the agenda on most courses.

Evaluating client-opinion studies

Respondents were next asked, in line with the comments in Table 4.1, what factors might account for positive results in a client-opinion study, other than the influence of professional intervention. A candidate answer list was in place regarding plausible factors such as passage of time; the 'placebo' effects of participating in the study; maturational factors; and changes in employment status, income or family circumstances (Figure 4.5). Only 13 per cent had knowledge of the potentially confounding influence of such collateral factors, with a further 26 per cent coming close. Sixtyone per cent had no knowledge at all.

Knowledge of experimental studies

The next area of investigation was respondents' knowledge of controlled trials. Only a tiny proportion of respondents could identify such a study, so respondents were much less sanguine than with the previous question. Although 5 per cent thought they *could* produce an example of such research, in fact less than 1 per cent of respondents managed to when the next question was asked: If *yes*, can you recall the title of such a study, or its authors and/or its subject matter? This left 99 per cent of respondents not able to identify an experimental study with their home discipline.

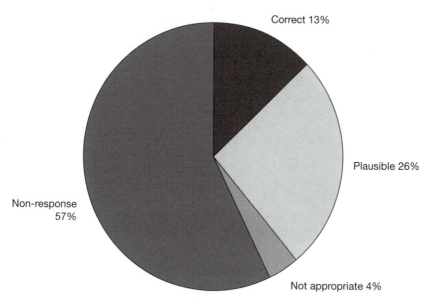

Figure 4.5 Respondents' ability to identify factors other than professional intervention that might account for positive change in a client-opinion study

Knowledge of basic statistics

When promising results from client-opinion studies or one group pre-post comparisons are tested using an experimental approach, the apparent effectiveness of the intervention often drops, because the control group minimizes or eliminates ('controls for') other influences on change. Nevertheless, even modest gains tell us what to reinforce in our practice and policies, and now and again we score. But it is important to assess whether the differenes that we observe, large or small, might have arisen by chance if there were in fact no difference between the two groups.

Thus the questionnaire sought to find out what basic knowledge respondents had of the term 'statistical significance'. The definition of this term used for rating responses was derived against descriptions given in seven key texts on research methods (Grinnell, 1981; Powers *et al.*, 1985; Grady and Wallston, 1988; Mitchell and Jolley, 1988; Greene and D'Oliveira, 1989; Whitaker and Archer, 1989; Herbert, 1990). From these sources, criteria representing three levels of understanding of the term were developed. The point here is that staff who have read, or have been taught about findings from research articles, need to know what is meant by 'statistical significance' and its place in drawing conclusions from comparative data. For example, it is necessary to understand this term when considering whether a reported difference between interventions or groups suggests a change should be made to current practices, or whether comparisons of effects are too uncertain to justify this, although understanding the difference between statistical significance and 'clinical significance' (does the one result in meaningful changes in practice?) is another, perhaps more important, skill (Figure 4.6).

Thus, knowledge of what is meant by the boring 'p-value' was pretty dismal across the sample. Remember that this issue was approached in two stages: first, via a measure of self-perceived familiarity; second, via a test of actual knowledge. One-third of the sample stated prospectively that they understood the term, though in fact only 4 per cent showed demonstrable understanding of it, with 13 per cent appearing to have a partial understanding. Some 64 per cent of those who said they knew what the term meant gave clearly mistaken answers. It is unlikely, therefore, that the majority of staff were equipped via their professional or subsequent training critically to appraise a research study pertinent to their work.

Implications for training

These matters can be disposed of quickly since the research findings are clear. The approach of evidence-based research and development units in both health and social care has typically been to undertake what is in effect remedial education with staff (CEBSS staff conducted 387 such courses over a five-year period). Meanwhile, university courses continue to pump out workers with no more knowledge of research methodology, effectiveness research or critical appraisal techniques than their predecessors. There were no significant differences between recently qualified and long qualified staff in these results.

The problem we face then is largely one of simple ignorance. What is taught instead – a bit of a puzzle, given the centrality of the issue – is something called 'theory' (see Chapters 2 and 4). Where appropriate teaching is in place (in just a few universities

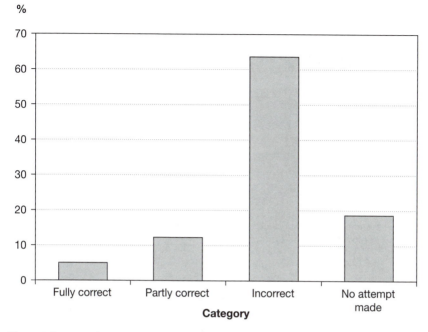

Figure 4.6 Respondents' actual ability to define the term 'statistical significance' having indicated familiarity

Note: N = 436.

at present) it is often confined to a day or half-day 'module', and is presented as an add-on specialism near the end of the course. It should be one of the very first things students hear about after the welcome speech.

Recommendations

1   Standard research methods courses, where they have been available at all, have switched off student interest for years. This is because they are largely taught by social scientists and statisticians who have limited knowledge of the social work literature and of the working conditions of staff. We recommend therefore that social work academics either take on this task themselves and integrate teaching about research with believable, non-artificial case examples; or that they run jointly taught courses (*taught*, note, not 'facilitated', with social scientist colleagues). When this happens it has marked effects on the rest of the course (see Gambrill, 1997; Macdonald and Sheldon, 1998). If the same principles are applied to training at post-qualification level the reception is very positive, and pre-post data on substantive knowledge gains are encouraging (see Figure 4.7 and CEBSS, 2003).

2   We have limited empirical material on 'what works' in dissemination projects (see CEBSS, 2003), though if we include the lessons from health (see CRD, 1999) we see that the signposts all point in the same direction, namely:

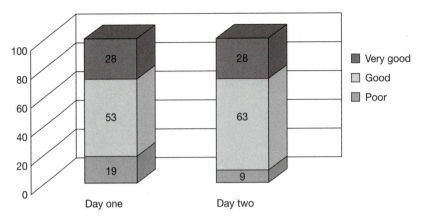

Figure 4.7 Example of satisfaction measures from the 'appraising the evidence' training –
pooled data (% of respondents)

Note: N= 300

- The work has much to remedy, and the approaches which show the best
  gains follow from the use of a broad approach (i.e. face-to-face work, conferences, training courses, site visits, projects, websites, user-friendly reviews
  and newsletters, and the development of an organizational *esprit de corps*).
- It is fatal to neglect workplace conditions if research-derived knowledge
  and skills are to stand a chance of encouragement. Bringing staff from
  the same offices and from different grades together in groups; working
  jointly with supervisors and students in seminars; getting service user/
  client representatives to produce simple, workable, implementation plans
  which anticipate obstacles; negotiating a little free time for private study;
  encouraging journal clubs and evidence-based practice groups which meet
  inside and outside working hours, have all be shown to have a positive
  impact.

There are many examples in print and in reports showing that staff have somehow
been taken by surprise regarding the idea of evidence-based practice and would like
more clarification. However:

1   Sometimes there is *never* enough 'clarity' to justify social workers changing their
    routine practices. We would argue that, above all, proponents of evidence-based
    practice have made clear exactly what is required and why.
2   There are *never* enough resources, despite the angle of spending increases
    in Social Services over the years. Nothing is ever perfect, but now we need to
    show that we have done something tangible with the sums of money sent our
    way.
3   There is, in the reactions of staff who feel that their professional *raison d'être* has
    been neglected, a worrying sniff of 'Stockholm Syndrome' compliance with new
    'initiatives' which distract them from what they want to achieve.

4   Access to research materials has been shown to be a problem for staff (see Sheldon and Chilvers, 2000; Sheldon *et al.*, 2004). Many do not have access to a library worthy of the name. Where there are good systems operating (Hampshire Social Services has an admirable rapid, delivery-to-desk facility) usage rises sharply. Librarians no longer regard themselves as mere keepers of books, but as expert information-retrieval advisers. Our experience is that when they are involved from the start in dissemination projects, and are briefed on workplace obstacles, they regularly come up with innovative, time- and trouble-saving solutions. Adopt a local librarian.

5   There is an increasing output of systematic reviews in our field and these comprehensive reports will, in future, probably meet most of the information needs of staff. Table 4.2 gives a short list of the sort of information available.

6   Thus, at present, if a social worker felt the need for pre-screened and sifted information on, say, the effectiveness of parent training (see Woolfenden *et al.*, 2001), on the effectiveness of psycho-social interventions to help people with Schizophrenia (see Cleary *et al.*, 2008), or wanted to check on the effectiveness of different approaches to the rehabilitation of elderly people following acute hospital admission (see Nocon and Baldwin, 1999; Lomax nd Ellis, 2002) then it would be relatively easy to find good guidance. This looks to us to be the way forward.

Table 4.2 A selection of systematic reviews of psycho-social interventions

Smith, L.A., Gates, S. and Foxcroft, D. Therapeutic communities for substance related disorder. *Cochrane Database of Systematic Reviews* 2006, Issue 1. Art. No.: CD005338. DOI: 10.1002/14651858.CD005338.pub2.

Rawlings, B.A. *et al.* Systematic international review of therapeutic community treatment for people with personality disorders and mentally disordered offenders. Report 17. University of York: NHS Centre for Reviews and Dissemination 1999.

Corrigan, P.W. Social skills training adult psychiatric populations: a meta-analysis. *Journal of Behavior Therapy and Experimental Psychiatry* 1991, issue 22, No. 3: 203–210.

Barlow, J., Coren, E. and Stewart-Brown, S.S.B. Parent-training programmes for improving maternal psychosocial health. *Cochrane Database of Systematic Reviews* 2003, Issue 4. Art. No.: CD002020. DOI: 10.1002/14651858.CD002020.pub2.

Macdonald, G.M., Higgins, J.P.T. and Ramchandani, P. Cognitive-behavioural interventions for children who have been sexually abused. *Cochrane Database of Systematic Reviews* 2006, Issue 4. Art. No.: CD001930. DOI: 10.1002/14651858.CD001930.pub2.

Macdonald, G.M. and Turner, W. Treatment foster care for improving outcomes in children and young people. *Cochrane Database of Systematic Reviews* 2008, Issue 1. Art. No.: CD005649. DOI: 10.1002/14651858.CD005649.pub2.

Cleary, M., Hunt, G.E., Matheson, S.L., Siegfried, N. and Walter, G. Psychosocial interventions for people with both severe mental illness and substance misuse. *Cochrane Database of Systematic Reviews* 2008, Issue 1. Art. No.: CD001088. DOI: 10.1002/14651858.CD001088.pub2

Cuijpers, P. Psychological outreach programmes for the depressed elderly: a meta-analysis of effects and dropout. *International Journal of Geriatric Psychiatry* 1998, Issue 13, No. 1: 41–48.

Evaluation research strategies

Eleven basic questions to ask of an evaluation research study

1   *Is the research question clear and unambiguous?* 'To investigate changing patterns in family communication in the direction of increased openness' is hopeless (we didn't make this one up by the way), and records the sort of defensive cosiness that has stalled family therapy outcome research for years (see Chapter 8).

   Most changes in thinking, communication patterns or in emotion have visible behavioural or circumstantial correlates which can usually be linked to plausible, qualitative reports from those using the service, always providing they are not distorted by persuasive questioning. Hypotheses are what is needed, but these must be so framed as to have a ready chance of failure; otherwise they are of no use. They must be 'risky' in the Popperian sense (see Chapter 2). These are simple defences against self-deception.

   For an authoritative source on this issue, look no further than the late Douglas Adams' posthumous collection *The Salmon of Doubt* (2003). His character, Dirk Gently of the Holistic Detective Agency, consults the Great Zaganza horoscope looking for predictions to guide him on a strange quest:

   > First he glanced at some of the entries under other birth signs, just to get a feel for the kind of mood the GZ was in. Mellow, it seemed at first sight. 'Your ability to take the long view will help you through some of the minor difficulties you experience when Mercury. . . .' 'Past weeks have strained your patience, but new possibilities will now start to emerge as the Sun. . . .' 'Beware of allowing others to take advantage of your good nature . . .'. He then read his own horoscope. 'Today you will meet a three-ton rhinoceros called Desmond'.

   Now *there's* a hypothesis.

2   *Are we dealing with a population or a sample?* An example of the former would be *all* the patients discharged from a given group of hospitals over the past year; or *all* foster-parents in a given region who have been exposed to behaviour-management training. We are still left with questions about whether this year's discharges are typical or whether they are just the last people thought suitable for resettlement. If dealing with a sample, are foster-children in rural areas typical of those who live in cities? Thus, if we are dealing with a sample (we usually are), how was it chosen? There are several approaches to this question. One could yoke together characteristics such as gender, ethnicity, income and categories of problems and so on, but these approaches, while not worthless, quickly become over-complicated when, having selected some allegedly telling factors, we then have to ponder a long list of out-of-the-frame factors (e.g. housing tenure, childhood experiences, personality, levels of extended family support). The best answer to this problem is to select large samples, randomize the individuals within them, expose half of them to the intendedly helpful regime

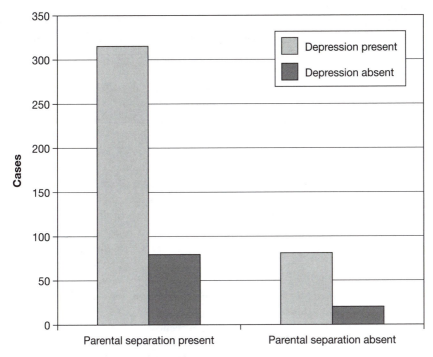

Figure 4.8 Hypothetical data regarding a possible association between parental separation in childhood and later depression

Source: from Sheldon and Macdonald (1999)

but not the other half – or allocate controls to waiting lists, of which we have plenty.

3 *Does size matter?* Appraisers of research are often led astray by visual differences in bar chart figures. An example is given in Figure 4.8, which we sometimes use at conferences to test perceptions of the significance of results. The majority (*c.* 65 per cent) opt for the conclusion that there is indeed an association between parental separation and a later diagnosis of clinical depression. They do so due to the presence of large numbers, and the tallness of the left-hand bars. However, it is the *ratio* of differences in the four cells to which they should be directing their critical attention: the proportions are the same.

While small is rarely beautiful in social research, *large* does not automatically guarantee methodological virtue. There was once a large telephone survey of voting intentions in the USA. It was conducted by the editors of a popular magazine, the readership of which was predominantly white middle class. Hundreds of thousands of people were contacted by telephone and the vast majority opined that Franklin D. Roosevelt would be defeated in his bid for the Presidency. He won a landslide victory on the 'new deal' ticket. He was voted in by the unemployed farm and factory workers who didn't have telephones, and hadn't the spare cash for magazine subscriptions.

4   *What is the claimed level of attributive confidence in the study?* Like social workers, researchers are not usually in it for the money. On the whole, they very much want to show a useful effect which could possibly be extended to others. The supplementary question here is, regardless of the attractions or disappointments of the reported results, can they reasonably be claimed from the methodology employed? In short, client-opinion studies cannot tell us whether improved well-being, functioning or satisfaction measured on a scale is 'plausibly due to us'. The data are at best suggestive and identify the agenda for future, stricter research.

5   *Are the outcome measures used based upon behavioural or observed circumstantial changes or are they limited to self-reports?* Some outcomes are unequivocally more definite than others. Although crime levels, rates of school exclusion, or figures on receptions into care are all subject to sociological and political influences, none the less, over time, with enough studies of the same issues and with large enough samples, we get a 'fix' on problems and what might help to ameliorate them, providing that we give preference to objective outcome indicators.

6   *Is it clear how much attrition there has been, either from the whole sample or differentially between the comparative samples?* Attrition, for example, drop-out rates, can seriously threaten the health of research studies since it interferes with end-representativeness and with the chances of a fair statistical tally. Often the most demanding or troubled clients fall out of the programme early, leaving behind better engaged, easier to help individuals. More damagingly, the drop-out rate between comparison groups can be uneven, as when most of the control group wander off since they are getting nothing following assessment.

7   *Are statistical tests used appropriately?* When discussing their findings, are the authors careful to refrain from spinning stories around effcts which (whatever their apparent size) are not statistically significant? Good practice is for authors to report probability levels, rather than rely on a simple cutpoint (since the cutpoint may move depending on whether we are weighing the information in exploratory or confirmatory mode).

8   *Are the findings professionally significant?* It is a maddeningly persistent feature of American clinical social work research wherein small, *statistically* significant findings are reported on problems that would never get past reception in British Social Services departments. Having decided whether or not the focus of a study is professionally relevant, we need to determine whether any statistically significant changes are 'clinically' meaningful. Medicine has a nice 'bottom-line' test of utility in the NNT (number needed to treat) measure; that is, within the confines of a given study, assuming that there are no major methodological or statistical distortions, how many people would have to be exposed to the intervention to get one clearly improved case: 3? 6? 20? 40? The significance of the results depend of course upon the nastiness of the condition, and what others have previously achieved. For example, a one in 18 complete abandonment of serial juvenile offending would justify a drinks party in the Home Office; a one in 35 complete recovery figure for a typically terminal form of cancer would be

regarded as a blessing. In our field, equally dire conditions are held to require much lower NNT figures, possibly because potential paymasters don't imagine they will ever contract them.

9 *Are any follow-up measures in place?* Some patterns of professional influence can look quite impressive from the beginning to the end of a project, but then trail off later. One reason for this is that we have not taken enough notice of the advice of respondents to client-opinion questionnaires and interviews, namely that we should consider not jumping completely out of their lives at the end of a specified service period, but should check upon maintained progress from time to time, or even offer 'booster' sessions.

10 *Is the intervention clearly described?* One of the commonest faults of social care research is that *what* exactly is being evaluated is written up in a general way. Sometimes the work going on within a project is described in terms of a summary of its 'mission statement'. What the clients actually receive, why it is thought on the basis of what literature to be an appropriate intervention, what checks, if any, were made to ensure that disparate staff were actually implementing best laid plans is often not stated.

11 *Does the research report contain 'weasel words'?* This is the 'most cat owners who expressed a preference [how many?] said their cats preferred Whiskas' (how do we establish the preference of cats?), 'most people with healthy hearts eat more wholegrain' problem. Words like 'substantial', where no back-up figures are produced; phrases like 'it was clear from the comments' should invite the question: How were the qualitative comments selected, and against what criteria? Phrases like 'a typical group of service users' – 'how many? and how were they selected'? – should always put our ears back.

Conclusions

1 Knowledge of 'what works, for whom, at what cost, in what circumstances, over what time-scale, against which outcome indicators, how, and why?' should surely be the main preoccupation of training courses for social workers. All other values and ethics considerations, however exciting to debate, are marginal unless such concerns predominate. Questions of values and ethics should therefore not be divorced from questions of service effectiveness. Consider this:

> If the characteristic patterns of risk and dependency confronting social workers were to spread to the majority of the population, the general public would very soon demand services of the highest quality from professional social workers of the highest calibre, and the idea of applying egalitarian principles to standards of knowledge and skill would be laughed out of court.
>
> (Pinker, 1980: 259)

Quite so.

2 Staff need to be immunized by training against accepting authoritative claims which they subjectively may or may not like the sound of through critical appraisal skills training courses. These *can* be made interesting.

3   Managers must be persuaded to allow their employees a little thinking, planning and reading time. This happens only in a few departments at present.
4   Another task for management is to regard library and information staff as indispensable colleagues and to give them their heads regarding the question on how best to promote ready access to articles, books and websites in busy workplaces.
5   Supervisors need to be trained to ask more why? and how? questions of their staff. When this happens it produces good results (see Sheldon and Chilvers, 2000).

There is nothing in these proposals which threatens the role of professional judgement. But such opinions need to be based upon wider knowledge than the last five cases which bear a passing resemblance to the one in hand.

All of the above strictures on the question of 'what shall count as evidence' depend upon an attitude of mind among staff; namely, that Social Services interventions are evaluatable in similar terms to complex interventions in health. Here, by way of illustration, are details of an experiment carried out within the CEBSS project at a large, multi-disciplinary mental health conference. The conclusion (see below) from a systematic review of the effectiveness of case-management approaches in the field was read out (see Marshall *et al.*, 1998), but with a mythical, second generation neuoroleptic medication for schizophrenia, Lususoproxine (*Lusus* is Latin for playfulness) replacing references to case management. Here is what the audience heard:

> Lususoproxine increased the numbers remaining in contact with services. Lususoproxine approximately doubled the numbers admitted to psychiatric hospital. Except for a positive finding from one study, Lususoproxine showed no significant advantages over standard care on any psychiatric or social variable. Cost data did not favour Lususoproxine but insufficient information was available to permit definitive conclusions.

They were then asked what they thought should happen in the light of these findings, and all suggested that the medication should no longer be used. However, when they were let in on the experiment, their views – accompanied by a 'Mexican wave' shrug – were that little could be done about social care interventions since they were embedded in national and local policies, and that different (unspecified) rules applied.

In conclusion, the most common negative reaction in discussions of the idea of evidence-based practice is that it is antithetical to practise wisdom and intuition. The following quotation sums up our views on this:

> Most contemporary scholarship on judgement concerns itself with how we might counteract biases that intrude on rational decision making. By means of rigorous training in (social) statistics and probability theory, this effort is designed to improve our judgement by strengthening our reason. There is much to gain from this endeavour, for intuitive biases are many and their influence in decision-making is often pernicious. An education in reason is all for the good. The

problem is that this education is generally portrayed as a means of *replacing* intuitions with conscious, rational thought, and that any such effort will prove counter-productive. The alternative, however, is not simply to give freer range to intuitions. The task is to educate them.

(Thiele, 2006: 120)

Part II

Social work methods, including assessment procedures

5 Assessment, monitoring and evaluation

> Everything is what it is because it got that way.
> d'Arcy Thompson

General points

We are taking these three stages together, conscious of the convention that chapters on evaluation usually come at the end of books. But what may be claimed at the end stage is dependent upon the quality of the original assessment, the goals arising from it, and the measures against which progress has been monitored. Working the other way, the accuracy of assessments can only be judged against measures of progress and, ultimately, by the outcomes which result. Otherwise, as computer programmers say, 'garbage in, garbage out'. There are some other general points to make about assessments and why they can be problematic:

1   First, we should be sure that there is one. Obvious as this point might seem, inquiry after inquiry in both the childcare and mental health fields have found, instead, case notes which amount to little more than collections of factual data intermingled with more speculative material, giving the impression that these comments were put there more for storage purposes than as the considered basis for a plan.

   The lack of a comprehensive assessment and consequent care and protection plan was a feature in the death of Victoria Climbié (see Laming, 2003), in the neglect, abuse and near deaths of three children in Sheffield (see Cantrill, 2005, and Chapter 10, this volume), and many others. That this issue should keep arising has stretched public and political patience to breaking-point. Even allowing for the deceptive power of hindsight, as Lord Laming remarked: 'this is not exactly rocket science'.

2   Increasingly the approach to assessment has been to standardize assessment and planning into 'tick-box', 'write-in' forms with too little regard for questions of validity and reliability. This may secure the gathering of information across a range of domains, but does not, in and of itself, secure an assessment, which entails the critical appraisal of the information gathered.

   The clients of social workers, given increasingly high eligibility thresholds, will usually be in a state of imminent crisis, and disinclined to sit down and run through an account of the long and winding road which led them to our door

– or we to theirs. Nevertheless, as consumers ourselves, say, of the health service, we expect to receive a medical assessment prior to intervention except in the most dramatic of circumstances. When we don't get one, as in the case of 'reflex prescribing' by GPs, we feel uneasy. In social work we have allowed 'something must be done' pressures from the media, from employers and from clients themselves to distract us from a technically necessary activity. This is vital for ourselves if we are to do our jobs properly, and necessary for our clients who usually have hopes about receiving effective aid – or at least of convincing us that they have no case to answer. In our experience, where the need to put together a 'map' of problems over a decent period of time (covering likely causes and effects, and usually involving more than 'the' identified client or intended beneficiary) is explained, then time and patience can usually be found. After all, most of the complaints against Social Services departments refer not to the *longueurs* of contact but to frustrations about short, glancing consultations resulting in clients being endlessly referred elsewhere.

3   Social histories entail establishing an overview of major categories of past events, mapping and exploring current relationships and so on, so that current events may be viewed within the context of a person's life. Social histories have fallen out of fashion of late, probably because they are time-consuming, and because in previous decades there never seemed to be *quite* enough information on which to proceed. So, a few years ago, we flipped to very quick 'appraisals', largely of risk (to the department as much as to clients themselves). These provide a limited picture of how problems have built up and therefore little information on potential leverage points.

4   There is a beguiling idea, long in circulation, that 'assessment is an ongoing process'. Well yes, it is, but it cannot be never-ending. Why not think of it as a substantial stage near the beginning of a case, with, one hopes, smaller modifications and reviews being undertaken as new information comes to light, and progress is or is not made? The reality is that it is very easy to postpone an assessment in the face of urgent or neglected problems with statutory implications. But then we know of many cases where once 'first aid' measures have been taken (the child is safely in foster care; the eviction has been forestalled; the violent partner has been barred from further contact) the other, slower burning aspects of cases are neglected, only to recur later in more threatening forms. The authors therefore advocate a definite 'diagnostic' phrase to work, focusing on the *aetiology* of problems by getting clients to 'rewind' the 'videotapes' of their lives and take stock.

5   However, this word 'problems' seems to give some social workers and academics semantic indigestion. Therefore they tend to coat the word with euphemisms such as 'unmet needs'. Euphemisms are lies and must be resisted; just say no when you are offered one, otherwise you will find yourself wanting more and more. Strangely though, clients who come our way, either directly or via research projects, usually see themselves as drowning in *problems*. After all, people rarely seek the help of social workers for trivial difficulties, nor do they have services thrust upon them unless their difficulties are threateningly high in the risk stakes. Recognizing this does not entail denial of people's strengths. A good assessment will identify, affirm and capitalize on these.

6   We would next like to reassure the reader that we do not take the view that subjectivity can be completely eliminated from assessments; or that given a detailed enough protocol, the case notes should contain only objectively verifiable 'facts'. Indeed, if you turn back to Chapters 2 and 4, it should be clear that we see human beings as rather pre-programmed towards noticing certain types of events and not others, to jumping to conclusions, and to sticking to them. However, given that we know we have these semi-automatic cognitive tendencies, does it not behove us to take precautions when the welfare of others is at stake? For example, we have seen (Chapter 2) that remembering is an active, socially constructed process, bearing little resemblance to any camera or tape-recorder-like activity. What we remember about ourselves and others and what we forget is strongly influenced by psychological factors:

> 'Memory is like a dog that lies down where it pleases'. (Vanloon). Nor does our memory take much notice of our order not to *preserve something*: 'if only I had never seen that, experienced it, heard of it, if only I could just forget all about it'. But it is no good, it keeps turning up at night, spontaneously and uninvited when we cannot fall asleep. Then, too, memory is like a dog, it retrieves what we have just thrown away, and returns with it, wagging its tail.
>
> (Draaisma, 2004: 1)

Such factors explain why those who have suffered sexual abuse in childhood, when memory was just forming, find their lives plagued with flashbacks of these events in later life. Precautions can be taken during the preparation of assessments to these and other distortions by requesting examples from clients, asking them to recount other, more positive experiences regardless of their dramatic content, and by gently probing unexplained gaps in narrations.

The above may seem a daunting concoction of things that can go wrong, but when pulled off sensitively but candidly (an awkward balance) clients often find assessment a therapeutic experience in its own right.

Stages in assessment (see Figure 5.1)

Referral and early engagement

The ideal shape for any assessment procedure is, metaphorically, that of the funnel or tun dish: wide open to start with and then tapering off. A small experiment once conducted with social work students learning communication and interviewing skills via closed circuit television exercises (Sheldon and Baird, 1982) demonstrated the need for such an approach. Students (n = 30) were given identical information about clients, written on cards, but with referral and case information placed in different orders. The students were then asked to play the role of interviewer or client. What was fascinating was that if the first item presented involved concerns by teachers, then the interviewer (reflexively) wanted to pursue education-related matters. If relationship problems between partners were placed first on the list, then the focus of the interview became communication patterns within the family.

People come forward for help, or are impelled forward, in complex ways. Therefore the *route to referral* is the natural starting point for assessment. Clients may have been to several agencies before receiving what they regard as useful assistance or none. Some will feel that they have already told their stories, and may be reluctant to go through the whole process again.

Previous contacts can also result in a 'shaping' process, whereby clients are persuaded that their difficulties are of a certain kind, with certain origins, and with certain preferred solutions in prospect. There is also a large literature in social psychology on the subliminal power of initial impressions and of reputation which, it appears, can be more powerful influences than the *content* of what is said or done (see Cohen, 1964; Zimbardo, 2000).

Another aspect of pre-assessment experience is the way in which clients are received when they seek help. Rooms give messages. They may be welcoming and homely, or impersonal and threatening. On placement visits we have experienced the full spectrum of these impressions, from the bizarre – walls plastered with posters testifying to the idea that bed-wetting is largely a medical phenomenon (it isn't) because the receptionist's son had such a problem – to pictures everywhere of children in a hospice (the receptionist was a volunteer in such a facility), but the overriding impression given was, 'so you think *you've* got problems'. We have encountered neglected décor, wobbly chairs and boxes of broken toys, Christmas trimmings still up in early February, and prominent notices detailing the action that will be taken in cases of aggression, racist remarks or drunkenness on the part of clients, as if such infringements were routine in that place (see Braithwaite, 2001). Staff must be protected from such threats of course, but should they not be trained as to how firmly to deal with them on a case-by-case basis? Research tells us that the more welcoming and normal an environment, the less likely is insult or havoc to occur. There is thus no substitute for social work staff taking an interest in the 'front-of-curtain' environment, for often this space simply does not seem to *belong* to those who work in the rooms behind it.

Social histories

Patterns of unfolding interaction and their consequences for individuals and members of the family as a whole are the stuff of a good family assessment (and may also be important when working with individuals). Tendencies to promote conflict or to sacrifice one's needs to avoid it; to seek dominance; to distance oneself; to play good person/child roles or bad person/child roles are often played out as a matter of 'reflex', and sometimes they are part of a 'game' which carries hidden reinforcement.

Staff should take notes during the conduct of an assessment because, as we have seen, memory is fallible; because clients' stories are full of dates, times and sequences which can easily get jumbled up, and because it is natural for listeners unconsciously to add in material to a narrative to round it off and make it 'coherent'. Yet sometimes it is the very 'incoherency' of accounts which make for the most interesting starting points. But also, imagine being interviewed by a financial adviser about your pension prospects with him or her nodding sympathetically throughout, but never writing anything down.

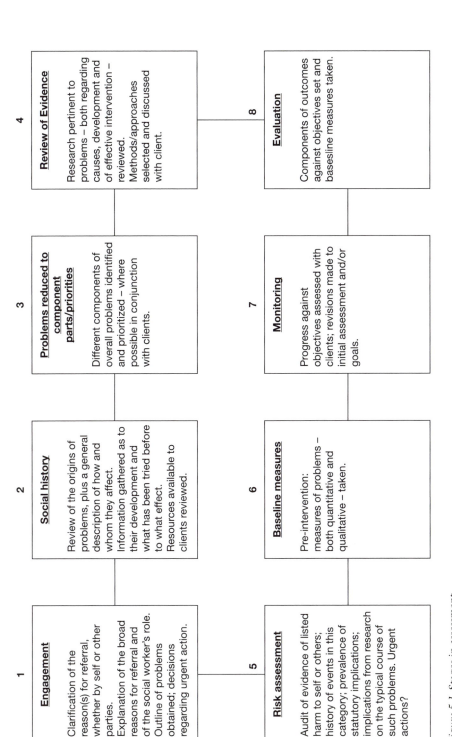

1

Engagement

Clarification of the reason(s) for referral, whether by self or other parties.
Explanation of the broad reasons for referral and of the social worker's role.
Outline of problems obtained; decisions regarding urgent action.

2

Social history

Review of the origins of problems, plus a general description of how and whom they affect.
Information gathered as to their development and what has been tried before to what effect.
Resources available to clients reviewed.

3

Problems reduced to component parts/priorities

Different components of overall problems identified and prioritized – where possible in conjunction with clients.

4

Review of Evidence

Research pertinent to problems – both regarding causes, development and of effective intervention – reviewed.
Methods/approaches selected and discussed with client.

5

Risk assessment

Audit of evidence of listed harm to self or others; history of events in this category; prevalence of statutory implications; implications from research on the typical course of such problems. Urgent actions?

6

Baseline measures

Pre-intervention: measures of problems – both quantitative and qualitative – taken.

7

Monitoring

Progress against objectives assessed with clients; revisions made to initial assessment and/or goals.

8

Evaluation

Components of outcomes against objectives set and baseline measures taken.

Figure 5.1 Stages in assessment

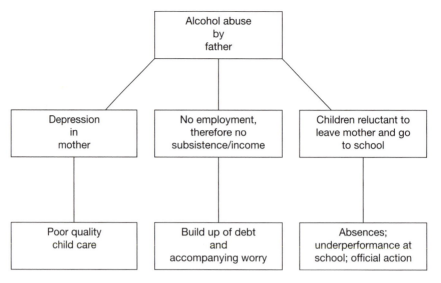

Figure 5.2 Interrelatedness of social problems

underlying emotional difficulties. Some are based on self-doubt and self-defence. We have seen a number of children who have spent long periods in care present with sharply different problems, showing, for example, aggression, self-centredness and serious risk-taking behaviour. Such children have learned to distrust the motives of others; they *expect* adults to let them down; they have few secure, counteractive relationships, and so they decide to look after themselves in whatever way seems safe at the time. As W.H. Auden (1994) observed, '*Those to whom evil is done, do evil in return.*' The 'evil' does not have to be intentional, by the way.

The trouble with the issue of presenting versus underlying problems, or of historical causes lying at the heart of current behaviour, is that it once got us a bad press (see Brewer and Lait, 1980). This was because of the then quite widespread belief, derived from psychoanalytical theory, that 'surface' manifestations of problems – regularly drinking away the grocery money, neglecting children, stealing – were ubiquitously the result of some long-buried conflict. One can still come up against only slightly less evidence-immune behaviour from family therapists today, who seem always to be able to trace equally manifest troubles to 'family system' pressures. Well, sometimes, perhaps, but sometimes talking more openly about problems rather than in code or avoiding them altogether can influence matters positively. This is so even in cases where later evidence suggests that their problems were not directly due to twisted communication patterns (but then headache is not caused by lack of aspirin in the bloodstream).

In the past, therefore, social workers were advised that there was little point bothering with such epiphenomena. Let us at this point make another plea for pluralism: in some cases relationships have failed and children suffer, and will make others suffer because of what happened to them. However, sometimes, whatever the direction of casual probabilities, it is sensible to start off by offering help with 'here-and-now' problems, and then to move backwards.

Risk assessment

Once the social worker has achieved an overview of current problems and has developed some ideas about their aetiology, it behoves her or him to undertake an assessment of any potentially serious risks posed. Given the high eligibility for service thresholds now in operation, most cases which come our way are likely to warrant this. We have to highlight this issue somewhere in the assessment sequence, but in reality it pervades all the stages under discussion, hence the vertical lines in Figure 5.1.

At the beginning we often have insufficient knowledge of the range and scope of problems to assess any risks that might attach to them or how these might be handled and so must return to the issue later. However, it is dangerous to regard risk assessment either as a postponable phase or as something done and dusted by a certain stage. In some cases we know at the point of referral that there is a real and present danger to self and/or others, and the circumstances giving rise to this perception will have to become the lead topic of conversation. In other cases, patterns of behaviour and/or circumstances may be deteriorating insidiously, and it is a mistake not to regularly review initial risk assessments.

Over the past few years a host of risk assessment instruments, national standards frameworks and departmental guidelines have been developed. However much comfort we allow ourselves to feel regarding these attempts, there are some provisos to enter about them.

1 We inhabit an organizational and political culture which sees risks as virtually always foreseeable by someone; which sees the (as it turns out) mistaken priority accorded to certain *other* allegedly risky cases (where nothing has yet happened) over the one where something did, as evidence of culpable misjudgement. In this fraught atmosphere we have – at a conceptual level – a difficulty in separating out risk that is *estimatable probabilities* from 'anyone's guess' *uncertainties*. This is an old problem:

> Uncertainties must be taken in a sense radically different from the familiar notion of Risk from which it has never been properly separated. If we do, it will appear that a *measurable* uncertainty or 'risk' proper . . . is so far different from an immeasurable one that it is not in effect an uncertainty at all.
>
> (Knight, 1921: 205 in Bernstein, 1996)

The tangible result of this confusion, and of the developing 'blame culture', is professional defensiveness, covert self-protection, and 'going-through-the-motions' behaviour by staff (ask any social worker in private). Take this example from the inquiry into the death of Kimberly Carlisle:

> I walked with the family to the door of the building and watched as they walked across the road to where their old car was parked. I still have a clear mental picture of the way they each walked across the road and got into the car, parents holding children by the hand, children leaping around in the car as they got in, laughing, shouting and playing happily with each other. It was almost an archetype of a happy family scene.
>
> (Blom-Cooper, *A Child in Mind*, 1987: 108–110)

The inquiry chairman's response was to observe that 'Far from being reassured, [the social worker] should have been alive to the risk of being manipulated. Plainly he had been deceived' (p. 112). Plainly? Certainly, with hindsight, we know that that family was not a 'happy family', though even with hindsight we do not know that 'manipulation' and 'deception' were present in that scene – even dysfunctional families can have happy moments. And the implicit criticism is sustainable only with the benefit of hindsight; the invited counterfactual (removal on the basis of this 'happy scene') is not plausible.

Where such wishful standards of professional prescience exist, the outcome is unlikely to be that social workers will be more careful; rather it will encourage them speculatively to record *absolutely everything*. Too much information, not properly sifted, not looked into sceptically, is a greater enemy of good assessment than too little.

2   Many of the risk assessment schedules in use, which are intended to guide staff towards greater objectivity and consistency, are the products of a retrospective identification of factors present in cases where death or serious harm has occurred. Only recently have such guidelines been subjected to validity and reliability testing. Validity raises the question as to whether an instrument actually measures what it purports to measure or just collateral factors. Reliability raises the questions as to whether two or more different people or one and the same person would, at different times, come close in their views as the result of using a given schedule (for a sober, evidence-based debate on such matters see Macdonald and Macdonald, 1999a).

It is worth remembering that the decisions taken to remove 34 children from their homes in 1990 for reasons of 'satanic abuse' (the children, when grilled by social workers, admitted to seeing fiery crosses and infant sacrifices) were made with the aid of 'The Satanic Abuse Instrument' thought up in the USA. When the press first got hold of it they castigated Social Services managers for their complacency. When the removals based upon it were seen to be a ghastly mistake, they did so again for overzealousness. If such brainstorms (and there have been many) do not suggest the need for 'a sober, evidence-based debate', then it is difficult to see what does.

3   There is another problem, this time regarding allegedly measurable uncertainties. Supposing we had a risk assessment schedule with an 84 per cent reliability level (which owing to a mental 'essay mark' effect looks first class in the prediction stakes) who would decline to use it? But we are usually dealing with very large numbers of people who fall within a given orbit: millions of children, thousands of mentally ill people and so on, and we know very little about the base rates of 'suspicious' collateral circumstances in these populations.

The problem, then, with all but *massively* accurate screening instruments (we have none, nor does psychiatry, nor does education), is that when applied to large populations they yield discomfiting numbers of false positives (not really a risk at all) and false negatives (not a risk on paper but one in actuality). Therefore the risk of harm through hyper-vigilant good intentions should be as much to the forefront of our thinking as the risk of harm through lack of watchfulness. Take, for example, the proposed National Child Database wherein every child in the

UK will have a computer file, and 'incidents' which might affect their development and 'circumstances' regarded as risky or adverse will be entered by the different professionals who come into contact with them. This scheme has raised doubts in the minds of some academics (see Munro, 2005) over what will be the level of decisional accuracy, or indeed, of accurate recording. The aim of this new scheme is that information about children will be easier to 'share' – a factor that inquiries regularly throw out as something to be improved upon. But sharing information does not tackle the equally important one of interpreting the *significance* of items in the wash of information that passes back and forth.

4   The next point concerns *types* of suspected harm – because risk is not a unitary phenomenon. Some bad events seem to come out of nowhere. For example, take a couple living in pleasant domestic surroundings who are seeking a little help with a parenting problem with their child who has Asperger's syndrome, and who suddenly snap and injure him. Then there are slowly developing risks where problems and provocations steadily mount and it is difficult for staff to appreciate the significance of the pattern. Then there is the occupational hazard of inurement to risks. Both authors have felt their hair gently rise when training childcare staff who have presented live case material. The reaction of participants to our discomfort usually takes the form of 'if you think *this* is a risky case, you should hear about some of my others' reassurances. However, they presume that it will be *these* apparently more difficult cases that will 'blow' first, and that the problems under discussion are somehow 'normal' in the neighbourhoods in which they work. Desensitization to squalid living conditions and threats to the development of children have featured in many inquiry reports and we need to guard against confusing weary acceptance of what seems chronic with non-judgemental 'acceptance' (see Chapter 6).

5   All the caveats discussed in this section aside, some risks *are* foreseeable; as when we have been told that the carer of a frail elderly person living at home is going abroad for a year because of her job, and her son, who has no track record in the matter, will be 'holding the fort' or when an ex-partner with a record of violence is due for parole; or when a new baby is on the way to an isolated single mother who is struggling to cope with the one she already has.

It is thus important to distinguish between the general watchfulness that most social workers adopt when working in risky areas and formal risk assessments undertaken at a particular point in time and designed to answer specific questions about the likelihood of harm. The former approach is an integral part of our responsibility to recognize, for example, children in need of protection, or older people at risk of falling. The latter entails using a formalized approach designed to improve the quality of decision-making by providing a clear framework for the collection, organization and interpretation of information. The most robust approaches are those based on established statistical associations between certain criteria and a specific outcome of interest (i.e. so-called *actuarial* models). These are the kinds of models that insurance companies use to assess risk and the subsequent cost of policies. As a general rule, they are better than those made on professional consensus (see Gambrill and Shlonsky, 2001).

The evidence thus suggests that improving risk assessments requires that we move from the latter to the former model, and in recent years there has been a growth in the development of such approaches (see McIvor *et al.*, 2002). Their effectiveness depends upon their being able accurately to identify and measure things which we are confident influence the probability of something happening; easier in some areas than in others. Given all these compromising factors, what then is the most secure way of approaching risk assessment?

1　First, get to know the risks associated with the problems you are dealing with, and their base rates. For example, what is the recidivism rate for juvenile offenders with a record of certain types of criminal behaviour? What is the probability of someone who deliberately harms themselves, or attempts suicide, doing so again? The tendency for social workers to focus on the uniqueness of individual cases means that we often rob ourselves of this appropriate challenge to our judgement and our (necessary) optimism. So, having been persuaded that someone who is remorseful and cooperative is not a serious risk regarding further violence, it is unlikely that we will pay much attention to statistics that tell us that 60 per cent of people with such a history are likely to do exactly the same thing again. It would be wiser to start from the position of 'what is most likely to happen on the basis of the broader evidence base?' and then adjust one's assessment in the light of factors that either add to, or mitigate, one's concerns. Knowledge of protective factors is relevant to the latter.

2　Piece together the chronology of events, including contacts with other agencies, and collect information from all relevant parties. This 'picture-making' is routinely undertaken in circumstances where people have died, and typically leads to a great deal of information known to a variety of people never before put together. We are less good at it with the living and the as yet uninjured.

3　Be explicit and transparent. Make it clear *what* information you have gathered, why you have gathered it, and what you think its significance is. Say what story you think it tells, estimate what it says about the likelihood of the risks you are concerned with, and over what time period. Spell out the things you think might contain the risk, including those services and supports that other agencies or other people can introduce. Ensure that they understand their roles and their scope to avoid diffusion of responsibility which can be a side-effect of the increased cooperation that all inquiry reports call for.

4　Monitor the impact of particular forms of intervention and consider the length of time it is taking to bring about a given level of change. Is this in line with, or at odds with, the interventions literature for this approach? The latter point is particularly important when the risks one is dealing with are cumulative. For example, when children are routinely neglected but are not necessarily at a specific risk today or tomorrow, although their development and future life chances may be in longer term jeopardy.

5　As new information comes to light, reassess – preferably with a supervisor – your estimates of likely danger. Even though we can rarely estimate the absolute probability of something bad happening, we can, and should, be able to make a stab at estimates of relative probability. If someone is seriously depressed and at risk of suicide or self-harm, then learning that the same person has been left by their partner, or that they have lost their job, should alert us to heightened risk and prompt us to reconsider whether current services are sufficient to contain it. For reasons of self-protection too, 'show your working out' regarding changing risk levels and anchor decisions in events as much as in conversations. *Invite* your supervisor to alert you to any logical 'jumps' or *non sequiturs* in your assessments. This process of active review is perhaps one of the most important aspects of risk assessment.

However, what is too little realized is that not taking considered risk can be the most hazardous option of all. 'Frozen watchfulness' is a condition that not only affects abused children, but whole organizations.

Case or problem formulations

These were once *de rigueur* but have fallen from fashion of late except in family therapy and cognitive-behavioural approaches. They have been replaced by summaries. The problem with these is that they are often, at least from our research on recording (see Sheldon, 1985, 1989: Macdonald, 2001), little more than assemblages of key phrases picked from the rest of the assessment. But a formulation is more than a summarizing description. It should contain best guesses as to the likely origins, patterns of development and present-day manifestations. Look at the following summarizing statements from case records:

> This case contains many interactive problems to do with finances, inconsistent parenting, and pressures within the family system.
>
> (Sheldon, 1989: 14)

This statement gives *some* information, but leaves largely unaddressed important questions of which? why? how? and so? It is difficult to get a clear idea of the social worker's thinking and plans from them. A good formulation is both a summary of main aetiological elements as seen by the social worker in negotiation with clients, but it has dynamic features too. That is, certain qualities should attach to problem formulations, the most important being clarity, unequivicality, and a sense that they could readily be overturned by subsequent information or experience, and none the worse for that. Here is an example of what we regard as a good formulation (it was written by a student, incidentally). It concerns a case where the referral to Social Services came via the school because teachers were worried that the children were tearful and fractious at going-home time:

> Because of his lack of experience with children and his anxieties about discipline, Mr A tended, on joining the family, to crack down severely on minor infringements of rules – what he calls 'starting as you mean to go on'. However, the children's relationship with him is not sufficiently well developed that they are willing to accept this as his legitimate role. They see it instead as a rejection of them; as a desire to dominate them, and to replace their natural father. Discussion of this problem with the family and the drafting out of a simple agreement describing the obligations and expectations of both adults and

children, may be a useful temporary measure to reduce the present high level of conflict (rows and slaps) between Mr A and the children. A separate series of meetings with Mr A and Mrs L aimed at teaching Mr A how to express his positive feelings towards the children in a way that they can accept (including how to deal with rebuffs) should enable him to cope better in joint activities. It would be a good sign if these increased beyond their present low level.

(from Sheldon, 1995)

Now it may be that this analysis is mistaken. It may be that the social worker's encouragement that Mr A should try to understand the children's apparent rejection of him and try to react differently *does not* result in him spending more time with them, or that it does, but that they continue to dislike it. It may be that the relationship with the natural father calls all the tunes. It may be that the confrontations between adults and children continue at their current level, or that there are fewer of them but when they do occur they are nastier. In which case, this formulation has proved inadequate and the social worker will need to think again. However, having 'placed the bet' on the possible dynamics of this problem, the social worker would have got to know about the need for revision quite readily.

Setting intermediate and longer term objectives

The word *goal* and the word *objective* tend to be used interchangeably in social work; the important point to emphasize is that, whatever term we use, we focus on the issue of how we will know when something has been achieved or not, and what standards of non-subjective proof are being used to determine this. Thus, if a family 'seems happier these days', what is it that happens or no longer happens that leads one to the opinion that this partly qualitative, partly quantative goal has been achieved? To concentrate only upon the qualitative (what *kind* of change) and ignore the quantitative (*how much*), or vice versa, is self-defeating in evaluation terms.

In social work, intermediate and longer term objectives, and qualitative and quantitative factors tend to get mixed up together. This is partly due to the complexity of the cases with which we deal, but it also results from inadequate training in these matters, and from a stubborn occupational attachment to the heart-warmingly all-encompassing. Therefore, it is wise to address the question 'How shall we know, and be able to show others that we have achieved this?' That is, how shall we know, over and above our subjective feelings, that something worthwhile has happened? Positive views from clients should by no means be neglected, but one should also expect to see tangible behavioural or circumstantial change to give these statements credibility.

Another problem is that the word *goals* is usually preceded in social work texts by the word *flexible*. This is to remind us that circumstances change and that we need to change with them. True, but in most studies of the process (see Sheldon, 1977, 1985; Gibbs, 1991) we find many more examples of vague, protean (i.e. anything that happens to happen can be slipped into the loose framework) goals than of style-crampingly narrow objective setting. There is a balance to redress here. Our recommendations are to follow the advice of Karl Popper (1963) on finding out that conjectures and theorizing can be as broad as one likes to start with, but then at some stage we must reduce opinions, hopes and expectations to statements designed to be vulnerable to refutation.

Goals are thus self-administered challenges to good intentions. To switch metaphors, they are points to steer by, and the last thing that any navigator or those on board need in a point is a *flexible* point.

Case example

One of us once supervised an able student who was working on a demanding case involving a couple who were unremittingly 'at war' with each other, but seemed in a strange way to enjoy this state of affairs. They had a young son who was caught up in these games, which the student likened to those of the couple in the play *Who's Afraid of Virginia Woolf?* The son was the main concern as he had long spells of something close to elective mutism. He was removed from the home and placed in a specialist children's unit, with work continuing with the couple while options for his future were considered. The approach used was a mixture of social casework and behavioural therapy. Thirteen interviews were conducted but at the end of the contact there was little sign of change. Therefore the focus switched firmly towards the welfare of the child and to the need to build a separate future for him. However, when the student had to compile case studies for submission with his placement report, he summed up this one in the following terms: 'At least all their hostility is out in the open now'(!). The view of the supervisor was that attempts to achieve certain goals in this case had failed. This did not constitute a failure on the student's part; nor was it evidence of a failure to select the approaches most likely to succeed according to the literature; it was a failure of influence. Better, surely, to admit this, to learn from the experience, and to realize that social workers cannot be of much help in the face of determined efforts to subvert. Later the couple split up and the child was successfully fostered; he regained his voice because silence was no longer the only safe course.

There is nothing wrong with the idea of a flexible *policy* in a case, it is just that when you come to goal setting these need to be highly specific statements; that is, *inflexible*. There is nothing to prevent us, in the light of experience, from substituting one set of clear goals for another. Better to fail clearly and early, and then to revise, than to drift.

It is our experience that most clients value interim feedback on progress, both with tasks that they have agreed to pursue themselves and in respect of those undertaken on their behalf. Here are the necessary steps:

1   Introduce early on the idea of the need to monitor key events, whether of a positive type (which it is hoped will increase), or of a problematic type (which it is hoped will decrease), or both.
2   Negotiate with clients as to what measures would best represent progress, and try politely to squeeze out vagueness of expression by asking for examples.

3   Introduce the idea of record-keeping regarding both hoped-for qualitative and quantitative changes. Diaries are useful.
4   Standardized instruments (see Fischer and Corcoran, 1994) may be used to assess change on a before-and-after basis.
5   Work with clients to produce estimates of the likely duration of attempts to change something. We know from the literature on task-centred casework (see Chapter 6) that this can have motivating effects. If the work is likely to be lengthy it can help 'pace' clients and immunize them against disappointment.
6   Do not be afraid to redefine goals and objectives, or to try out new approaches to problems; just restart the monitoring scheme each time.
7   Give positive feedback to clients on any progress made. Many live lives where there is little encouragement available, only inspection.

Evaluation

We have four recommendations to make:

1   Do one. Most case records contain nothing worthy of the name. In place of evaluations we tend to get summaries at the end.
2   Evaluation should be given a *much* higher profile on qualifying courses and in-service training than it currently has. Live case material is an excellent teaching medium in this regard. Unless social workers know *how* rigorously to evaluate their own work, they become at best mere consumers of academic and departmental exhortations.
3   Pre-post follow-up approaches probably represent the optimum level between rigour and practicability, whether qualitative comparisons are being made (e.g. handling family disputes through discussion and negotiation rather than dictation and threats) or quantitative comparisons (e.g. weight gain, attendance at eating disorder groups). This means that we need *baseline information* before proceeding, and we regard the routine absence of this information from Social Services' records as a serious fault.
4   Single case designs have been around for years, and relevant books and articles are full of practice examples of their use (see Sheldon, 1983, 1995); yet social workers seem to suffer from a kind of graph phobia, and prefer to rely on purely verbal reports instead. In our experience clients like to use these devices, but in any case they are for *us*. An example of a simple, single case design will be found on p. 146. There are many more advanced versions though, some of which have the rigour of small controlled experiments.
5   The strictures discussed above apply to projects as well as cases. We were once involved in the evaluation of a purpose-built mental health hostel/day centre. It was deliberately built prior to the surrounding houses, its main aim being to integrate residents into the local community, but discrimination against the people living there did not fall as a result. Thus commissioners of evaluations should be aware that their investments 'can go down as well as up'. The reaction of the local authority to the news in this case was 'at least the local community felt able to complain'(!). Remedial measures with much greater involvement of community groups and local politicians helped.

Conclusions

We have tried to set down what we think are the characteristics of a good assessment, and make no apology for it being an 'ideal type'. That is, we know well that organizational factors, crises, shortage of time, uncooperative clients and changing caseload priorities will probably hinder the completion of stages in any neat order. The point is that if the social worker has a structure in her or his head, or better still in his or her notebook, then they will know that some information is still missing, and can pursue it if the opportunity arises.

6 Social casework and task-centred casework

Which words
Will come through air unbent,
Saying, so to say, only what
they mean?
       Peter Porter, 1982: 771

Social casework

Social workers cannot not do social casework (*discuss*). This blend of individual help, taking account of the life histories of clients, their current problems, both psychological and practical, and their family and community circumstances, is just in the nature of the job. The phrase is rarely heard today though (perhaps because it does not contain the word 'management'). Nevertheless, it long described the essence of what social workers did – they worked with people and their problems (cases), and they still do.

Biestek (1960) provided an influential conceptual framework for the approach, but it was more concerned with ethical principles than with methods, because what one did back then was largely determined by the dominant psychological hybrid of the times: dilute psychoanalysis blended with 'humanistic approaches' as espoused by Carl Rogers (1951, 1961).

Biestek was a Catholic priest who went native among welfare workers without abandoning his rather absolutist views on ethical matters. His work therefore, when read today, seems to avoid some of the awkward complexities and moral compromises of practical social work. Biestek's ideas thrived in the rarified atmosphere of graduate courses, predominantly in the USA, but also among an influential minority of British academics and the elites of the psychiatric and medical social work specialities.

Like Rogers, Biestek was primarily concerned with the *process* of helping, in contrast with the present, where social work is often seen as a commodity. Yet if one talks to students or staff on in-service training courses, discussions quickly turn to questions of how best to engage disaffected clients and of the kinds of working relationships they are trying build with them. The new official version of these encounters is that they are a 'supportive', 'enabling', 'transparent' pursuit of outcomes; this as a corrective to an alleged previous tendency for social workers to dawdle along with clients, admiring the interesting psycho-social views, but forgetting about the destination and who was sponsoring the excursion.

Biestek and Rogers produced separate accounts of relationship – mediated attempts to influence the choices, motives and problem-solving capacities of clients – and their work will form the framework of this section of the book. However, as well as describing their views, we also offer a critique of what is proposed and supposed by them, informed by empirical research.

Here are the key principles of social casework presented in the order that they have been most influential:

1   *Individuation and non-directivity.* You might think that there is no such word as the former and that the Americans have been messing around with the language again, but the word was in use in the seventeenth century: '*Individuate (verb) distinguish from others of the same kind; to single out*' (*OED*). This principle reminds us that whatever our needs for shorthand categorizations, all people are in some respects like *all* other people; like *some* other people, but, ultimately, like *no* other person. That is, they are unique in their personal histories and aspirations – so long as we remember that their aspirations might include subverting a court order or obtaining a really secure supply of hard drugs. For Biestek and a generation of writers on social casework, worthwhile change comes from within the individual as a result of a set of insight-building, trust and confidence-enhancing dynamics which are deliberately fostered within a special therapeutic relationship. Biestek, Rogers and their contemporaries drew on each others' work, forming a 'school' which attracted members from across the helping professions. Above all they argued for non-directive therapy tailored to individual histories. Such principles still loom large on training courses for counsellors and social workers. The key ideas: (1) that externally imposed solutions are easily abandoned when obstacles are encountered – which is in line with cognitive dissonance theory being developed at the time in social psychology (see Festinger, 1957); (2) that (somewhat romantically we think) clients already have solutions to their problems inside themselves; they need only to be released by invitations to 'explore' in a safe environment. Advice, based on some expert knowledge, was largely ruled out by this principle, and here is a quote from Florence Hollis' influential text (1964: 21) which may explain why this was tenable:

> To a certain extent the official position of casework has been more extreme than in actual practice. Workers have probably recognised that there needs to be some guidance and have developed subtle ways of exercising such influences.

The word 'subtle' amounts to a justification for *covert* persuasion: if so, there is uncomfortable research from social psychology showing it to be an under-estimated influence. But how ethical is the idea? Since change is usually what helpers are after, how subliminal can we afford to be and still get it? Here are the reflections of Paul Halmos (1965: 90), a friendly critic:

> One of the central ideas of the counselling ideology is 'non-directiveness'. According to this ideal, counsellors must do their work without ever violating the personal initiative of the individual patient or client. It is necessary to stress at the outset that this 'must' does not follow from the psychological theories

of the counsellor and, indeed cannot follow from them, for there can be no logically derivable entailment from the propositions of a theory about factors, about what 'is', resulting in the confirmation of what 'ought to be' and 'must be'. It is a commonplace in philosophy that one cannot divine an 'ought' from an 'is'.

Sophistry aside, the problem is that the 'is' is itself a doubtful notion because: (1) robust studies have long shown that helpers of all professional stripes detectably influence their clients' thinking, feeling and behaviour without always realizing it; (2) it is easy to identify their theoretical leanings simply from a blind reading of samples of their case notes, and (3) that some of these covert influences are non-verbal, and sometimes unintentional. In a discussion with Skinner, Rogers acknowledged this: 'We are all deeply engaged in the prediction and influencing of behavior, or even the control of behavior' (Rogers and Skinner, 1956).

Social workers cannot behave like plumbers or electricians: 'What's the problem?'. 'It's over there', 'Oh! You need a . . .'. So it is best to acknowledge influence, both overt and covert, and to take out only a part share in the effectiveness of any solutions negotiated with clients. Otherwise, in adopting the non-directive position, if the attempt to help fails, then this is always ultimately down to the client. The best advice is to tread lightly (for you tread on their assumptions, history, culture, habits and appetites) and try to build a therapeutic alliance, drawing on the resources of 'insider' knowledge from the (expert) client and one's own research-derived knowledge and professional experience.

To illustrate the sort of process we have in mind, here are the words of a recent client who had a long history of domestic abuse, rape, attempted murder, and consequent serious depression. She was asked at the end of a series of interviews to say what she thought she had got from them:

> Well at the start, it was all new to me because I've spent so long hiding the truth from other people – I was ashamed I expect. But I learnt in our talks that I could say *anything* – what I mean is that you wouldn't fall backwards off the chair if I told you something awful or something I was ashamed of. But then I also liked it when you didn't let me get away with anything. I had lots of complications in my life and you got me to think more clearly about them. You never *made* me do these things, but I soon got an idea of where you thought I should be heading. Somehow I got it into my head that all the knocking about was something to do with me; that I must have 'asked for it'; made it happen somehow. Now I know that I must have been mad to put up with it and that *nobody* should be treated like that. But it's only when you stand back and start to say to yourself, hey, I'm a person too, what about bloody *me*?
>
> (Interview transcript, 2004)

2   *Self-determination.* This principle overlaps with both *individuation* and non-directiveness and proposes that the caseworker should (again on both ethical and technical grounds) attempt to create a relationship which at every stage reinforces

the decision-making capacity of the client and holds that he or she is sovereign judge, 'subject to terms and conditions', as they say. A liberal position then, but likely to flood the minds of anyone working in social services with scores of urgent exceptions. But here is the case for the stance:

> The only purpose for which power can be rightfully exercised over any member of a civilised community, against his will, is to prevent harm to others. His own good, whether physical or moral, is not a sufficient warrant. He cannot rightfully be compelled to do or to forbear because it would be better for him to do so, because it will make him happier, because, in the opinion of others, to do so would be wise, or even right. There are good reasons for remonstrating with him, or persuading him, or entreating him, but not for compelling him, or visiting him with any evil in case he do otherwise. To justify that, the conduct from which it is desired to deter him must be calculated to produce evil to someone else.
>
> (Mill, 1859: 73)

The principles enshrined in the above quotation were intended to defend the individual against the (then) new-found appetite of governments for ever more detailed state intervention in the lives of individuals (J.S. Mill must now be turning in his grave).

Self-determination should not therefore be seen as a moral gift bestowed upon clients in the interview room. It exists in a context of law, regulation, and in the complex social interactions we have with each other – which include good withheld and harm done, sometimes with insight and forethought, sometimes not. So this is a much tougher view to hold now than in 1859. In complex, industrialized societies, people are much more interconnected and inter-dependent. Mill put forward many exceptions to his rule, for instance, children, 'the insane' and 'mentally infirm', and some of these categories defy close definition. However, although this principle of not doing things to 'help' people if they do not themselves wish it is hedged around with all sorts of marginal cases, it stands nevertheless as a profound truth. The Dutch have a nice, cautionary, word for it: *bemoeizorg* ('meddling care').

But let us now get on to the territory of the exceptions and marginal cases, because this is where social workers live.

Virtually all the empirical research we have on what it is like to be mentally ill, to have a learning disability, or to be a frail elderly person living at home and dependent upon services, shows that the maintenance or passing back of as much control over their lives as is feasible, including considered risks, results in improved functioning, greater life satisfaction, and greater satisfaction with services. It is the 'as far as is feasible' (whose risk is it anyway?) caveat that causes ethical difficulties:

> People who seek assistance may find their problem re-defined by those who feel they know better, and attempts may be made to deprive them of a freedom which they had before – a freedom to learn by their own mistakes. . . . Such a conviction of knowing better than the client is as true of those who seek to 'politicise' clients as it is of those who want to offer them therapy. Both approaches can devalue clients' own perceptions of their lives and of their goals. Self-determination must

mean the right to try to achieve something for oneself (and fail if need be), subject only to the restraints of the laws which govern everyone's actions.

(Campbell, 1984: 38)

Laws, regulations, national standards and 'benchmarks' cover all the above client groups, but how do they help, say, when a patient no longer under a section of the Mental Health Act decides to stop taking his or her medication and, apart from some mild disorders of thought, *currently* exhibits no antisocial behaviour? What influence might reasonably be brought to bear in the case (one of ours) of a teenager with a moderate learning disability who is spending increasing amounts of time with a group of youths who poke fun at him and exploit him, but whose *apparent* friendship he values? How free from professional interference should a frail, semi-housebound and socially isolated elderly person be to decide that, after all, she doesn't like the warden popping in, and would rather do without the inedible meals on wheels?

In light of the above criticisms, what should we attempt to retain of the casework ideal? Well: (1) we should remember that even if advice is given it may be ignored, so there is not always as much to lose as we might think; (2) it is part of our code of values that we do not abandon people who do not see sense as we see it, we stay with them (if we are allowed to) in the hope of later influence or of finding another way through. This is not a pious point: respondents in client-opinion studies regularly ascribe value to the way in which social workers stay the course with them, even though there are underlying disagreements or failures to carry out plans; (3) we can go part of the way with Beistek and try to keep the 'locus of control' as near to the client as possible without playing Rogerian word games. So, instead of pushing in with advice which can make clients feel 'done to', we can try to create a relationship in which emerging rules are: contemplation before action; clarification of any goals that the client has; testing out what might go wrong, and persuading clients to look at problems from more than one perspective.

However, frankly, given the evidence from empirical studies of outcomes in social work and related disciplines, it is probably time to ditch some of the ideas of social casework, but to consider retaining some of the relationship-building factors in modified form. We personally see nothing wrong with considered advice or direct interpretations, so long as they are used in due proportion and put forward tentatively for the client to think about 'You have ears and eyes and a mouth – use them in that preportion', a wise supervisor once observed. Thus the contrast between a manifestly caring relationship which recognizes the client's independence, and within which contrary views based on some expertise can be debated but no attempts made to impose them, can create the motivation to think again, and to experiment with changed behaviour, or to see one's circumstances differently.

The non-judgemental attitude

'*Cum dilectione hominum et odio vitiorum*'. Literally: with love for mankind and hatred of sins.

Opera Omnis, Vol. 2, col. 962, letter 211

Judge not, that ye be not judged.

St Matthew

So here we have textual authority on this adopted principle, but what happens when people try to put it into practice? The journalist Bernard Levin (much missed purveyor of good sense to the nation) once asked whether Lord Longford, who campaigned for the parole of the child killer and co-torturer Myra Hindley after many years of incarceration and (apparent) repentance, was barmy. He concluded that *yes, of course* he is barmy, but the question is, is he right?

Social workers come in for quite a bit of stick when they try to understand the origins and motivation for conduct which the rest of society finds abhorrent or stupid. Yet they are charged with the task of social redemption: helping young people to give up crime, stopping drug-taking, encouraging people to bring up children well, and so forth. Going around trying to do good is a risky business. Clients often don't want it done to them, and the general public balk at our sin-eating activities whenever they amount to anything that might be mistaken for understanding, sympathy, or lack of due condemnation.

The community has its rights too of course, and we are not soft on these. We question, though, whether stern moral lessons and rather suspect training schemes are not likely further to alienate the young, who tend to come from poor, broken families, are often functionally illiterate, and have been thrown out of most of society's normal institutions. Many of them already know quite a lot about shame and disapproval.

It will be seen, therefore, that given the histories and predilections of some of the clients who come our way, maintaining a non-judgemental attitude towards them is a tall order. But this pessimism – or realism as critics would have it – is partly based on a misunderstanding of the concept. Neither Beistek nor Rogers, nor any of the other writers on the ethics and politics of helping, are recommending the recruitment of a corps of soft-headed people to do social work. Rather they are arguing that (1) for ethical reasons – because unless you believe in congenital evil, persistent wrong-doing does not emerge from *nowhere* as an uncaused set of events – few, if any, *suddenly* become depraved; and (2) for practical purposes – since a helping relationship based on regular doses of disapproval is unlikely to get very far – we should recognize that social work is a special calling, and just do our best with this idea.

Non-judgementality as a concept is quite close to Carl Rogers' principle of *unconditional positive regard*, which is itself based on two propositions:

1 Human beings are valuable in their own right as an end and not just as a means. They are equipped with great capacity for change, adaptation and even redemption if positive counter-influences are brought to bear.
2 That in most cases a trust-building relationship backed up by a genuine desire to understand offers a better chance of change than punishment or restriction alone.

However, the question is, is it *achievable* for human beings to separate out the person from the person's behaviour? Some clever authors have doubted the validity of trying so to do:

> If this principle were applied in child-rearing, parents would respond approvingly and affectionately when their children appeared with stolen goods, behaved

unmanageably in school, physically injured their siblings and peers, refused to follow any household routines etc. 'Unconditional love' would make children directionless, impossible to live with, and completely unpredictable.

(Bandura, 1969: 79)

But Bandura may be taking too narrow a view of his own 'social learning theory', in that surely it is the duality of social disapproval and action taken against misconduct *plus* the availability of a benign, rational, listening, future-directed relationship that is more likely to prevent repetitions of the behaviour in question. After all, few of us take much notice of disapprobation from someone we classify as 'them'.

The argument from increased understanding, '*tout comprendre et tout pardonaire*' (to understand all is to forgive all), serves a little as a shield against being taken advantage of, but there is always the occupational hazard of desensitization to manipulation to take into account. Madame de Stael (1807) put it differently: '*Tout comprendre rend très indulgent*' (to be totally understanding makes one very indulgent). However, we may take comfort from the fact that few social workers end their careers without being able to produce examples of people who have overcome the most depressing and challenging of circumstances.

Acceptance

Social workers probably undervalue their willingness to try to understand and advise upon events, thoughts and feelings of all kinds arising from desperate circumstances, but clients in surveys do not. They regularly report that being listened to without apparent prejudgement by someone to whom they attribute a sympathetic desire to understand what most people would regard as non-understandable is what gave them hope or dissuaded them from giving up (see Maluccio, 1979). Social workers in mixed occupational company underestimate the extent to which the complexities of their jobs makes them come across as rather woolly-sounding (though sometimes of course it is because their thinking *is* woolly). Many people one meets believe (1) that social problems are simple, and the solution to them is just a matter of more legal constraint, better enforcement, stricter penalties; and (2) that social work fails because we try to deal with a minority of people who simply do not deserve our patience and tolerance. Try this one on for size though.

Case example

This case involves a young man with two children. To say that he was estranged from his wife is to distort the facts, yet he did live away from home and was something of a recluse. Nevertheless, he loved her and by all accounts, she loved him. He had decided to separate 'for the good of the children' – but this was not the usual sort of 'good'. He suffered from a severe form of obsessive-compulsive disorder (see Chapter 11) which involved excessive attention to hygiene; and various rituals which dominated his life, but above all, from

---

ruminations about 'bad thoughts' and a strong feeling that one day he might act upon them. The worst among these involved the sexual abuse of his own children. The case records contained no example of anything of the sort happening, but there was an ever-present fear that it *might* if he lost control.

The history revealed persistent attempts to secure help. The *dramatis personae* were two GPs: the first one could not hide her revulsion and found a way to remove him from her list; the second confessed himself 'baffled' but nevertheless prescribed cocktails of medication which either sent his client to sleep or made him even more agitated. Enter a consultant psychiatrist, who did not think he could improve upon the existing regime, but regretted the fact that he could no longer procure aversion therapy. (Even if it were valid on ethical grounds, it is ineffective.) The consultant saw him at three-monthly interviews for 'reviews' but was useful only in referring him on to other specialists. These included a psychologist who gave up after one session and referred the client back to the psychiatrist, who recommended a course of ECT (he was not depressed but deeply unhappy). The patient undertook this almost as a form of deserved punishment or 'exorcism'. Apart from memory loss, there was no effect. Meanwhile, someone in the surgery, which was in a small village, leaked the story of the reasons behind the separation, and a campaign of 'outing' this client as a potential paedophile began. He was ostracized by many, and became even more reclusive. Eventually the possibility of cognitive-behavioural therapy was hit upon (more by chance than from a reading of the research) and he was referred to one of the present authors, who saw him on seven occasions. What emerged was a childhood history of buggery at the hands of his stepfather, with, he suspected, the partial collusion of his mother, and the fact that his obsessions began in his early teenage years and grew worse later.

The patient reported finding the CBT approach useful, particularly discussions of his childhood experiences, and of the non-rational aspects of his patterns of thought. The contents of his history that concern us here are: (1) a feeling of *despoliation* arising from his sexual abuse and a feeling of betrayal by his mother; (2) a feeling that he had been 'chosen' for a bad life and had come from 'bad blood', and (3) the steady onset of his obsessional preoccupations with the *worst thing that could happen* and the fear that these impulses could attach themselves to just about anything. Therefore there was a consequent preoccupation with suicide; (4) fantasies about a 'cure' that would not involve him too much in trying to understand his illness, but would take the form of something *done to* him, ideally involving surgery; and (5) a strong feeling that however much support he was given, 'something' would soon 'snap' and would lead him to 'his destiny'.

The patient had more understanding and self-forgiveness by the end of the CBT sessions and thought he had made some progress with deflecting obsessive thoughts. He also went out more, and sought and received the support of two old friends. Then, one evening, after a sleepless night full of what he always referred to as 'the worst thoughts', he drove into a nearby wood and gassed himself with exhaust fumes. The message he left explained that it was 'best' for his children and for his wife, and that although 'people' had been very helpful, he now realized there was no real cure and that he would have to fight his demons for the rest of his life and was too tired to do this.

The priest at the crematorium chapel gave a brisk, coded sermon about the perils of mental illness, and how much more (unspecified) help should be available to sufferers. Then he hastily left. From his behaviour one found it hard not to think that he saw himself as committing a potential sinner to judgement thankfully sooner rather than later.

Not all cases are as dire as the one described above, but it does provide an example of the need for acceptance and how people can be affected by its withdrawal. We view this as primarily an ethical stance, but think that if it can be managed it is a therapeutic good in its own right. Forgiveness is not our preserve but understanding surely is.

Controlled emotional involvement

> Better by far for Johny the bright star
> To keep your head and see his children fed.
> A Battle of Britain poem
> by John Pudney, 1940

We have no pills to dispense and no devices into which to plug our clients, so social work requires the use of the self alongside the knowledge provided on training courses. By this we mean it requires that we draw also on life experiences and that we make considered use of the resources of our own personalities. It is surely true that when dealing with a case involving a child in difficulties we naturally think of our own childhoods; when dealing with the problems of older clients we naturally think about the effects of ageing on our own parents or grandparents or upon ourselves. These experiences are not just a memory store of happenings, they are (unless we have led a *very* sheltered life) coloured by emotions. These range from the joyful to the abject, and, when they are filtered through our capacity for rational thought, are a source of empathy – an ingredient essential for the job. But personal experiences can also distort encounters with others (see Salzberger-Wittenberg, 1970) since both parties bring hopes, fears, misgivings, no-go areas and 'most favoured solutions' with them into the interview room.

As a student one will be lucky to escape the experiences of enthusiastically putting more and more into a case to try out new-found knowledge, and disattending to the fact that the client is putting in less and less. Ardent desires to meet expectations from clients that someone else should *do something* to sort out the mess can distort professional relationships. Entrants to the profession (or seasoned hands for that matter) will not escape the experience of finding the praise and thanks of clients flattering and not wanting to spoil 'good progress' by raising awkward questions too soon.

Close involvement with people in the worst of difficulties (the following example of a student placed in a hospital for very sick children comes to mind) invariably carries personal costs.

Case example

A second-year postgraduate student placed in a children's hospital was allocated a case involving a very ill toddler whose bedside his young parents hardly ever left. They had other practical difficulties in their lives too. After two or three contacts, the medical diagnosis was changed to one which was terminal. The parents were filled with anger and despair. Such cases can tap into our own worst fears as *momenti mori*. This was certainly the case here; the student needed more and more reassurance from the child's parents that she was being useful in the face of something she could do nothing about. Other cases and the academic side of her course were virtually abandoned. With more active supervision and joint interviews the necessary balance was just about recovered. Indeed, something was learnt from the experience. However, there were no flashes of personal insight, only a slow realization by the student that she was getting sucked into a problem and was therefore of limited practical use. This was remedied, but at some personal cost.

The term 'controlled emotional involvement' obviously has two components: *control*, and *emotional involvement*. One comes across colleagues who defend themselves by not getting too close to clients; by 'switching off' on the way home, for example. We all have our own devices, but the maintaining of mere social distance will not suffice since clients pick it up and think that this would-be helper cannot handle their pain. Some emotional involvement is vital in an effective helping relationship. On the other hand, workers who are drawn into what eventually become (as in the example above) mutual support groups are also unlikely to be effective in helping clients to manage overwhelming emotions. For managed they have to be, as any bereavement counsellor will testify. Perhaps the best advice comes from the old booklet produced by the Royal Humane Society on saving people from drowning. Rule 1: usually, 'don't jump in'.

Controlled emotional involvement is therefore best demonstrated by the clarification of strong feelings, and by an affirmation of their (justifiable) normality. In the case above, hardly rational anger at the medical staff for having 'misled' them and getting the diagnosis 'wrong' was the focus. The couple later became ashamed of these feelings, and the focus had to change.

The social worker must retain the role of someone able to analyse and be gently objective about such thoughts and feelings, not in any sense by arguing stridently against them, but capable of guiding clients towards a more balanced point of view. Picking up on the life-saving analogy used above, much can be done by exploiting whatever nearby 'buoyancy aids' are available to clients. In the present case, grief had greatly isolated the couple, although they did have an extended family willing to offer support, if only someone could tell them how. In addition, much of the best work done in this case was practical: talking to medical staff about the psychological complexities of the case and acting as a go-between.

Confidentiality

Biestek and his contemporaries were working mainly in voluntary sector projects. They, he in particular, since his employer was effectively God, took the view that private information confided by clients was confidential and, as in the confessional, all but inviolate. This 'pure' view of confidentiality translates into the idea that what passes between a social worker and his or her clients is preferential, and no business of the state. This claim is sometimes on ethical grounds and on grounds of protected professional status (doctors today are fighting the erosion of this principle). But it is also made on practical grounds (i.e. that nothing would work otherwise, and that, if a chance of change is forgone, others nearby, and eventually the public itself, might be the losers). But this too throws up dilemmas; for example:

1   We are citizens first and professionals second, and therefore in a democracy, we are bound by laws just like everyone else. Therefore, however beguiling the idea of special professional status regarding the duty to pass on information about wrongdoing or potential threats to the safety of others, our licence to practise comes from the state via the regulations of the agencies that employ us. Of course it is true that the state, through its policies and through its bureaucracies, creates many of the problems of which clients complain. Should we not therefore regard law and policy as blunt instruments which we have a duty to sharpen up in the interests of a more inclusive type of social justice? We have all done it, but consider this dialogue between Sir Thomas Moore and his son-in-law from Robert Bolt's play *A Man for all Seasons* set in the (much more) dangerous times of Henry VIII:

    'The Law, Roper, The Law. I know what's legal not what's right and I'll stick to what's legal. . . . What would you do? Cut a great road through the Law to get after the devil?'

    (Roper) 'I'd cut down every law in England to do that!'

    'Oh? And when the last law was down and the devil turned round on you, where would you hide, Roper, the laws all being flat? This country is planted thick with laws from coast to coast – man's laws, not God's – and if you cut them down – and you're just the man to do it, d'you really think you could stand upright in the winds that would blow then?'

    Social work textbooks with a strong theme of eugenics circulated in the USA until the 1940s. Social workers stationed on Ellis Island took part in 'reviewing' potential immigrants for evidence of recidivist genes – which, under the influence of Lombroso, meant 'don't like the cut of your gib'. The New York Charity Organization Society lauded the eugenics programme as 'one with which social workers may sympathize and in which they should clearly cooperate'. They envisioned a reduction of the 'social burden' if the 'feeble-minded', the insane, the 'incorrigibly criminal' were prevented from breeding.

Meet your ancestors. Weeding out the 'biologically impure' was current theory and became state policy; it was struck down, *not* by campaigning social workers, but by the law.

2   We take payment from the state or from some state-regulated body; we therefore have contractual obligations. The situation may be different in oppressive, non-democratic states such as China, Zimbabwe or North Korea. They also have 'laws from coast to coast' but they are ideologically inspired and corruptly administered so as to suppress legitimate dissent. It is interesting to note that the more totalitarian the regime the less likely it is to employ social workers, since their very existence is an acknowledgement that all is not perfect in the realm. Those who think it is not are obviously suffering from 'false consciousness', a phrase taken up in some influential radical social work texts (see Freire, 1973; Corrigan and Leonard, 1978; Langan and Lee, 1989). 'Freedom is the ability to recognize necessity' was one of the more chilling phrases of Lenin. Therefore, social workers, who are regular users of the law for the protection of clients and others (e.g. the Human Rights Act; the Disability Discrimination Act), cannot flout other bodies of law of which they happen to disapprove. The best social workers *use* the law as skilled advocates.

In social work education students are often sensitized to questions of ethics, including confidentiality, but are left with the dilemmas. Indeed, in some textbooks, the fact that these are very difficult to resolve is a cause for celebration: 'Look at how *complex* our field is.' A common format for ethics textbooks is the presentation of dummy case examples, the pros and cons of certain courses of action are set out, and the reader is left to make up his or her mind. But probably the best way to teach ethics is as a thread running through all other aspects of the curriculum. Otherwise ethical principles tend to hover above particular cases and exist only as desiderata.

Case example

Jane C, aged 12, was referred to Social Services by a (somewhat exasperated) child psychiatrist. The problem was that she regularly urinated and defecated on the floor of her bedroom and sometimes spread excrement across its walls. Family interviews with the psychiatrist had produced blank denials that anything was wrong in the family, and interviews with the child alone produced only the sense that she was equally puzzled by her behaviour but that she 'just couldn't help it'. The family tried the tactic of selective reactions to the behaviour, some based on rewards, some on punishments, but they failed to affect it much in either case. A puzzle.

Interestingly for the first time, it was decided to gather information from other people who knew her (e.g. schoolteachers and one or two youth groups to which she belonged). The contrast in these reports could not have been sharper. The school regarded her as a model pupil; she was a Girl Guide with a noteworthy interest in bringing along younger members; she attended Sunday School regularly, where the Pastor described her as a 'polite, helpful girl, mature beyond her years'. So why was she continuing to shit in her bedroom? As a protest against, as yet, undiscovered sexual interference – an obvious candidate theory? However, sympathetic interviews with a child specialist produced no evidence, and a strong sense of embarrassment on her part.

A medical examination having already been carried out without finding any physiological reasons for her behaviour, it was decided to abandon further forensics and to treat the behaviour. A reward-based behavioural scheme of more robust design than the parents had put into practice themselves was drawn up in the hope that her reaction to it might at least yield more information as to causes. She agreed to the scheme with alacrity but the soiling and smearing grew worse.

Then, one day, a haunted-looking Mr C (father) came into the office to discuss 'something' which he declared he would only talk about if he could be promised that it would 'not go any further'. He tried hard to swear the social worker to confidentiality, but when informed that information which affected the rights of his daughter would have to be attributed, he still went on to tell his story. Some 18 months previously his wife had discovered that he had been having a long-term affair with someone at the factory where they both worked. His life had been made 'hell' since that day, and his wife, allegedly in thrall to a local Pentecostal church, had developed the idea that 'sparing the rod was spoiling the child'. In the interview with Mr C it became apparent to the social worker that the real motivation for his wife's change in behaviour was to punish him by punishing his daughter. It also emerged that the behavioural scheme had been hijacked by the mother, and that her negative-image punishment regime coexisted alongside it. Mr C was clear that humiliation was the goal of his wife's behaviour, but it was difficult for him to think of leaving home without his daughter.

A case conference was called and the details which had come to the social worker's attention were revealed. This was an explosive affair, but the couple did agree to attend sessions with relationship counsellors while their daughter went to live temporarily with relatives. One and a half sessions were held; then the mother walked out during the second session.

Mr C did leave home without his daughter. Thus the focus of the case moved firmly to child protection, and it was decided to seek a place at a state boarding-school for the daughter, which is what she said she wanted. She settled in immediately, and never soiled again. Mr C went to see her on a few occasions and invited her to live with him. She always politely refused and, against the trends in childcare outcomes, never went home again. She turned instead into a happy and academically able teenager.

Had Mr C's request for even partial confidentiality been respected in the interests of preserving a relationship which *might* have improved over time, then not only would this have transferred an injustice to the child, but there is no guarantee that the facts in this case would ever have emerged.

As a general principle social workers should advise clients – as soon as a compromising subject is broached – that they are perfectly willing to listen to complicated stories, but that anything which threatens the welfare of another person, or is a serious breach of the law, cannot stay within the interviewing room. In our experience clients rarely clam up at this point, but seek help to remedy matters. In the current case, the revelations led at least to a *controlled* explosion.

It is thus vital that social workers have a clear sense in a case as to 'who is the client?' Most cases contain multiple claims for support. In the case example above, the original referral was made by the *parents* requesting 'advice'. If we look past this administrative category to the questions of whose rights and needs were most in jeopardy, whose natural development was most at risk, who was least free to speak about the problems, then the 'client' in this case was clearly Jane C. But note that her parents *lied*; they were not 'misunderstood'; nor was it the case that the 'conditions were not right for them to confide'; they lied.

Social casework today

The potential power of social casework stems from the setting up of a planned therapeutic encounter governed by certain ethical and technical principles, so that individuals come to feel that there exists a motivating contrast between how they might have been treated in the past and how they are treated in these exchanges – which may add up to a more empowering, optimistic set of possibilities for the future.

Social workers try every day to form relationships of trust with their clients, almost always in unpropitious circumstances. We try to build up a history and an aetiology of problems, and struggle to individualize services. We try to engage with people who the rest of the community has given up on. We try to pass as much control over the direction of help to clients as possible so that they are encouraged to take their own decisions. We are willing to listen to stories which would be threatening to most ordinary social relationships and in as confidential a way as is compatible with the rights of others. Publications in the 1970s and 1980s about the death of social casework were therefore a little premature. Politicians and managers abhor an intellectual vacuum, but this is what has confronted them about what social work is in general, and social casework is in particular. It was/is as if we were/are inviting them and the taxpayer to invest money in a scheme that no one was/is prepared to define. A historical example springs to mind: 'An opportunity for investing in an undertaking of great advantage, but nobody is to know what it is' (South Sea Bubble Prospectus, 1719). However, an attempt to bring casework methods into the scientific fold *has* been made, and we should examine its credentials.

Task-centred casework

BS' (then) 8-year-old daughter once caught him reading Reid and Epstein's *Task-Centered Casework* (1972) and asked what it was about. She paused after the explanation and, in Alice in Wonderland fashion, replied: 'But what *other* kind could there possibly be?' Well, the foregoing paragraphs provide something of an answer.

Here is a description of this hybrid form, followed by a list of defining characteristics.

> Task-centered casework is a system of time-limited treatment for problems of living. Since this system makes use of much that is familiar in casework practice, some readers will not see it as remarkably innovative. But since we call for these familiar methods to be used within a rather novel structure, others will view task-centered casework as a decided departure from classic principles.
>
> (Reid and Epstein, 1972: 1)

The above quotation testifies to the (still little realized) fact that early experiments did not try to alter the *content* of what was done with clients, only the framework (i.e. the structure) within which the service was to be delivered. The first, matched comparison study (Reid and Shyne, 1969 – see below) entailed a comparison of short-term casework, still with a decidedly psychoanalytic flavour, with the standard long-term version, and containing much the same therapeutic ingredients.

The results of this experiment were rather positive, but despite being one of the first to show defendably positive results for social work intervention, it evoked strongly defensive reactions. Why? Well, because time-scale and the directness of the method threatened existing orthodoxy, which argued for long-term, gradual, pragmatic, non-directive approaches. All else was dangerous heresy. We shall examine the results of the research later, but first let us explore the defining features of the method.

1   It grew out of three sets of findings in the research literature: (1) the fact that many clients remained on the books of agencies for years, and that professional optimism was tolerable only because someone else was paying the bills; (2) that the goals of such services were rather vague and hard to evaluate; (3) that the results of casework approaches when examined via scientific methods had proved disappointing (see Chapter 3). Therefore something new and more cost-effective was required. William Reid's collaboration with Ann Shyne provided the empirical justification for change, and his work with Epstein produced the 'recipe book' on how to replicate the results of the trial. However, recommendations to make more use of this approach do not depend solely on this original work, because the principles have been widely incorporated into welfare schemes to the present day. Task-centred approaches are used with a wide range of psycho-social difficulties where a variety of different service priorities exist. See, for example, the case management study of work with elderly people by Malepa and Reid (2000), the group work study featuring people with long-term psychiatric difficulties (Garvin, 1987), the review by Ford and Postle (2000) on applications to care management; and see also Reid (1992) for a summary of the range and scope of the approach based on recent research.

2   The main characteristics of task-centred casework are derived from the realization that, especially in complex cases, social workers cannot do *everything*. But if you visit any place where social work training has recently taken place and examine the leftover flipcharts, you are likely to find diagrams consisting of a series of overlapping circles which resemble the Olympic symbol. Within the circles will be headings such as 'goals', 'process', 'culture', 'outcomes', 'community',

'family', 'society', 'peer group', 'economics', and so forth. These sketches look impressively all-inclusive, and testify to the complexities of the job, but they can also induce staff to throw up their hands in horror at the impossibility of serving all these interlocking needs. But it gets worse: these diagrams probably give a truer picture of the range of influences operating in all but the simplest cases than any flowchart. The problem is that we rarely have the influence or the time to address all these factors together. Therefore, it is sensible for us to prioritize, to try to concentrate our influence where it will do most good. Because of this realism the approach was called 'mechanistic' in its early years, in which regard it was in good company, since most of the things shown to work well have earned themselves such criticism (see for example Chapter 7).

3   The hallmark of the task-centred approach is the introduction in the early stages of contact of the need for a time limit on future work, typically eight to ten weekly interviews. Reid and Shyne referred to this approach as 'planned, short-term service' (PSTS), and there were three elements to it: (1) encouragement to help develop motivation for change via structured, problem-solving consultations with a known end-point; (2) encouragement for cooperation with 'experiments' to test out new problem-solving approaches; and (3) close monitoring of the results with the client(s). Thus the contract does not expand to match slower than credible progress – though research studies show that agreed short-term extensions so that something extra and specific can be achieved is valued.

4   The next distinguishing feature is open, contractual negotiation with clients about their long- and short-term goals, with discussions as to how these might be achieved in 'bite-sized' pieces. Thus, as in cognitive-behavioural approaches (see Chapter 7), larger problems are broken down into their separate parts and addressed in piecemeal fashion, each gain building upon the last. Such approaches also carry a 'desensitization' effect in that clients grow used to the idea of approaching tasks which carry an emotional charge in a stepwise fashion.

5   Assessments in task-centred casework are directly related to the origins and development of *current* problems, and considerable effort is put into priority setting.

6   Attempts are made to influence small clusters of problems, and counselling and practical advice focus on the here and now.

7   As the name implies, this approach has at its core the delineation of a series of particular tasks; pieces of work to be carried out within a given time-scale. Emphasis is placed upon bridging the gap between insight or knowledge of what needs to be done and behavioural and circumstantial change. Some of these tasks will be self-assigned to the social worker and amount to advocacy; more often they are assigned to the client who, with support, learns, say, how best to address a meeting with his or her creditors; how to put into operation a plan to ensure that the children are in bed by a reasonable time without fights, and so get up in time for school, how to prepare for a job interview, and so forth. These tasks are circumscribed and are chosen for their positive reinforcement effects.

8   Direct advice is not eschewed; nor is the provision of information; nor are suitably adapted versions of research findings on how things have worked out for other people. Proponents tend towards the view that, within the dynamics of a

helping relationship – one which cannot be allowed to take *forever* to establish itself – trust is usually built through small increments of success.

9   Finally, social workers using this approach adopt a progress-chasing style and take seriously the need to monitor and evaluate their work. Therefore, if completion of a set of tasks is proving difficult for the client(s) and needs to be scaled down, this can take place before motivation atrophies.

Research on the effectiveness of task-centred casework

Task-centred casework had its origins in the pioneering research of Reid and Shyne (1969). These researchers recruited 120 families who were seeking help from the Community Service Society of New York to take part in an other-treated controlled study (there was no randomization, though attempts were made to match clients according to type and severity of problems). The sample size is reasonable. The target groups were people with moderate to severe family and relationship problems, and/or problems with their children – all sufficiently threatening to bring them to the attention of this agency.

The experimental group in Reid and Shyne's study received planned short-term service (PSTS) in the form described above, while the control-condition clients received longer term, standard services which, from the case records made available, resembled the psychoanalytically flavoured casework widely practised at the time. We have some methodical misgivings about the study: (1) the outcome indicators, although clearly scaled, are ratings from tape-recordings and questionnaire returns. These were undertaken by independent people but we cannot be sure about the extent to which they were 'blind' to the conditions under test. If, however, therapeutic 'politics' and 'demand effects' did play a part in evaluating the results then they did so in the opposite direction to that which one would have expected (see below); (2) non-randomized trials tend to flatter the approach under test – this is generally true, but not here; (3) our most serious concern is that clients were directed to one condition or the other according to their presenting characteristics. Here is how clients heard of the approach to be used with them:

> In PSTS cases the worker necessarily had to face the clients with the limits of service at the beginning. This was usually done in the first interview after intake. Case-workers generally informed their clients that treatment would consist of 8 interviews within a 3 months period. The family was not led to believe that their problems would be solved within this period but was given the impression that meaningful changes for the better would be achieved.
>
> (Reid and Shyne, 1969: 55–56)

The mean number of interviews for PSTS was eight; for CS it was 26 with a maximum number of 100 interviews. If we compare the total number of interviews in the two conditions we see they are 422 for the PSTS condition and 1,562 for the CS sample.

The results were adjudicated by an independent research body of good reputation, using material from questionnaires designed to measure improvement, stasis or deterioration. The unexpected result was that CS failed to produce better results in terms of the alleviation of problems than PSTS. The differences were statistically significant ($\chi^2 > 0.2$) (see Table 6.1).

Table 6.1 Task-centred vs. continuing service results

	PSTS	CS
Considerably alleviated	27	27
Slightly alleviated	57	37
No change	15	20
Aggravated	1	17

It will be seen then that this first good news came from a study that was really a research project looking at *efficiency* gains rather than the effectiveness of content differences. Both groups improved; although there is clear evidence that the task-centred group improved more definitely and tangibly than the CS group, and that clients were more satisfied with this approach.

Task-centred casework does not rely for its reputation on just this early study. A number of studies have been conducted since with similar results and in adjacent fields (e.g. psychology and psychotherapy) (see Bergin and Garfield, 1994). Given the ubiquity of the approach, the total output of good-quality research, particularly of controlled trials, remains disappointing. Nevertheless, since the structures under investigation in the few experiments that we have in social work are almost exactly the same as those in the larger literatures of the other helping professions, we can say with some confidence that the approach is probably better than many longer term approaches, certainly cheaper and certainly quicker, and so potentially allows us to see more people (see Reid, 1978, 1992; Doel and Marsh, 1992). It is not a panacea, however, and there are circumstances in which other, longer term interventions are necessary (e.g. in supporting parents who find it difficult to provide adequate care, perhaps due to a learning disability, or young people involved in antisocial behaviour) (see Henggeler *et al.*, 1998). Too often it has been used as a means of rationing services.

Conclusions

Social casework and task-centred casework have been an important test-bed for the ethical framework which social work has tried to develop for itself regarding therapeutic interventions. In our view, the principles of social casework still provide a meaningful and, if interpreted pragmatically, a workable model of how we should go about trying to engage clients caught up in complex personal and social difficulties. We regard them as a necessary but not a sufficient condition of useful change: something more specific needing to be added in many cases. The evidence from therapeutic effectiveness research in general (see Chapter 3) is that warm, genuine, empathic, accepting, non-judgemental relationships are highly valued by clients, but then if one has a chronic drink problem, a serious mental illness or a debt problem spiralling out of control, the literature contains many more pointed methods which need to be brought to bear. The results are equally good whatever kind of professional uses them (see Nathan and Gorman, 1998). Task-centred approaches require that we give continued attention to the process factors developed by the social casework movement (see Doel and Marsh, 1992; Marsh, 1997; Stepney and Ford, 2000).

To sum up, in our everyday lives we all value efficiency and up-to-date knowledge, but we rather like it mixed in with believable reassurance, positive regard, and an avoidance of unnecessary compulsion. Task-centred casework goes a long way towards fulfilling these requirements. We have much to learn from the casework tradition and have not fought hard enough against the forces of corporatism to retain its best elements:

> Reformers are always said to love people, though, often what they love is tidiness.
>
> (Blythe, 1964)

7 Cognitive-behavioural approaches

> As more and more of the behaviour of the organism has come to be explained in
> terms of stimuli, the territory held by inner explanations has been reduced. The 'will'
> has retreated up the spinal cord, through the lower and then the higher parts of the
> brain, and finally, with the conditioned reflex, has escaped through the front of
> the head.
>
> Skinner, 1953: 48–49

Well, possibly, except that yesterday's experiences and their consequent predispositions *are* inside us. But, more practically for now, Chapter 4 identified the use
of cognitive-behavioural methods as one of three key developments in the upturn of
our fortunes over the past two decades regarding research into the effectiveness
of social work. This chapter is a guide to these approaches which follows the 'logical
fit' point made between pp. 302 and 306. Thus it presents a review of the research
on how we acquire patterns of behaviour (whether pro- or antisocial or self-defeating)
in the first place, and on what experiences are known to affect these patterns. We then
discuss how social workers can make routine use of these techniques (see Roth and
Pilling, 2008).

Learning theory and research

Most of what makes us truly human, most of what makes us individuals rather than
'clones', most of what gives us a discernible personality – made up of characteristic
patterns of behaviour, emotion and cognition – is the result of learning. We also get
a little help (or hindrance) regarding what we learn and how easy or difficult this is
from genetic endowment. These influences affect such dimensions as temperament,
personality, gender identity, and various aspects of intelligence. Most recent findings
in developmental psychology support the view that babies and children are far from
being *tabula rasa;* they are actively involved in the learning process in a biologically
pre programmed way:

> At a very early age, human babies show signs of a strong urge to master the
> environment. They are limited in what they can do by the slow development of
> their skill in controlling their own movements. Thus it is fair to call them
> 'helpless' in the sense that they cannot manage the environment well enough to
> survive unaided. This makes it all the more interesting to discover that the urge

to manage the environment is already there at the time of this helplessness and that it does not appear to derive from anything else or to depend on any reward apart from the achieving of competence and control.

(Donaldson, 1978: 110)

Longitudinal studies of temperament (see Thomas and Chess, 1982) show remarkable stability in personality characteristics from shortly after birth onwards. Indeed, we now have several large twin studies with 1000+ samples, comparing identical and fraternal participants, showing that behavioural problems in childhood and adolescence have inherited components via such factors as impulse control and sociability (see Koenen *et al.*, 2006; Tuvblad *et al.*, 2006; Onofrio *et al.*, 2007). These studies show not 'genes for' but complex interactions between environment and trait heritability, requiring individually tailored approaches (see Chapter 3). Here are two different mothers from such a study talking about their children. The first is every parent's idea of what they deserve to get when they have a baby:

> John was my touchy feely baby. From the first day in the hospital he cuddled and seemed so contented to be held that I could hardly bear to put him down. We took him everywhere because he seemed to enjoy new things. You could always sit him in a corner and he'd entertain himself. Sometimes I'd forget he was there until he'd start laughing or prattling
>
> (Heatherington and Parke, 1986: 85)

The second testimony is closer to some people's reality; let us call this child Damien:

> Nothing was easy with him. Mealtimes, bedtimes, toilet training were all hell. It would take me an hour and a half to get part of a bottle into him and he'd be hungry two hours later. I can't remember once in the first two years that he didn't go to bed crying. I'd try to rock him to sleep but as soon as I'd tiptoe over to put him in his crib his head would lurch up and he'd start bellowing again. He didn't like any kind of changes in his routine. New people and new places upset him so it was hard to take him anywhere.
>
> (Heatherington and Parke, 1986: 85)

Child 1 might do well in less than adequate circumstances, child 2 might be all right in tolerant, secure, loving circumstances; but what if child 2 is born in adverse circumstances? This is how 'the fruit machine of life' operates. Outside these general predispositions and the possession of a few, universal 'hard-wired' drives towards what Dennett (1991) has called 'the four Fs': flight, fight, food and procreation, our actions and their internal, emotional concomitants are largely the products of experience.

Natural selection has, to a unique degree, favoured *Homosapiens* with immense behavioural flexibility, with memory and with foresight. The advantage of these gifts for an otherwise physically unpromising primate is that we are less caught out by environmental change – either over time or through shift of location – and that we can multiply our influence many times over through advanced forms of social cooperation.

Archilocus observed in 650 BC that 'the Fox knows many little things – the hedgehog one big one'. Fine for *Erinaceous Europeanus* over several millennia until, in the late nineteenth century, Herr Benz decided to pursue the production of horseless carriages. Human beings, on the other hand, know very many little things – some of which make us safe and happy, some of which get us into trouble.

Learning enables us to live in the past, the present and the intended or feared future simultaneously. The lessons of yesterday's environments, still inside us as a result of conditioning, affect today's behaviour and also influence the direction and valiency of our goals and anticipations. There is nothing 'mechanistic' about this idea, since the patterns are immensely rich and complex. However, if we are to understand their origins we need to start by investigating the simpler mechanisms of learning. We should bear in mind, however, that outside controlled laboratory conditions these rapidly extend themselves into long, chain-like sequences of stimulus associations and stimulus–response association. Such quantitative extensions lead to *qualitatively* different patterns. With our large and complex brains (upward of 100,000,000,000 nerve cells and interconnections between them which strain mathematical imagination) we are consequently neither the prisoners of physiological reflexes nor of current environmental contingencies. Nature has in us favoured *conditionability* or *programmability* or *learning*: the ability to profit from experience. The most basic form of learning is classical conditioning.

Classical conditioning

Ivan Petrovich Pavlov won the Nobel Prize for his work on the *physiological* processes of digestion. He and his colleagues embarked upon a project to map the range and effects of conditioned reflexes from a sense of frustration, because no matter how great the care they took to control the circumstances in which they conducted their experiments, certain psychological phenomena always interfered. In other words, the laboratory animals developed associations and anticipations about food, as they do in domestic life. These effects fascinated Pavlov, who saw them as a challenge to scientific method:

> In our 'psychical' experiments on the salivary glands, at first we honestly endeavoured to explain our results by fancying the subjective condition of the animal. But nothing came of it except unsuccessful controversies and individual, personal, uncoordinated opinion. We had no alternative but to place the investigation on a purely objective basis.
>
> (Pavlov, 1897: 183)

We are trepidatious about introducing discussions of animal experiments into social work textbooks because of the Pavlovian reactions these discussions tend to produce. They are however necessary to the debate because they make clear the 'psychological grammar' of learning processes, so that when we come to investigate the more complex learning of human beings the framework is already in place. However, there is nothing contained in the following paragraphs which does not also apply to human beings.

Pavlov's procedure (the right pictures will probably be in your head as a result of conditioning) was to collect saliva directly from the cheek gland of a dog, held in place by a harness, in a sound-proofed laboratory. Here is the sequence:

- A tone is sounded (*Neutral Stimulus: NS*); no salivary response occurs.
- The tone is sounded and meat powder is deposited into a dish in front of the animal or directly into its mouth (an *unconditional stimulus: UCS*) in that it produces salivary flow as a matter of innate reflex. This procedure is repeated several times.
- The tone (CS) is presented without the meat powder (UCS) and salivary flow occurs to this stimulus alone – the dog has learned a new response.
- Stimuli resembling the CS will tend to produce a similar reaction.

Classical or respondent conditioning is, then, a pattern of *stimulus association* learning. In the natural world, stimuli impinge in *clusters*, and there are spatial and temporal connections (features of place, circumstances and time) which through-out evolutionary history have proved useful for animals (including humans) to respond to interchangeably, since one, or one class, might predict the likelihood of another. Thus anything that might reliably signal the possibility of satisfaction of a basic drive, or the avoidance of danger, conveys an advantage on 'better-safe-than-sorry' principles.

In the case of salivation this operates by ensuring that the elapsed time between first prospect of food energy being available for use is shortened – as is the feeding episode during which we would once have been vulnerable to predation (the best time to invade Britain is still 1.30 p.m. on a Sunday). In the case of learned fear reactions the advantages operate through the flight/fight mechanism of the body: changes in muscle tone, heart rate, blood pressure and blood-clotting speed, sweating, breathing rate, pupil size, and so forth, all of which prepare us for more effective escape or for combat. With a little imagination the reader should be able to work out the precise advantages conveyed by each of these physiological changes – think brutal.

However, while it is useful to remind ourselves of the power of fierce drives and emotions, it is a mistake to forget the powerfully pleasurable feelings which (through the limbic system in the brain) exert a telling influence on our behaviour and thinking. Praise from an admired friend or mentor can produce such warm feelings that all our day-to-day doubts are washed away. It has long been known that the brain contains dedicated centres for pleasure as well as for pain (see Olds, 1956). The physiology of all this is not our particular concern, but the environmental effects certainly are, since decision-making, namely our own and that of our clients, is not the desiccated intellectual process represented in some textbooks on cognition; it is powerfully influenced by emotion, by chains of conditioned predispositions, and by intrusive memories of past successes and failures (see Domassio, 1995).

Let us look at another classic experiment in this field, that of Watson and Rayner (1920). These pioneers were keen to see whether Pavlov's experiment applied in human cases of unreasonable fear and anxiety. 'Little Albert' (so called in parody of Freud's celebrated 'Little Hans' castration anxiety' case), a 6-month-old child (who today would be subject to the sterner provisions of the Children's Act) was volunteered for his study by his mother. He was placed in a playpen and introduced to a tame white rat (NS) – no reaction beyond curiosity occurred. A gong was then struck loudly (UCS) every time the animal was introduced. Next, the animal (CS) was repeatedly released *without* the accompanying noise, but it still gave rise to fear and avoidance reactions. The child had learned a new fear (a conditioned response, CR), purpose-built in the laboratory. What the rat learned about toddlers is open to speculation. Interestingly, 'Little Hans' saw a large brewer's dray-horse collapse and die in the street right next to him, but Freud was little interested in this event, preferring the view that horses represented for the child rampant symbols of male sexuality which threatened his love for his mother. But then working horses in nineteenth-century Vienna or anywhere else would have been geldings or mares, scope for a whole new theory there.

Two clinically important phenomena were demonstrated in Watson and Rayner's work. The first is *generalization*. Pavlov noted from his experiments that anything resembling the CS would eventually, in chain-like fashion, come to produce the same CR. Little Albert came proportionately to fear a whole range of similarly furry objects bearing decreasing resemblance to the original CS. We see this phenomenon of stimulus generalization in our own cases, where clients have a bad experience in one setting but then adverse responses spread to a wide range of only vaguely similar circumstances. This is a notable feature of post-traumatic stress disorder (see Joseph *et al.*, 1995) and of social phobias, leading to increasing withdrawal and isolation. The details are usually more complex in clinical cases, but the basic mechanisms are much the same as those encountered in laboratory studies.

This is an ethically unsettling experiment but it was conducted a long time ago and standards are different now. However, it is a study we can learn from, and it should be remembered that the researchers were simply re-creating circumstances that often occur naturally; otherwise there would be fewer phobias. Shortly after Watson and Rayner's experiment, useful clinical applications of their findings appeared in the literature (see Cover-Jones, 1924).

Let us return now to the point about generalization. Happily, it can produce therapeutic benefits in the opposite direction, as in a study of a few years ago (Sheldon and Macdonald, 1996) where modest investments by a local authority in sponsored day care for the children of poor single parents (many of the children presented with behavioural and developmental problems) was seen to result in a range of improvements under home conditions too. Therefore, in cases where morale is low, small initial gains can spread to increasingly more demanding circumstances through a feeling of competency being reacquired.

The second important phenomenon demonstrated by Pavlov, and confirmed in many studies since, is that of *extinction*. In one sequence of trials, the bell (CS) was rung again and again without the accompanying UCS, the result being a gradual disappearance of salivation on cue. Some kind of 'unlearning' of the conditional response had taken place. One can see the evolutionary advantage of this ability to de-associate in that some loose clusterings of signals – either of potential danger or potential satisfaction – would always have been 'expensively' unreliable. No point therefore in wasting energy on what might be unreliable harbingers.

In summary, classical conditioning is the associative mechanism through which we learn what to fear or to approach, which circumstances reliably predict danger, and which opportunities for satisfaction. It works through emotional arousal. Both pleasant and unpleasant emotions are involved, and cognition (that is, expectations and attributions) come in a little later. So far we have represented it as a useful, adaptive ability able to give us an 'edge' on once very hostile or ambivalent environments; as the environmental-programming mechanism which, long ago, allowed us to increase our chances of raw survival. However, it also carries costs, particularly in today's more complex and settled environments where (however tempting sometimes) attacking an adversary, a bank manager, say, or running away from a 'performance review' meeting will seldom prove to be socially effective.

Many of our clients who have emotional problems in the form of unreasonable fears or undue anxieties have learned to avoid what would be better squared up to, and have learning histories containing what appear to outsiders to be 'irrational associations'. Here is a set of such maladaptive connections (all explainable through the Pavlovian model) which we have encountered in our own practice:

- An 8-year-old, physically abused child, whose drunken father, having seen her grizzling about having her hair washed, had thrust her head under a hot water geyser, and who once in care responded to virtually *any* situation of routine dependence on an adult (particularly a male adult) with fear and aggression.
- A young man trapped in a crowded lift for 20 minutes, who panicked and thereafter regarded *all* confined spaces as threatening, including his room at work if the door was shut.
- A man who frequently exposed himself in public places, who had learned to associate expressions of revulsion with sexual pleasure; the more of one, the more of the other.
- A man who, as a child, was ridiculed by a teacher for feeling queasy after a routine vaccination procedure, and for a time developed a somewhat self-fulfilling fear of fainting in any formal, enclosed situation.
- A teacher with a substantial record of achievement over 14 years, whose newly appointed Head (who had 'previous' as most bullies do) thought his poorly disguised concerns about endless SATs tests and other 'accountability' measures 'off-message' and sacked him on a pretext. He was given a reference which could have been written by a Dalek. He became depressed as a result – since he had accepted this version of his worth over that of years of positive evaluations.

Case example

Mrs Wood, aged 40, was referred to the Social Services Department for 'support' by her somewhat exasperated family doctor. In his view Mrs Wood suffered from agoraphobia, a 'dependant personality' and a number of unspecified 'psychiatric difficulties'. Knowing how to motivate social workers, the doctor also said that he had some worries about Mrs Wood's young son, because not only had Mrs Wood barely left the house in the previous three years or so, but very little had been seen of the child – a stimulus which is reliably associated with being grilled before a child abuse inquiry (UCS).

During the first interview Mrs Wood was wary of discussing her problems and still reacting to her doctor's 'washing his hands' of her case and passing her on to Social Services and the outpatients department of the local psychiatric hospital – which, of course, she could not possibly reach. During the second home visit Mrs Wood was more forthcoming, and the following patterns in her problems emerged.

She described herself as 'always having been a nervous person'. She recounted stories about dismounting from her bicycle as a child whenever a car came up behind her, going some distance out of her way to avoid a dog, feeling very shy and conspicuous as a teenager, and so forth – a range of normal enough fears, but noteworthy in their combination and extent. She reported a strong and persistent fear of hospitals and of all medical encounters, probably stemming from her mother's blood-curdling account of the birth of her younger sister. Her mother had apparently nearly died in childbirth, and had filled the early years of her children's lives with graphic stories of medical mismanagement. Mrs Wood became pregnant 'by accident' comparatively late in life. In order to persuade her to have the baby in hospital, the doctor had played up the dangers of a home confinement, raising her already high level of anxiety about the birth.

One hot summer's day, when she was seven months' pregnant, Mrs Wood had fainted while crossing a footbridge spanning a small river near her home. 'I was sure I was going to fall in, and when I came round, people said an ambulance was on the way and I panicked. People were trying to hold me down, covering me with clothing.'

She fought to get free: 'I knew I had to get away; I got very upset, and eventually I persuaded someone to take me home. When I got in I was shaking all over. I shut and bolted the doors, back and front . . . I was sure that the ambulance was going to call at the house . . . I hid out of sight of the windows and eventually [it took about an hour] I calmed down, and sat waiting for my husband to come home from work.' 'Catastrophic' or even 'paranoid' thoughts of this type are an important feature of panic reactions.

Mrs Wood had her baby at home, against medical advice, painfully, but without serious complications. She tried to go out several times after the birth but never got further than the front garden, or, if at night, as far as the front gate. She reported the feeling at each attempt: 'Shivering, awful feelings in the pit of my stomach; pounding heart; light-headedness.' In the daytime everywhere seemed 'very bright'. She felt conspicuous out in the open, 'almost as if I might be struck down'. Her breathing felt loud in her ears and her biggest fear was that she would collapse again.

Mrs Wood eventually gave up these attempts and remained indoors for the next four years. For the first two years she reported that she did not really miss going out: 'The family were very good, they took the baby out, got the shopping, they are marvellous, so are the neighbours.' Later, however, Mrs Wood began to experience feelings of dissatisfaction and frustration with her confined existence and felt shame when she could not attend her mother's funeral. When Mrs Wood felt she *had* to go out, for example, to peg out washing, she reported making a quick dash, hoping no one would see her or try to talk to her, and 'great relief' when she got back inside. 'I think there must be something seriously wrong with me . . . in my mind' was initially her best idea as to the cause of all this.

If we examine this case in the light of classical conditioning theory, the following pattern emerges:

- Mrs Wood may have possessed a predisposing personality for strong fear reactions (see Claridge, 1985); certainly her accounts of her previous life showed her to be eminently conditionable to a range of not objectively threatening circumstances.

- Against a background of heightened anxiety about pregnancy, dreading the thought of having to go into hospital, Mrs Wood experienced a traumatic incident (UCS) which aroused in her a powerful fear reaction (UCR).

- This incident, when paired with the previously neutral stimulus of the footbridge and other stimuli associated with being out of doors (CSs), produced a conditional response to these stimuli. Even after the incident itself had passed, the pregnancy was over, she was perfectly well, and the crowd no longer in sight, she still experienced fears associated with this context.

- Mrs Wood reported that her panic state was made worse by the attempts of would-be helpers to restrain her until the ambulance came. Natural escape behaviour was prevented, thus intensifying her fear.

- This conditioned fear response quickly generalized to virtually all outdoor circumstances. Furthermore, every time Mrs Wood tried to go out of doors she was punished for the attempt by powerful emotions (setting up a 'fear of fear' reaction) – even though she saw such feelings as annoying and irrational.

- Every time Mrs Wood managed to escape from the outdoor circumstances that elicited the conditioned fear response, her strongly aversive feelings were reduced or terminated. This strengthened avoidance behaviour and made future experiments less likely.

- This client's family and friends unwittingly rewarded her long-term maladaptation to her phobia by relieving her of many of her responsibilities regarding her child, and by reassuring her that they did not mind her staying behind. The impression grew, strengthened by early non-cooperation with the treatment scheme, that Mr Wood rather liked having his wife at home and dependent upon him.

It will not have escaped the reader's attention that as we move from the laboratory to examples of conditioning in the natural environment, it becomes more difficult to specify the key stimuli combinations with the same precision. Was it the already learned fear of hospitals which became connected with particular outdoor circumstances? Or was it, perhaps, loss of consciousness, embarrassment at this, or fear of loss of control? Or was it, perhaps, fear of falling helplessly into the water? All of these possibilities were mentioned during the interviews. To what extent did fears for the unborn baby play a part? To what extent did the unsympathetic words of the family doctor predispose Mrs Wood to what happened? It is likely that *all* these factors were influential in producing the fear and panic response. In the natural environment stimuli tend to come in untidy bundles, as do responses, and it is often difficult to tease out their different effects. Mrs Wood remembers in particular the idea of being 'a prisoner of the crowd', the fear of hospitals and the narrowness of the footbridge. She also had a vivid recollection of the brightness of the day, of being helpless out in the open. Her memories cover the key stimuli, but have only a limited idea of their relative importance. The analysis is not as neat as the one provided by Pavlov in his carefully controlled experiments, but it is one made within the framework he constructed, and is dependent upon exactly the same general principles (see Sheldon, 1998).

In the case of this agoraphobic client, an extended hierarchy was constructed (see Figure 7.1) – without this 'softly, softly' approach she would not have continued with the process of trying to confront her anxiety-provoking circumstances. She was taught progressive relaxation and deep breathing during these assignments and spent several sessions on each item, sometimes accompanied by the social worker and sometimes deliberately not. If the next step seemed too large, the progression from one to the other could be bridged by spending longer completing the task. The procedure was labour-intensive, but was completed in three months.

Classical association is, however, an insufficient explanation for any of the problems referred to above, since it should be noted that once an emotional link has been established it leads to new patterns of *behaviour*, either to diminish aversive arousal (guilt, anxiety) or to increase pleasurable emotion. Such actions rapidly attract reinforcement through the temporarily positive or relief-inducing consequences

17	Stand alone on footbridge for 10 minutes	*High anxiety and*
16	Stand alone on footbridge for 3 minutes	*avoidance*
15	Stand near footbridge for 10 minutes	
14	Stand near footbridge for 3 minutes	
13	Stand 100 yards from footbridge	↑
12	Walk to town (unaccompanied)	
11	Walk to edge of town (accompanied)	
10	Walk to shops	
9	Cross the road	
8	Walk 20 yards down road	
7	Stand on pavement	
6	Stand at front gate	
5	Clean windows	
4	Put out washing	
3	Stand in garden	
2	Stand on front step	*Low anxiety and*
1	Stand in porch	*avoidance*

Figure 7.1 Schedule for contact with fear-provoking stimuli

Source: from Sheldon (1995)

which follow. Cognitive factors also play a part in such problems in the form of unreasonable beliefs and selective perception. These are not just clinical phenomena. In everyday life advertisers know well how to exploit our ability to associate one thing with another. *Question:* How best to sell cubes of rusk and dried cow's blood for cooking purposes? *Answer:* find a positive set of stimuli with which to associate this unlikely product (vegetarians should look away now). 'OXO', thanks to the advertisements, now conjures up images of traditional, secure family life when everyone still ate together at table.

An interesting question is: Why do the processes of extinction and habituation (reviewed above) not lead to a natural weakening of troublesome emotional, behavioural and cognitive connections? The answer is that this does happen to a degree via natural exposure. Most of us, after all, have had fears and anxieties which we have lost through counteracting experiences (the fourth case in the series on p. 136 – do count carefully – was BS, who later went on to train as a nurse). The problem is that *some* patterns of acquisition involve either (1) painful, dramatic pairings of stimuli, or (2) regular repetitions of less aversive experiences so that connections are re-established again and again. For example, someone with anxieties regarding groups of strangers is unlikely to perform well socially in such situations and is therefore likely to attract puzzled or critical responses which rekindle the fear. But the major reason is *avoidance*. In the example of the claustrophobic person on p. 136 little or no natural exposure occurred because he would *never* go in a lift or enter a confined space, preferring to pant his way up fire-exit stairs in tall buildings or to feign sickness if asked to accompany someone on the Tube. All of these avoidant responses tend to attract reinforcing consequences in their own right through a process of *negative reinforcement* (see p. 142).

There are yet further complications to a simple paired-association model of classical conditioning:

1   The possibilities for conditioning are endless, yet phobic and anxiety-avoidance reactions tend to form clusters. There are millions of electric sockets in the world, but few electrophobics; there are thousands of arachnophobics in Britain, yet spiders here pose no risk – though the situation in Australia or Borneo is different. The concept of *preparedness* throws some light on such strange patterns of emotion and behaviour (see Seligman, 1971; Shanks, 1995). We appear to be particularly prone to acquire fears of certain *classes* of things: heights, enclosed spaces; small, scurrying organisms; anything large and looming, sudden, noisy or fast.

2   Some individuals are more conditionable to certain circumstances then others. We have met many people suffering from phobic reactions, but few who did not have a history of minor episodes of the same sort of thing. Eysenck (1965) demonstrated this difference years ago in the laboratory. The apparatus was simple: a machine generating a mild shock, plus a galvanic skin response (GSR) recorder (which measures arousal via the sweating reflex). Subjects were preassessed on the introversion/extraversion scale of the Eysenck personality inventory and divided into two groups. The pairing of signals and aversive stimuli, then later the presentation of the signal alone, produced significantly higher GSR for introverts than for extraverts. Therefore, there are some neuro-

physiologically derived personality configurations on the shoulder of a curve of distribution for these tendencies, who are either more 'punishment-sensitive' and easier to condition (probably by reason of central nervous system differences) than those on the opposite slope, who are harder-to-condition, relatively punishment-insensitive individuals. An analogy might help: some people are closer to having a 'Ferrari nervous system', namely very sensitive to stimulation; some are closer to having a Citroën 2CV nervous system. It may seem paradoxical, but the 'Ferrari' group are the introverts, and the 2CV group are the extraverts. The former manage the environment to avoid over-stimulation; the latter prod at it to enhance stimulus input. Most of us are Ford Foci.

3   Cognitive factors also play a part in the acquisition of 'unreasonable' fears. Human beings do not simply respond to stimuli, they interpret them. Thus, above and beyond the simpler, classically conditioned fears based upon direct experience there is a range of not entirely rational thoughts about such problems: that if sufferers confront their *bêtes noires* they will die of a heart attack as a result; that such stresses will make them mentally ill, and so on. Users of cognitive-behavioural approaches seek to dispel such interpretations via an educational, reality-testing approach.

Having given an outline of stimulus-association conditioning and its effects, we now turn to another major theory of learning, this time concerned with *stimulus–response* associations; that is, with the influence of consequences on behaviour.

Operant conditioning

As we have seen, the more we learn about child development, the more we are forced to abandon the environmental determinism of the 1960s and acknowledge that much of child development unfolds from within. Very young babies show signs of a strong urge to explore, to *operate upon* (hence the word operant) and to manipulate their environments (not a fancy new term; see *Hamlet*, Act III). Such exploratory activities rapidly attract consequences of a positive, an aversive or a relief-producing kind. Some of these consequences just happen, some are desired (e.g. in withdrawal of attention from bad behaviour in a child). Thus, from the earliest years, by accident and by design, human beings are exposed to sets of *contingencies* (if you, then . . .), which experiences amount to a sub-Darwinian process of the natural (and unnatural) selections of behavioural patterns. Some sequences are 'stamped in', others 'stamped out' (see Thorndike, 1898). Nothing new here, but once again the contribution of behavioural psychology has taken the form of charting the dynamics. The towering contribution in this field is that of the American psychologist B.F. Skinner (1953, 1973) whose project was to develop an entire psychology without reference to interior goings-on. If you now find yourself thinking of rats, do remember that this is a Pavlovian reaction.

Adopting the earlier principle of 'simple first, complicated later', let us start with Skinner's animal experiments. He gave his name to a glass-sided box equipped with a food dispenser and a release lever or disc which the animal (usually rats or pigeons – never both) could operate from inside. All other factors are under the control of the experimenter. The following is a summary of Skinner's procedures:

- A rat which, let us say, has missed its breakfast is placed in a glass-sided box equipped with a food release lever, and engages in exploratory (operant) behaviour, eventually bumping into the lever and hitting the jackpot. The rat tries this again and clumsy initial operation quickly gives way to expert tapping. The rat's unlikely behaviour (for a rat) has been *positively reinforced* and so it is repeated, or rather the other way around. It has learned a new pattern of behaviour. Thus, *a positive reinforcer is a stimulus, which strengthens, amplifies, or increases the rate of the behavioural sequence that it follows.*

- Next imagine a Skinner box with a wire grid for a floor, capable of delivering an irritating and continuous level of electric shock *until* an encounter with the lever turns this off for a period. As in the previous case the rat spends a lot of time operating the respite lever. This process is called *negative reinforcement.* It also leads to an increase in new behaviour, but with the object of removing an aversive set of conditions. Thus a *negative reinforcer is a stimulus, the contingent removal of which strengthens, or increases the frequency of the behaviour pattern which led to it.*

- Next consider a situation where depressing the lever in the Skinner box leads every time to a loud noise. Behaviour is decreased, probably extinguished. The animal quickly learns an avoidant reaction. Thus a *punishing stimulus decreases or extinguishes a behaviour pattern which it follows, or rather this is what we call something that does this.*

Why do we need such technical terms to describe what we recognize as analogues of everyday happenings? Well, another way of making the point that human beings can learn practically *anything* (that trust is usually repaid; that people can change; that aggression pays; that tight, vigilant control equals safety) is to say that almost any set of stimuli can acquire reinforcing or punishing associations through the consequences they bring, or have brought in the past. Some examples follow to illustrate the point. Most people would identify physical pain as a punishing stimulus, but through classical and operant association it can come for some people (masochists) to cue and strengthen sexual arousal to the point where it becomes an end in itself. Most of us in our lives have received approval from someone whom we dislike. It is hard to think of such compliments as 'punishing', though they may satisfy the technical definition and make cooperative behaviour less likely in the future, as this World War II reminiscence by the historian Richard Cobb (regarding his commanding officer) illustrates:

> He displayed a watchful and petty hostility to all university graduates under his command, and a positive loathing for those who had been to Oxford or Cambridge, as if they had gone there on purpose, in some mysterious fore-knowledge that they would be meeting him at some point later in life. From the start, I could not help feeling rather flattered that he should have taken such an active, vigilant dislike to myself; I thought that it did me credit; it was a sort of tribute. There is something very satisfying about being disliked by the right sort of people.
>
> (Cobb, 1997: 86)

Good advice for social workers, perhaps?

Thus the only scientific basis on which the valency of stimuli can be decided is through a close study of their *effects* – not on any prior classifications of intent. If you doubt it, try giving your GP a tenner for his trouble next time you visit the surgery. Here are a few more examples from our own practice regarding the way in which reinforcement contingencies have led to the development in problems:

- A lonely man with a serious drink problem who had learned that brushes with the police after altercations in public houses usually resulted in his daughter travelling a long way to stay with him until he was 'better'.
- A learning-disabled child whose experience had taught him that running away from his foster carers typically led to a period in police care (exciting), a car ride home (interesting), and a kindly reunion (comforting).
- A 12-year-old boy who felt his needs came a poor second to his parents' troubles discovered by accident (operantly) that a random, peer-inspired episode of fire-setting had the effect of jerking his father out of the depressed state he had been in since a serious industrial accident, and produced some concern for *him*. More fires broke out.

Or, imagine this:

- A newly qualified social worker who discovered that her standing with management was rather more dependant upon up-to-date records and attendance at meetings than on the quality of face-to-face work with clients. She reluctantly embraced 'virtual reality social work' and spent more time at her word processor.

A case example showing the use of contingency management techniques

Mark, aged 9, was referred to Social Services via the education social work service (the department held a supervision order on an elder brother following three instances of theft). Junior school staff were greatly concerned about Mark's disruptive behaviour in class and were beginning to use psychiatric terminology to describe this. Expulsion was likely unless something could be done and there was concern regarding the amount of physical punishment used at home.

Mark's childhood, in common with that of his brother, had been somewhat troubled. A history of marital difficulties between parents, and two lengthy periods of separation from them while in the care of relatives, had been the most distinctive features. Family life seemed to have settled down of late and the social worker handling the case had filed increasingly optimistic reports about this. However, it was known that the parents had often disagreed about the enforcement of rules, but the father, when present, followed a 'boys-will-be-boys' philosophy – this, perhaps, to excuse some of his own wayward behaviour. In addition, Mark was not a bright child and had reading difficulties requiring remedial teaching – with which he rarely cooperated.

With the somewhat hesitant cooperation of the school authorities, an investigation of Mark's disruptive behaviour began in its natural setting. A student social worker observed what happened in lessons. She was introduced just as 'a student' and spent periods sitting unobtrusively at the rear of the classroom to observe and record his behaviour. This revealed the following: (1) 'disruptive behaviour' usually meant Mark leaving his desk or group activity and refusing to return; but after that he would occasionally make loud noises, slamming down objects, teasing, hitting and pinching other pupils, and generally interfering with their work; (2) some teachers had more difficulty with Mark than others; (3) the most common methods of dealing with Mark were: reasoning with him, or speaking sharply to him, both of which seemed to have only a marginal and temporary effect; trying to distract him, which again only worked in the short term; or placing him outside the door – to which he did not seem to object at all, and which, again, had little effect on his subsequent behaviour. By and large teachers ignored him when he was not being disruptive, most operating what the headteacher referred to as a 'sleeping dogs policy'.

The working hypothesis developed in this case was that Mark's classroom behaviour was largely a product of the following contingencies: (1) when he was at all well behaved (which records showed was a fair proportion of the time) he was left alone; (2) conversely, when Mark caused or threatened a disturbance he received immediate attention from teachers; (3) attempts to punish Mark were ineffective, not only because they were admirably half-hearted, but also because of his immunizing exposure to much more serious forms of it at home; (4) Mark's reading difficulties sometimes made it hard for him to join in lessons – he was bored and a little embarrassed by this and escaped from these conditions by amusing himself with other, more dubious pursuits. The reinforcement patterns thought to be operating in this case are as follows:

- Mark's behaviour was *positively reinforced* with attention for bad behaviour (a commodity in short supply at home for any behaviour). A further contrast between consequences of good and bad behaviour was provided by the fact that his teachers saw all too little to reward in what they called 'his attitude'. Thus his teachers were only prepared to reward extended runs of good behaviour, and these occurred rarely.
- Mark's tendency to get out of his seat and his disruptive behaviour were also *negatively reinforced*. School work was difficult for him to succeed at because he did not possess the skills required and so became bored. If called upon to contribute to class activities, he usually tried, but often made a mess of things. Thus, leaving his seat and his disruptive behaviour had the effect of terminating or reducing boredom, embarrassment and worries about failing.

Results from the attempt to reverse these reinforcement contingencies – to provide positive reinforcement for remaining seated and concentrating on school work, and none for disruptive or aggressive behaviour – are shown in Figure 7.2. The compendium term for the approach used in this case is 'contingency management' which breaks down into the following components:

- *Extinction:* In practice, this meant that disruptive behaviour (as defined above) was to be ignored by teachers whenever possible. If other pupils complained of Mark's behaviour, they were told in a matter-of-fact way to ignore it if possible.
- *Positive reinforcement:* Any short period in which Mark's behaviour did *not* contain disruptive features was to be responded to as quickly as possible by the teacher, as a useful opportunity positively to reinforce behaviours incompatible with the target behaviour. This category included sitting still, working at an exercise, trying to read, neat work, and so on. Where Mark joined in a group task – such as answering questions put to the whole group, or reciting an exercise – first the group would get the teacher's praise, and then Mark would receive a special mention for trying harder and showing progress.

This classroom programme was complementary to a scheme already running at home. The daily progress card was used to link the two so that three initialled entries per day earned Mark a coloured star on his home progress chart, praise from his parents, 10 minutes' extra TV time per entry, plus a small pocket money reward for every three entries. A bonus scheme was introduced to reinforce good weekly averages so that, initially, four stars a week resulted in an outing with Mark's father or mother (they were not keen but proved persuadable).

An important part of the programme was an augmented remedial reading scheme implemented by teaching staff. This was carried out by a favourite teacher of Mark's who did not normally fulfil this function.

- *Problems:* The programme's most vulnerable point was the extinction contingency for aggressive behaviour. Some behaviour was simply impossible for teachers to ignore, either because of the risk of injury to other pupils, or because of the bad example set for the rest of the class. Existing approaches, such as standing him outside doors, or sending notes home, had proved ineffective. Similarly, if sent home, Mark would be free to play on his own for the rest of the day, and his mother's aversion to contact with the teachers was also strengthened. A further difficulty lay in persuading his teachers to show interest in Mark if his *current* behaviour justified this, and not to dwell upon either what he had recently done, or upon what he might do in the near future.
- *Time out:* A time out from the reinforcement scheme was tried and proved to be successful, bridging the gap until the positive reinforcement scheme took control of Mark's behaviour. A half-empty room opposite the secretary's office with the door left open was used for this. A desk was placed there together with reading and writing materials. Extremely disruptive behaviour was first responded to by a form of words, which gave Mark an option to sit quietly and get on with his work. If this failed, he was unceremoniously removed by his teacher without comment. This occurred on eight occasions during the course of the early part of the programme; each episode lasted for about 15 minutes.

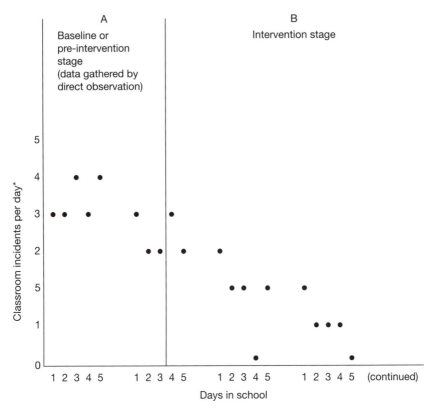

Figure 7.2 Example of an AB design with a stable baseline

Baseline data from classroom management scheme for a 'disturbed' 9-year-old boy under threat of exclusion from school.

Note: *Predefined with teachers as any combination of: interfering with the work of others; causing physical pain to others; leaving his seat and failing to return within one minute of first being asked; making loud noises or noises continuing long enough to distract other pupils.

Source: from Sheldon (1995)

Follow-up of the home and school programmes at six months revealed substantial and well-maintained gains in school, and less dramatic, but still useful gains at home. However, the main achievement in this case was that Mark continued to be taught at his ordinary school and, at the time of closure, was seen, in the words of the headteacher, as 'still a bit of a challenge to discipline' rather than as a 'disturbed boy'. Figure 7.2 contains the evaluation data from this case.

Schedules of reinforcement

One of Skinner's most important discoveries was that *patterns* of reinforcement affect the acquisition of new behaviour (see Ferster and Skinner, 1957). In other words, the rate and the sequencing of reinforcement strongly influence performance. In Skinner's animal experiments, *continuous reinforcement*, that is, 'one-for-one' patterns of reward, led to the most effective sequences of behaviour acquisition until satiation effects took over. However, regarding efficiency, it was possible to shape behaviour towards an acceptance of lower but still predictable patterns of reinforcement via the introduction of tolerable 'piecework' rates – say, one reinforcer per four presses. In human terms this is the equivalent of working hard all month for a delayed but predictable pay cheque. However, behaviour under the control of continuous reinforcement is easily extinguished. Apart from a brief 'spurt' to test out the contingencies, responsiveness falls off rapidly if reinforcers are withdrawn.

The natural environment of both animals and humans rarely delivers reinforcement on a continuous schedule. It is far more likely that rewarding breakthroughs will happen occasionally and after considerable effort. Skinner and his colleagues experimented with such *variable ratio and intermittent* patterns of reinforcement following the shaping up of a behaviour pattern. The best way to envisage what happens is to think of the behaviour of gamblers. All of us fall into this category from time to time, when by luck, chance or random experimentation life delivers unexpected sweetness. So we then try to work out exactly what the contingencies were, occasionally resorting to 'superstitious' interpretations – the lucky pen for the exam; the tie worn the last time one got a job. Such patterns of hopeful persistence in the face of delayed gratification are extremely resistant to extinction – which is bad news, given that most troublesome behaviour is shaped up in this way; it is good news for would-be helpers however if they build this knowledge into their practice as a means of sustaining gains already made.

The main message of these experimental findings (well replicated in therapeutic-outcome studies) is that reinforcement contingencies need to be *very* reliable if they are to hold sway over the problem-reviving power of occasional, unpredictable reinforcement which 'immunizes' responses against extinction ('one more go might just do it').

To sum up, the main therapeutic techniques derived from this model of learning are as follows:

1   Encouraging clients to take note of *discriminative* stimuli (Sds), i.e. the signals which predict future trouble (SΔ) or pleasure (Sdr), or which are known to elicit certain patterns of behaviour. Anyone who has tried to give up smoking will be aware of the power of these cues – a cup of coffee, the end of a meal, a drink. But it is also necessary to help clients to identify more complex, external prompts (e.g. what is it about the behaviour of others which signals that it is time to curl up or withdraw, and to consider what other options might be available?).

2   Where a problem results mainly from an *insufficiency* of certain behaviour, it may be possible simply to identify and *positively reinforce* a low-level adaptive responsible so that it can be 'amplified', and its place in the individual's repertoire strengthened. In other words, we can work to enhance the positive consequences for desirable behaviour. A good starting point is simply to raise the question with oneself: What actually pays off for this person, in this setting, group, family or organization?

3   A performance may be *shaped* by the selective, positive reinforcement of approximately similar behaviours until they become progressively more like the performance desired. Research shows this happy idea to be the most powerful approach available to us (see Sheldon, 1995; Cigno and Bourne, 2000).

4   Where the problem results mainly from an *excess* of unwanted behaviour, it may be possible to identify and positively reinforce a response which is *incompatible* with existing responses.

5   Again, in respect of an excess of troublesome behaviour, it may be possible to apply *negative reinforcement*, so that whenever the individual stops this behaviour and performs some desirable alternative, aversive stimuli (e.g. disapproval or social isolation) are terminated.

6   It may be possible to reduce the frequency of undesirable behaviour by *extinction*; in other words, simply by removing the reinforcement currently available to it.

Learned helplessness

It is difficult to know where best to place this discussion, since researchers working in both the classical and operant paradigms have contributed to our understanding of the phenomenon, well known to social workers, of collapse of morale and the inability of individuals to engage their troublesome circumstances even though help to do so is at hand.

One of the most damaging things to learn is that one has little or no control over one's circumstances and is helpless in the face of unpredictable, external forces. The primary function of the cerebral cortex is to aid adaptation to wayward circumstance; the primary purpose of the long period of socialization which humans undergo is to equip them to track, to model, to predict, and then to adapt to or change their circumstances. What happens when this proves impossible? This interesting question was first investigated in Pavlov's laboratory by Shenger-Kristovnakova in 1921. She conducted a series of experiments to investigate how animals cope with being conditioned to respond to stimuli which are then made contradictory or ambiguous. Such situations are prevalent in the complex social environments of human beings, and so the findings have relevance outside the field of animal behaviour (see Gilbert, 1992; Peterson *et al.*, 1993). The experimenters taught animals to anticipate food on the presentation of a circle but not an ellipse (which signalled an aversive stimulus). It was then made increasingly difficult for the animal to distinguish between these figures by arranging for the circle to become narrowed at the sides, (and for the ellipse to fatten out. Another variation (Masserman, 1943) involved the random substitution of consequences – so that the animal was unable to predict whether food or discomfort would follow a given action.

The effects of these studies were that the animals' behaviour first became agitated and uncharacteristic – hence the term 'experimental neurosis' – but that later (and this is the important point), even when the original and obvious stimulus discriminators were replaced, the animals remained immobile rather than taking an easy escape route.

Evidence from similar studies with human participants suggests that there is more than a metaphorical relationship between such experiments and what social workers encounter in their day-to-day practice with clients who, frustratingly for would-be helpers, seem to prefer the devils they know.

Vicarious learning and modelling

Many of the difficulties which come our way are due to learning deficits; that is, they result from gaps in the behavioural repertoires of individuals. For example: how to manage difficult behaviour from a child; how to negotiate about rather than fight over conflicts of interest; how to cope with living again in the community after a period in a psychiatric unit; how to be calmly and rationally assertive when put upon. Solutions to these problems are largely a matter of social skills which may not have been acquired naturally, or which may have atrophied owing to intervening experience. The problem is that the natural behaviour of helpers is verbally to review such problems, and then to hope that new understandings will by some 'osmotic' process translate into new patterns of behaviour. This, as studies of the effectiveness of social work, clinical psychology and psychotherapy have been telling us for many years, is a rather optimistic assumption. No one ever learned to swim or to cook or to bring up a child by attending tutorials on these subjects.

Vicarious learning (i.e. learning by imitating the behaviour of others) is a 'wired-in' tendency which emerges in early infancy. Three-week-old babies will readily copy facial grimaces (see Plate 7.1).

Mothers have known this for centuries but, as you can probably tell from the hairstyles, experimental psychology only caught up in the 1970s (see Harris, 1972). You

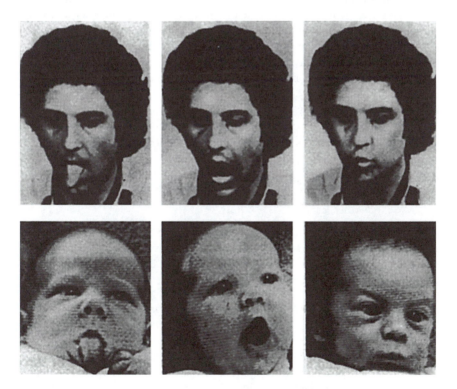

Plate 7.1 Imitation of facial gestures by two- to three-week-old infants.

Source: Harris (1972) *The Scientific American*

can confirm it via personal experience. On public transport, one is often confronted with small babies slung over their mothers' chests and facing backwards, wide-eyed, over the seat. If you smile or pull a face, the baby will struggle to copy this, although it is too young to have learned the behaviour. (Try it, but don't get caught, since it can cause consternation among fellow passengers.)

Think once again of the evolutionary advantage that this ability to observe, interpret and learn from the experience of others was. It means that we do not ourselves have to suffer to avoid suffering. We do not always have to repeat a long series of trial-and-error experiments, chancing occasionally upon a favourable outcome (or not). We can simply watch how others approach problems, break down the performance mentally into steps and, if it seems to work, try it out – either piecemeal or wholesale. But, as always in the field of learning, we must remember that while this capability may lead usefully to, say, the ability to look confident when we are fearful, it is also the process by which we can learn to intimidate or deceive with style. Learning itself is morally neutral, and ethical judgements about it have to be made later.

We must now turn to the stages and the mechanism involved, since it is from these that we can acquire an appreciation of the therapeutic possibilities. Vicarious learning can account for the following patterns of behavioural change:

1　The second-hand acquisition of completely new *sequences* of behaviour. Remember adolescence when, being stalled somewhere between childhood and adulthood, most of us experimented *gauchely* with strange new ways of walking, dressing, talking, and so forth, behaviours largely gathered from others or from images in the media. Such symbols of changing identity are tried on, kept, adapted or discarded according to the internal and external reinforcement they produce. Another problem is that sometimes there are no suitable models available.

2　Emotional reactions may also be learned vicariously. As children we learn what to fear by watching others behave fearfully, or how to cope by watching others approach threatening circumstances with sang-froid.

3　Thought patterns, more particularly problem-solving styles, may be acquired by watching how others cope with challenges and then inferring (not always accurately) what processes of mental computation and interpretation might have led them to a given course of action.

There is a substantial literature on which to draw here (see Bandura, 1969: Hall *et al.*, 1997). It recommends that, whatever the nature of the problem in view, modelling and social skills training programmes should be organized according to the following common stages:

1　Identifying specific problems resulting from gaps in the client's behavioural repertoire and deciding what new patterns of behaviour could be shaped up to fill these.

2　Dividing the target responses into their component parts. For example, for a chronically shy person, practise walking confidently into a room full of people (you don't have to feel it – just to look as if you do); deciding who to stand next to and what to say; introducing oneself; getting in on the conversation, and so forth.

3   Identifying with clients any patterns in their thinking (images and inner speech) which may encourage misinterpretation of the motives of others and/or avoidance responses (e.g. 'people are looking at me; they can tell I don't belong here').

4   Demonstrating to clients what a competent performance might look like; rehearsing any problematic parts of the sequence or going through it slowly and deliberately, emphasizing options and decision points.

5   Developing more complex performances by linking together different sequences.

6   Paying attention to any problems of discrimination; that is, identifying any difficulties the client may have in knowing whether a certain piece of behaviour is appropriate for a given setting.

7   Gradually introducing difficulties likely to be found in real life as the client becomes more able to cope with its vicissitudes (for instance, not getting an immediate answer when trying to make friends; meeting increased persistence after saying no to something).

Outcome studies in this field point to modelling as an effective technique providing that it focuses on explicitly defined behavioural deficits; the results from more general-purpose programmes are less good. As a result of the above trends, textbooks in the field now regularly refer to a 'cognitive revolution' having taken place. For the following reasons we are just a *little* cautious about these developments. There is much supportive research and it is methodologically respectable, but confined to areas where the addition of a noteworthy cognitive component produces marginally better results – but more importantly, longer lasting gains (see Blackburn *et al.*, 1981; Hollon *et al.*, 1991 – but see also Stuart and Thase, 1994). These results in no way justify taking our eyes off the tried-and-trusted factors of behaviour-rehearsal, reinforcement contingencies and controlled exposure, all of which have regularly been shown to be influential in cases such as are contained in this volume (see Feske and Chambers, 1995). The danger stems perhaps from the reinforcement contingencies that operate upon would-be helpers. That is, that less direct means of influence somehow signify greater skill or prestige: the 'look-no-hands' effect identified by B. F. Skinner in 1971.

Behavioural approaches are inconvenient; they take one out of the interview room and into the rain; to the school gates and into the classroom – if that is where problems manifest themselves. They require being there at bedtime if that is typically when dangerous fights between parents and children break out. Furthermore, using these approaches one can fail to achieve one's goals clearly and publicly. Thus there are many short-term reasons for avoiding them and 'going cognitive'; we have skipped down this primrose path before. However, behaviour therapists have always had to take account of the way stimuli are filtered, over- or under-responded to and eccentrically interpreted, though until recently they have not always done so systematically. Similarly, cognitive therapists have always had to look at whether changes in understanding translate into more positive patterns of behaviour, though again, they have not always done so systematically. The recognition that there was thus scope for a pooling of findings and techniques – providing that the gold standard outcome criterion of changed behavioural performance in line with case objectives is retained – has led to unprecedently positive results across a wide range of problems, so much so that the National Institute for Health and Clinical Excellence (NICE) now considers that CBT should routinely be made available to people with mental health problems.

There are thus four sets of influences on behaviour: environmental consequences, emotional associations, background genetic predispositions influencing temperament and conditionability, and cognitive factors which influence the way in which stimuli are recognized, categorized and interpreted in the first place. These cognitive influences may be further broken down as follows.

- *Perception:* This is an old topic in psychology, and we have already studied it in Chapter 2. The more we learn about it the less it comes to resemble any simple camera or tape-recorder-like process and the more it is seen as an active, constructive process, strongly influenced by cognition and previous experience. Consciousness gives us our very being. A number of brilliant attempts at an empirically based conceptual analysis exist (especially Dennett's *Consciousness Explained* (1991) – it isn't; and David Chalmers engaging, *The Conscious Mind, In Search of a Fundamental Thesis* doesn't *quite* make it either). Yet this does not make it a mystical phenomenon, only deeply mysterious. Sydney Harris' delightful cartoon still sums up where we are (Plate 7.2).
- *Attributions:* Human beings search actively for meaning when confronted by complex stimuli. We seek to attribute causality (sometimes making mistakes) as we try, like amateur scientists, to evaluate potential threat, rewards or sources of relief. Attributive cognitions fall into two main patterns: the external (circum-stantial) and the internal (dispositional). The typical direction of causal attribution tends to vary with personality, with experience, with psychiatric illness, with regularly encountered contingencies, and according to emotional state. Some of us are statistically more likely to look to our environments for explanations of our failures; some of us are more likely to blame ourselves, and the same may be said of our successes.

    Social workers often encounter individuals whose patterns of self-blaming or self-excusing cognitions seem implausibly unidirectional. Here are a few case examples:

    - A young woman, worried and preoccupied by memories of persistent sexual abuse in childhood, who felt that she 'must have done something' to encourage her stepfather.
    - A client with a string of different psychiatric diagnoses to her name living in a hostel, who attributed the sound of nearby laughter to cruel jokes being made at her expense, and silence in the house to a wish by her critics that they should not be overheard when discussing her failings. Therefore she could never win.
    - A young man with 14 convictions for petty theft who complained that if only shopkeepers and householders would take greater precautions he would not be so cruelly tempted.

    The point about misattribution is that we all do it. We regularly go beyond the evidence; we 'join up the dots' of our observation and experiences and turn them into a meaningful but not always accurate pattern, and it is these reflexive

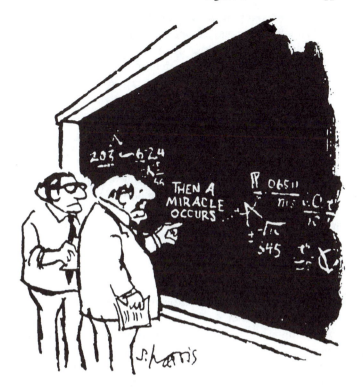

"I THINK YOU SHOULD BE MORE
EXPLICIT HERE IN STEP TWO."

Plate 7.2 Sydney Harris cartoon

Source: By permission of *American Scientist*

and over-general predispositions and tendencies (in either direction) that users of cognitive behavioural psychology seek to analyse with their clients and with which we try to get them to experiment.

- *Catastrophic thinking:* The next feature of cognition of interest to us is that of 'awfulizing', i.e. over-reacting to situations. It is easy to see how people with emotional troubles and learning histories filled with bad incidents might be shaped into hyper-vigilance for the first harbingers of trouble, and how, under the influence of anxiety, they might fail to develop proportionate responses. The clue to the presence of catastrophic thinking patterns lies in the selection of descriptions clients use to sum up their circumstances (e.g. 'awful', 'impossible', 'total', 'gutted', 'devastated').

  Here is a favourite example of an interviewer picking his way through a set of similar reactions and offering a gentle, evidential challenge to such self-defeating beliefs. Note the unthreatening directness and explicitness of the questioning. By the way, the client had attempted suicide before.

Therapist:	Why do you want to end your life?
Client:	Without Raymond, I am nothing. I can't be happy without Raymond, but I can't save our marriage.
Therapist:	What has your marriage been like?
Client:	It has been miserable from the very beginning . . . Raymond has always been unfaithful . . . I have hardly seen him in the past five years.
Therapist:	You say that you can't be happy without Raymond . . . have you found yourself happy when you are with Raymond?
Client:	No, we fight all the time and I feel worse.
Therapist:	You say you are nothing without Raymond. Before you met Raymond, did you feel you were nothing?
Client:	No, I felt I was somebody.
Therapist:	If you were somebody before you knew Raymond, why do you need him to be somebody now?
Client:	[puzzled] Hmmm . . .

(Beck, 1976: 289–290)

Sixteen lines, five minutes, and she has nearly another hour with him.

Vicious circles and emotional tangles are common enough in the lives of our clients (to say nothing of our own). Sometimes they form themselves into closed, self-sustaining, 'cat's-cradle' systems of belief, emotions and action. R.D. Laing's rather neglected book *Knots* (1972), perhaps more important than his other work, provides many interesting examples of this:

She has started to drink
As a way to cope
That makes her less able to cope
The more she drinks
The more frightened she is of becoming a drunkard
The more drunk
The less frightened of being drunk.

(Laing, 1972: 29)

Case histories reveal that the triad of influences – thinking, feeling and behavioural experience – operate in different combinations and strengths. It makes sense therefore for would-be helpers to adapt their approaches according to which of these appears primary.

Notes on assessment in CBT

Cognitive-behavioural approaches have a well-deserved reputation for evaluative rigour, but this attribute depends upon adherence to certain guidelines. Some features of cognitive behavioural assessment and evaluation overlap with more general approaches (see Chapter 5), and these paragraphs should be read with that in mind:

1   This form of assessment is mainly concerned with *who* does *what, where, when, how often*, and *with whom*. It is also concerned to identify the *absence* or with-holding of behaviours which it would normally be useful and reasonable to perform. It deals with the *consequences*, whether intended or not, which actions have for all the parties involved – those who are said to *have* the problem and those for whom someone else's behaviour is said to *be* a problem. The emphasis here is on both visible, problematic behaviour, and the absence or the inadequacy of adaptive behaviour.

2   Contra stereotype, it is also concerned with internal sensations, such as thinking patterns, doubts, persistent worries, fear, frustration and depression, but prac-titioners in this field try to keep the level of inference low, and are rather more likely to make use of standardized assessments to bolster intuitions (see Fischer and Corcoran, 1994).

3   Considerable emphasis is placed on *contemporary* behaviour and the thoughts and feelings which accompany it. Usually history-taking is limited to attempts to establish the *aetiology* of given problems and to emphasize to clients that trouble is often reactivated every day by what people do or fail to do, and by self-fulfilling expectations.

4   This concern for contemporary events is part of a wider attempt to establish the influential conditions that surround a given problem. Thus we are concerned here with such things as *where* things tend to happen and not to happen; what happens around the client or to him or her immediately *before* a sequence of the unwanted behaviour occurs; what happens around the client or to him or her *during* the performance of the behaviour; and what happens *after* the performance of the behaviour. Any natural correlation or variance in these factors provides useful extra information.

5   At some stages decisions have to be made with clients about which sequences of behaviour need to be increased in frequency and/or strength and direction, and what sequences usefully decreased in these ways. A further question is: what new skills would be required in order for the client to behave otherwise?

6   This focused approach, which accounts substantially for the greater impact of cognitive-behavioural methods in the outcomes literature, depends also upon a clear sense of *priorities* being established during assessments (see also Chapter 6).

Conclusions

Well, there aren't any spectacular ones. We have tried to make a case for a greater respect for research evidence in deciding how best to help the clients who come our way or who are forced to deal with us. At present, studies strongly indicate that we should not allow our traditional therapeutic role to be further eroded, nor allow our concern to prevent rather than merely contain to be further displaced. However, as regards the psychological underpinnings of these roles (by no means our only ones), we should, as a matter of urgency, invest more in training social workers in CBT. The government has invested £177 million in this proposal – something worth reinforcing.

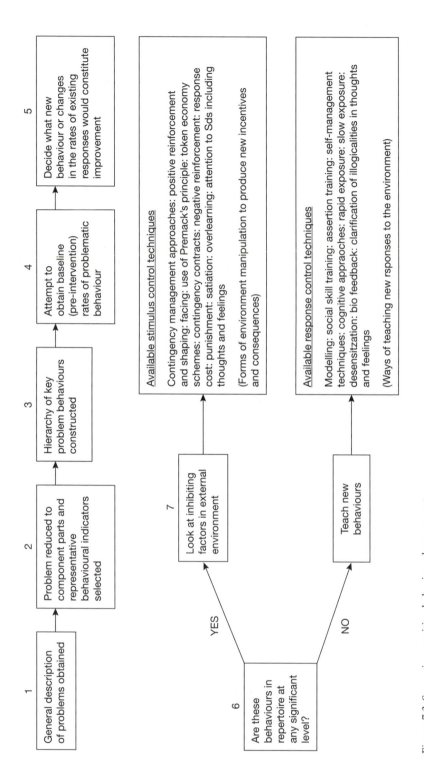

1
General description of problems obtained

2
Problem reduced to component parts and representative behavioural indicators selected

3
Hierarchy of key problem behaviours constructed

4
Attempt to obtain baseline (pre-intervention) rates of problematic behaviour

5
Decide what new behaviour or changes in the rates of existing responses would constitute improvement

6
Are these behaviours in repertoire at any significant level?

YES

NO

7
Look at inhibiting factors in external environment

Teach new behaviours

Available stimulus control techniques

Contingency management approaches: positive reinforcement and shaping: facing: use of Premack's principle: token economy schemes: contingency contracts: negative reinforcement: response cost: punishment: satiation: overlearning: attention to Sds including thoughts and feelings

(Forms of environment manipulation to produce new incentives and consequences)

Available response control techniques

Modelling: social skill training: assertion training: self-management techniques: cognitive appraoches: rapid exposure: slow exposure: desensitization: bio feedback: clarification of illogicalities in thoughts and feelings

(Ways of teaching new rsponses to the environment)

Figure 7.3 Stages in cognitive-behavioural assessment

Source: from Sheldon (1995)

8 Systemic approaches including family therapy

> Happy families are all alike; every unhappy family is unhappy in its own way.
>
> Leo Tolstoy, *Anna Karenina*

It is increasingly difficult to maintain neat distinctions across the therapeutic approaches used in practice. There is now so much borrowing of both concepts and techniques that some would argue that the similarities outweigh the differences. Insofar as theories are ways of helping us understand complex social phenomena there may be some truth in this, but as we argued earlier, both theories and interventions should be assessed on their evidential merits (see Chapters 3 and 4). Among the most eclectic therapeutic approaches is family therapy, embracing a variety of 'schools' with different emphases. Fundamental to each of these is the concept of the family as a social system and the proposition that effective intervention necessitates locating individual problems within that context and – in many circumstances – directing intervention at the family, rather than simply the pre-labelled individual. Systemic analyses may also be applied to other social systems such as groups or organizations.

In this chapter we discuss the origins and core concepts underpinning systemic approaches to family therapy and their implications for assessment and interventions. We highlight the distinguishing features of some key schools of family therapy and then look at the wider applications of systemic approaches within social work.

Origins

> There appear to exist general system laws which apply to any system of a particular type, irrespective of the particular properties of the systems and the elements involved.
>
> (Bertalanffy, 1968)

Bertalanffy was a German biologist who proposed that in order to understand how an organism worked one needed to examine the transactional processes that could be identified within it. He argued that the ever greater specialization in the sciences and social sciences would not lead to greater understanding of how things work unless attention was also paid to the interrelationships between them. His general system theory was taken up and developed by, among others, Gregory Bateson in the USA (Bateson, 1973). Bateson combined Bertalanffy's ideas about systems with those emerging from cybernetics to develop a framework for thinking about family relationships. Cybernetics was the term applied to the investigation of feedback processes in complex systems (Weiner, 1948/1961). Bateson proposed that – as with mechanical systems – families were systems that used feedback mechanisms to regulate themselves, sometimes to maintain stability and sometimes to facilitate change and adaptation.

A developmental perspective

There is no doubt that systems theory has influenced the ways in which researchers and practitioners think about the relationships between the individual, the family and the community or wider society (Cox and Paley, 1997). In particular there has been a growing appreciation of the influence of family and other systems on child development and our approach to the problems and challenges of childhood. It is now widely accepted that relationships among family members are transactional rather than unidirectional, with each member influencing the others in both direct and indirect ways (Minuchin, 2002):

> Families as units change across development in response to changes in the individual members, life circumstances, and scheduled and unscheduled transitions. Families develop distinct climates (Moos and Moos 1981), styles of responding to events (Reiss 1989), and distinct boundaries (Boss 1999), which, in turn, provide differing socialization contexts for the developing child. Reiss (1989) argues that the family regulates the child's development through a range of processes, including paradigms, myths, stories and rituals. According to this perspective, the stability and coherence of these processes reside not within individuals, but in the coordinated practices of the entire family.
>
> (Parke, 2004: 375)

With the development of ecological theory (see below) Bronfenbrenner drew attention to the impact on families of the wider social systems, particularly formal and informal support systems (Bronfenbrenner, 1979; Repetti and Wood, 1997). Increasingly, recognition is also being given to the historical contexts of family interaction, both in terms of the life course (parental and marital roles are affected by age, employment status and self-identify) and in terms of wider social events (e.g. mass unemployment, war) (Modell and Elder, 2002).

A useful overview of these and other developments is provided by Parke (2004). His paper looks specifically at what we know about their influence on child development and highlights areas where our knowledge is seriously underdeveloped but recognized as of growing importance. The latter include: our understanding of cross-cultural variations of family life and family theory; our limited knowledge of the experiences of children brought up by gay or lesbian parents; the impact of secular changes (such as the decline in fertility and family size, changes in the onset of parenthood and work patterns, rates of divorce) and reproductive technology (e.g. surrogate parenthood); the influence of biological factors on family functioning (see Plomin, 1994; Geary and Bjorklund, 2000), and the recognition of affect as a core family process (Dix, 1991; Gottman *et al.*, 2002).

The importance of a systemic approach to a range of social, emotional and behavioural problems is therefore clear, and increasingly informs the development of therapeutic approaches. What is needed is a comprehensive approach to the wide range of factors that influence family dynamics, culture and relationships, including an appreciation of the interplay between biological, individual and social systems.

Salient features of systemic approaches to work with families

Carr (2006) provides a good summary of the theoretical propositions made about families that are derived from general system theory and cybernetics, organized around six key domains. These are as follows.

Boundaries

1   The family is a system with boundaries within which there are subsystems, most notably the parent subsystem and the child subsystem.
2   The family is a subsystem of the wider social system in which it is located (community, society, professional system). This proposition is reflected in the ecological frameworks of Bronfenbrenner and underpins multisystemic family therapy (see p. 158).
3   The boundaries around a family need to be semi-permeable in order for it to adapt and survive. Chaotic families are those whose boundaries are too permeable. Isolated families are those whose boundaries are impermeable.

Patterns

4   The behaviours of individuals and subsystems within the family are influenced by the pattern of interaction that connects all family members.
5   Patterns of family interaction are governed by rules, and families repeat patterns of interaction (patterns are *recursive*).
6   Because everyone's behaviour is influenced by those of others, systemic propositions of causality are appropriately circular rather than linear. This approach avoids blaming an individual (for example, a child with behaviour problems) for problems that are relational in nature (scapegoating). More recent formulations have noted the need to take into account power relations within families and the need in some circumstances to locate responsibility clearly with particular individuals (e.g. in domestic violence or child abuse).

Stability and change

7   *Processes supporting and preventing change.* Within families there are processes that promote change (*morphogenesis*) and those that prevent it (*homeostasis*). Rules, roles and routines all help to promote stability. Families have to make important adaptations at a variety of transition points (e.g. becoming a couple, becoming a family, teenagers leaving home, divorce). Families referred for professional help include those who are unable to negotiate these transitions unaided.

Stability

8   Sometimes, when the family is under threat (for example, from marital discord), one family member may develop patterns of behaviour which, while problematic, also serve a positive function in terms of maintaining the family's stability. Thus, a child's problematic behaviour may draw parents' attention away from their own problems and unite them in trying to resolve their shared difficulty with the child.

9   Because of the role that symptomatic behaviour can play in families (promoting homeostasis), negative feedback (i.e. improvement in the symptomatic family member) can result in responses that effectively undermine improvement.

Change

10   Positive feedback (feedback that amplifies deviance) can result in changes which can have a 'snowball effect', i.e. getting families to achieve small changes can set a chain reaction in process.

11   Certain patterns of interaction can lead to the fragmentation of relationships. *Symmetrical* behaviour patterns are those in which one person elicits a similar pattern of behaviour from another (e.g. blame for marital dissatisfaction). *Complementary* behaviour patterns are those in which one person increasingly occupies one role and the other a complementary one. Carr gives the example of an increasingly care-giving husband and an increasingly depressed wife, whose relationship eventually becomes untenable owing to mutual anger and disappointment (Carr, 2006). This may also occur in the relationship between the professional helping system and the family (e.g. the social worker doing more and more and the client needing more and more). Such dysfunctional patterns of interaction can be one of the triggers that elicit 'problem' behaviour in another family member in an endeavour to 'unite' two people who are otherwise occupying symmetrical roles (see above, 8).

12   Both positive and negative feedback are sources of new information for families. New information throws a spotlight on difference, and itself can help families to adapt. Techniques such as circular questioning help to introduce news of difference to families (see below).

13   Family therapy is generally concerned with bringing about *second order change*, namely changes in the rules that govern family life. *First order change* (in the application of existing family rules) may be sufficient in some circumstances but not in others, for instance, at transitional points (e.g. adolescence).

Complexity

14   Systems theory distinguishes between first order and second order cybernetics. In the former, it is assumed that a therapist can operate independently of the family system. The latter assumes that when a therapist engages with a family a new system is created, of which the therapist is a part. In this case he or she becomes subject to the same sources of influence and patterns of interaction that characterize other systems. Different schools of family therapy adopt different positions on this.

15 Recursive patterns can replicate themselves within and across systems. Thus, patterns of violence may be seen in subsequent generations, and problem-maintaining relationships can be mirrored across systems, such that dysfunctional alliances within the family can be replicated in professional systems.

Most of us will have met couples who fit the 'symmetrical' or 'complementary' proposition (see 11 above). The tendency for improvement to be followed by deterioration (what psychoanalysts would call 'symptom substitution') is also commonplace in therapy. But one should not confuse familiarity with validity.

Key stages of systemic approaches to work with families

Because of their differing theoretical underpinnings, different schools of family therapy are characterized by particular emphases in assessment and methods of intervention (see below). None the less, they share a number of common features which we describe first. A detailed account of each of the stages of family therapy may be found in texts dedicated to this approach (see Walker and Akister, 2004; Carr, 2006).

Family therapy interventions typically comprise four stages:

1 *Planning.* This covers deciding who to invite to the first meeting and what should be on the agenda. Depending on the reason for referral it may be appropriate simply to invite the family, or circumstances may indicate the need to involve others in the family's network such as involved professionals, members of the wider family or the social network. Sometimes key people will be reluctant to attend, or others will object to their attendance. The worker needs to consider how best to involve people in such circumstances, either by meeting initially with certain people individually (to ascertain their views, or to explain why their involvement is crucial) or using early meetings to persuade 'objectors' of the same. In planning early sessions therapists typically formulate a hypothesis about the nature of the problems (and the family's strengths). Hypotheses will reflect the theoretical principles underpinning the therapist's approach and his or her previous experience (see p. 164). These will be shared with the family who will be invited to comment on their appropriateness.

2 *Assessment.* Like other phases in family therapy, assessment begins with the therapist engaging participants, followed by an explanation of what the purpose of the assessment is and what it will entail. This minimizes disappointment and frustration, and orients participants to the process. If there is more than one therapist, or a team providing advice (perhaps behind a one-way mirror), this will also be discussed and – if relevant – permission sought (e.g. for use of video-tapes). Many of the areas covered by family therapy assessments are similar to those covered in cognitive-behavioural assessments (see Chapters 5 and 7).

Genograms are often used (see McGoldrick *et al.*, 1999). These help to engage people, are a useful way of representing complex relationships, and provide an opportunity to ask relevant questions and identify family strengths. Exactly what is included or noted on a genogram will vary and families are often invited to say what they think should appear. Genograms can allow families to talk about things 'one step removed' (they are talking about a diagram on a piece of paper). This can help them share what otherwise might be difficult information or feelings, and provide an opportunity to recognize issues and patterns they may previously not have noticed, or that they may have been resistant to seeing. Assessment concludes with a problem formulation (see p. 107).

3   *Treatment.* This phase encompasses goal-setting, contracting for treatment, interventions and managing resistance. The process of goal-setting is very similar to that described on pp. 108–109. Goals need to be specific and realistic, and agreed upon by all family members. Carr suggests giving families information about the 'costs' of intervention and the likelihood of success (see also Chapters 5 and 6). The contract that family therapists seek to establish is acceptance of goals and a commitment to working towards them over a time-limited period (see also Chapter 6).

The precise nature of intervention will depend upon the theoretical focus of the therapist (whether it should or should not is another matter; see Chapter 4). Typically, though, these will comprise a range of techniques designed to alter problem-maintaining patterns of behaviour and the beliefs that underpin them (see below for examples). Homework tasks are a common feature of family therapy and serve a number of purposes. Intervention does not always deliver the planned changes. Often homework is not completed. As with cognitive-behavioural approaches, the therapist can sometimes underestimate the skills that family members possess or overestimate their commitment to the plan. Their assessments may not have identified values or cultural beliefs that are incompatible with what they have been asked to do. Most family therapy texts provide advice on how resistance can manifest itself and what strategies may be used to deal with it.

4   *Closure (or recontracting).* In this phase therapists schedule sessions less frequently and begin the process of fading out professional support. The extent to which goals have been achieved is typically reviewed with the family, and the therapist helps family members to understand the process they have been through (reviewing the work overall), troubleshooting future problems and relapses and how to deal with them. For those who find the prospect of 'going it alone' somewhat daunting, therapists might offer follow-up sessions, telephone back-up (perhaps to manage relapses) and a 'session in the bank' which families can use if and when they feel the need.

Case example

Mr and Mrs D got together in their late thirties via a contact agency. Both had been divorced previously as a result of infidelity by their partners, and both were watchful in their later union. An unplanned pregnancy produced identical boy twins, and whether partly as a result of inborn temperamental factors (see Chapter 7) or as a result of their own inconsistent parenting (both used the excuse of their age and the 'unexpectedness of the boys' arrival') both children were fractious, easily bored, and mischievous at home and at school.

However, one child was said to be the main offender, leading on the other. Thus Mrs D referred one of her children (aged 6½) to a child and family guidance clinic, saying that his behaviour was an intolerable strain on her marriage. Three impressions dominated the assessment at this stage: (1) both of the boys' behaviour was disruptive at home from time to time, but for longish periods one would lead off and the other would became a 'diplomat'; (2) the behaviour problems got worse the more their parents tried to discipline them; (3) the behavioural problems – dogged disobedience, hurling parents' possessions around, low-level stealing – were not *so* challenging, but they were pervasive.

Noting the rather negative nature of the parents' efforts at control, a simple positive reinforcement-based behavioural scheme was put into place (see Chapter 7). The referred child's behaviour improved steadily, and the case was quickly closed. Then a new referral was received for the other twin. When the social worker asked about his brother the mother said that he was 'good as gold' and that it was 'really' this other child about which she was worried. More as a test than a treatment plan, the behavioural scheme was then applied mainly to him. His behaviour quickly improved while the behaviour of his brother deteriorated sharply.

A series of family interviews were held, plus interviews with the children alone. This is what emerged: (1) the parents' somewhat obsessive attitudes towards their own 'rebound' marriage, their jealousy of each other and feelings that they were 'too late' having children spilled over into family functioning much more than had been supposed; (2) long sulks and frequent rows occurred which they tried to 'hide' from the children (children always know). Neither parent expected their relationship to survive long, but were trying to stay together 'for the sake of the children'.

Interviews with the twins were fascinating. (1) They were worried about their parents splitting up, knowing that they were unhappy (there were fears about 'orphanages'). (2) They had talked together endlessly about what to do about this and had come up with a 'parent trap'-type scheme to deflect their mother and father towards concerns about them. They did this deliberately but felt 'naughty' about it. They therefore managed this preoccupying disaffection by working shifts. One would give the adults something to occupy their minds while the other offered support, and then they would switch roles. It was almost as if in this family there was not enough love for two children at once.

Conjoint family therapy with the parents concentrating on the unresolved feelings that they had brought to their marriage had the most effect in this case; second came getting the parents to talk to the children about their troubles in simple terms. The positive reinforcement scheme was reapplied alongside but quickly came to be used informally. Naming the 'family games', though hotly contested, eventually brought visible relief to all.

It will be seen that, in this case, taking a family history was no simple process of assembling facts and impressions, but rather of establishing what events meant to the various actors involved. In this example, the history and its revisions, by adding in the separate psychological viewpoints from each member and a few 'I didn't know that you thought that I thought that . . .' breakthroughs, *was* the therapy.

Histories are for *use*, not just for the file.

Schools of family therapy

Carr groups 16 schools or traditions of family therapy (far too many, and some consolidation is overdue). These orient themselves according to whether their main organizing principles are concerned with (1) problem-maintaining behaviour, (2) problematic and constraining belief systems, and (3) historical, contextual and constitutional predisposing factors (Carr, 2006: 69). Most other therapeutic approaches appear in his list, including attachment theory and cognitive-behavioural approaches as applied to helping families change, begging the question what – for family therapists – is not family therapy? In this section we highlight some of the key aspects of one of the most commonly encountered of each of the three groups.

Strategic family therapy

Strategic family therapy starts with the assumption that the problems that bring families to the attention of professional helpers serve a purpose. Presenting problems can distract attention from other, potentially more threatening, relational problems within the family, such as marital conflict. They may reflect power struggles within the family. Family members are thought to be strategic in how they behave and in how they predict others will respond. Not surprisingly, families can therefore be ambivalent about change and even resistant to it.

Most families are clear about 'who is who' and boundaries are appropriately defined and maintained. For example, parents are in charge of their children, who know what is expected of them and what they can expect from their parents. Sometimes these boundaries are not clear, as when a mother and child collude in 'managing' the father, excluding him from important decisions, or when one parent undermines the authority of the other. Alternatively, family hierarchies can be too rigid to accommodate the changes that all families need to make when negotiating serious life events or new stages in the life cycle (e.g. changes in the exercise of power that inevitably come with adolescence). Finally, family hierarchies can be undermined by patterns of interaction which interfere with the family's ability to function. Typically cited examples are couples who each blame the other for the poor quality of their relationship (symmetrical behaviour patterns) or the couple in which ever more dominant behaviour by one partner elicits ever more submissive behaviour from the other.

Haley (1976), a founder member of this approach, argues that family problems are often attributable to these kinds of hierarchical problems. He also points out that social hierarchies manifest themselves in two forms, overt and covert, and both can contribute to the development of problems. Thus parents may ostensibly (overtly) set the rules, but in fact one parent may not follow through on rule-breaking, thereby covertly undermining it. If discrepancies between the overtly stated hierarchies and those covert hierarchies that manifest themselves in how people actually behave are denied, then problems can develop, such as marital conflict and child behaviour problems. It is these 'pathological triangles', as Haley calls them, that get in the way of families making important transitions in their life cycles. Haley also emphasized the role that people and units outside the family can play in the creation and main-tenance of problems, including the therapist him- or herself, or other colleagues such as residential care staff or psychiatric nurses. In other words, when thinking about problems and how to solve them it is important to recognize that the relevant social unit may include more than just the family (see Haley, 1976).

Assessment in strategic family therapy

The *de facto* hierarchy that exists within a family can be identified by therapists observing the sequences of behaviour that occur between members of the family. Assessment is typically conducted during the first interview which has four stages:

1　*A social stage.* Here, the therapist welcomes and engages *all* members of the family present (and ideally all family members would be present, though this is not always possible), finding out basic information such as who is in the family, and observing their mood, where and how they sit, their patterns of interaction and so on. In one case, when a child was asked to place himself physically to represent his place in the family, he walked out of the clinic and sat on the outside stairs.

2　*The problem stage.* Here, the therapist moves the focus from the social to the purposeful, enquiring as to why the family is there, what the problem is, or what changes the family is seeking. Typically the therapist will share what he or she knows so far (the referral perhaps, which may have been from a family member), will say why he or she has asked to see the whole family (e.g. in order to get everyone's ideas about the problem) and what his or her role is. Keeping the focus fairly general leaves room for family members to reveal their points of view. Haley suggests that, in general, the therapist starts with the person who appears least involved with the problem and treats the person most able to 'bring the family back' with the most concern and respect (Haley, 1976: 23). This stage is predominantly 'fact-finding' in that the therapist gathers the views of all those present without interpreting or commenting on them. Observation of the family's interaction remains crucial as this also provides important information, though not shared with the family. The articulation of the problem is left at a 'metaphorical' or rather general level: 'Many things cannot be said directly, or there would probably not be a problem' (Haley, 1976: 31). It is an opportunity for the therapist to acknowledge that things have been 'heard' without putting anyone 'on the spot', as this may result in someone withdrawing or feeling blamed.

3　*The interaction stage.* At this point the therapist asks the family to talk to each other about the problem. While remaining in control he or she gently but firmly keeps family members talking to each other rather than to the therapist, bringing in different family members as and when appropriate (e.g. if two people are disputing something, the therapist might invite a third or fourth person to share their views on the topic). On the principle that 'actions speak louder than words' the therapist may ask an individual who is seen as having a problem to engage in the problematic behaviour and for family members to show how they respond. If well conducted, this stage will provide good information about the family's structure (hierarchy). The strategic family therapist is looking in particular for evidence of 'pathological triangles' (distorted hierarchical relationships), difficulties in adapting to life cycle transitions, relationships that are overly symmetrical or complementary (see above), difficulties in giving and receiving love and control, and what substantive problem the presenting problem may be a metaphor for (e.g. child behaviour problems may be a metaphorical expression of marital problems).

4   *Defining desired changes.* This stage of the interview essentially forms the basis of a therapeutic contract. In this stage the therapist seeks clear, concrete formulation of the changes the family want to see. This means they have to be framed in a way that people will know when they have occurred (see pp. 108–109).

5   *Ending the interview.* If another appointment is made, the family may be asked to bring along someone whose absence was deemed to be important. The family may be asked to undertake a task ('given a directive') before the next meeting (see below).

Intervention in strategic family therapy

A key concept in strategic family therapy is that change occurs by means of the therapist 'joining' the system and bringing about change through the ways in which he or she participates in it. In doing so, it is argued that the therapist can effect changes in the ways in which family members relate to one another because of the ways in which they must respond to the therapist. Therapists align themselves temporarily with one member or subsystem in order to bring about change, while overall not siding consistently with anyone.

The therapeutic team will first agree a formulation of the family's problems (see p. 107). This will identify where changes are needed and how these might best be brought about. Key strategies used by strategic therapists are reframing, giving directives and reviewing progress. Reframing entails finding a positive way of describing the negative ways in which families typically experience and present their problems. So, in noting high levels of anger and frustration with the problems parents may be facing with their adolescent child, the therapist might reframe this as evidence of their concern for them. This is generally a good strategy, not least because of the association of negativity in families who drop out from therapy (see Robbins *et al.*, 1998).

Giving directives is probably the most central facet of strategic family therapy. It recognizes that for change to take place it must happen outside of the therapy sessions. Families are therefore given directives (homework tasks) designed to bring about change, particularly in relation to distortions in family hierarchies. Haley describes two ways of giving directives. In both the therapist tells people what to do, but in one instance he does *not* want them to do it because the change that is sought is brought about through the family's rebellion against the request. These directives are commonly referred to as paradoxical injunctions – but they can be confusing to decipher and need to be made with caution (see Sheldon, 1989).

Straightforward directives, where the therapist wants the family to do what he or she is asking, need to be precise and, wherever possible, should involve everyone (someone might be asked to do a job, someone to help, someone to plan). Attention to detail is important so that there is no room for family members to say they misunderstood what was required or forgot to organize life to ensure that it happened. Tasks should be achievable and, when designed to address a presenting problem, often focus on changing the sequences of behaviour that occur. For example, there is often a predictable sequence of events in the case of a child who is refusing to go to school and becomes distressed at the prospect of being excluded. One could 'write the script' of what happens between the parents and between the parents and the child every morning. Having ensured that there are, in fact, no problems at school, the strategic family therapist may first take steps to ensure the parents are motivated to work together (they may disagree about how to handle the situation but may agree that the long-term consequences are serious) and then give a directive in which the parents are clearly instructed how to handle the child. The 'how' will depend on the particular family. As with cognitive-behavioural approaches the therapist will review the process in a step-by-step fashion, troubleshooting what might go wrong and how it should be handled.

Paradoxical injunctions are targeted at families who are thought particularly resistant to change, or at points where resistance becomes an issue. They may be directed at the whole familiy or at just one part. If effective, it is because the family have set out to prove the therapist wrong, and in so doing have in fact solved their problem, or undertaken the task the therapist set as part of the means of bringing about change. Writers should note the therapeutic skill that is required if this strategy is not to backfire, and the responses that might be instrumental in ensuring it is not short-lived.

Other approaches that focus on problem-maintaining behaviour include brief therapy (MRI), structural family therapy, functional family therapy and cognitive-behavioural family therapy.

Brief, solution-focused therapy

Some schools of family therapy focus primarily on the beliefs people have about problems and the stories they tell about them. These are thought to underpin problems in relationships and therefore provide potential levers for change. Different theorists and therapeutic schools have developed different frameworks for understanding the role of belief systems (e.g. Campbell *et al.*, 1991; Freedman and Combs, 1996). Solution-focused therapy draws on ideas from a social constructivist perspective. Our individuality comprises a unique physiology and psychology, and a unique belief system – products of social interactions. Constructions that are deemed to be useful are adopted and retained. Those that are not useful are dropped, but then 'useful' can mean many things.

Solution-focused therapy differs from other schools of family therapy that draw on theories of language and communication (social construction) in its future orientation. Rather than starting with the problems that bring people to professional helpers it moves directly into what people see as solutions.

Intervention in brief, solution-focused therapy

Iveson (2002) has summarized the tasks of the first session as follows:

1   Find out what the person who made the referral, or was the referral, hopes to achieve from contact with the therapist.
2   Obtain a picture of what his or her life would be like if these hopes were realized.
3   Find out about things the person is doing or has done in the past that might help to realize these aspirations.
4   Find out what would be different if they took a small step towards realizing their hopes (see also Chapter 6).

The hallmark of solution-focused therapy is the use of a small number of techniques. Task 1 above provides the foundation technique of focusing the client on the prospect of a solution to their problems. In tackling the second task one of the most important techniques is used, namely asking the 'miracle question'. This could take a variety of forms, but is essentially the 'magic wand' question used by behaviourists. The therapist might say, 'Suppose you were to go home and go to bed. Sometime in the middle of the night a miracle happens and the problems that led you here today are solved – in the twinkling of an eye. The thing is, because you are asleep you don't know this. When you wake up in the morning, how will you find out that the miracle has occurred?' He or she would then go on to elicit a detailed account of how the world would be different. The main aim is to establish the possibility of change and introduce new potential futures. By using the language of miracles the worker also avoids sterile debates about whether or not the problem is solvable, or indeed whether or not it has been properly understood.

'Finding exceptions' is anther 'task 2' technique. However small or rare, the therapist prises examples of times when life has provided a taste of what it would be like if the problem were resolved. In other words (though the terminology of 'problems' is eschewed), the therapist seeks examples of when problems do not occur and what was different. The aim is to use this information to encourage the client to do more of the same and move towards realizing his or her aspirations.

Coping questions and compliments help people focus on their strengths and resources, both of which may have dropped off their radar or indeed never been noted. The therapist seeks to find examples of the client's ability to cope, or of their resilience. Without negating the difficulties they experience, the therapist might comment on the tenacity someone has shown in 'keeping going' in the face of adversity.

Finally, in addressing task 4 the therapist may well use a 0–10 scale to elicit information about different dimensions of their lives, and how near they are to achieving different parts of their solution. People are asked where they would place themselves on the 10-point scale in terms of their proximity to the solution (where '0' is nowhere near and '10' is the solution has happened) and to think about what incremental steps would take them nearer to '10'.

Other schools of family therapy that focus primarily on belief systems include Milan systemic family therapy (e.g. Campbell *et al.*, 1991), narrative therapy (White, 2000), constructivist (e.g. Proctor, 2003), and social constructivist (e.g. Cecchin *et al.*, 1993).

Multisystemic therapy (MST)

Multisystemic therapy is one of six schools of family therapy that Carr (2006) identifies as focusing on the role of historical, contextual and constitutional factors in the development of particular ways of thinking, feeling or behaving. It is probably the most sound, empirically based family treatment, though whether the developers would describe it as family therapy is a moot point. It is a multi-faceted, short-term, home- and community-based intervention for families with young people who have severe psychosocial problems. Its focus is on all those systems that impinge upon family and on the target child's behaviour.

Theoretically it draws on both social ecological and family systems theories, marrying this to research on the causes and correlates of serious antisocial behaviour among adolescents (Henggeler *et al.*, 1998, 2002). MST is designed to provide alternatives to out-of-home placement for young people. Out-of-home placements might be psychiatric inpatient services for adolescents with mental health problems, custody or secure accommodation for teenagers who are offending, or placements in foster care or residential care for young people at risk of abuse and neglect. It is commonly described as a family preservation service model that provides time-limited services (four to six months) to the whole family and that includes all those social systems whose involvement is necessary to finding solutions to problems. MST focuses on the 'here and now' and on the future, and the focus of the work is problem-maintaining patterns of interaction.

While each programme is unique in its implementation, it differs from most family therapy schools in being a 'manualized' treatment. In other words, the programme developers have written a detailed treatment manual that therapists are trained to use and to which they are expected to adhere (Henggeler *et al.*, 1998). Teams consist of three or four professional MST therapists, supervised by a clinician with advanced training and considerable experience. These workers have small case loads and they (or at least the team) are available to programme participants 24 hours a day, seven days a week.

Assessment in MST

MST includes a comprehensive assessment of child development, family interactions, and their interactions with other social systems such as school or peer groups (see Chapter 5). The aim is both accurately to understand a young person's problematic behaviour and what is maintaining it, and where the points of leverage or influence might be. Interviews with family members usually take place in the family's home, and may include individual interviews as well as with the whole family.

Intervention in MST

MST is not characterized by a particular set of intervention techniques. Rather, 'intervention strategies are integrated from other pragmatic, problem-focused treatment models including strategic family therapy, structural family therapy, and cognitive behavior therapy' (Henggeler, 1995: 121). It is not confined to systemic interventions or to interventions that are directed at the family. One-to-one cognitive-behavioural work designed to help young people manage peer pressure is common, as is dealing with issues that render adolescents particularly vulnerable to school exclusion or antisocial behaviour (e.g. remedial education, social skills training). In short, multisystemic family therapy tries to effect changes in a young person's social environment that will help him or her to change their behaviour and maintain those changes.

Summary

This brief overview of three major schools of family therapy demonstrates how diverse an area of work 'family therapy' is. While some schools originate with a focus on a particular set of problems such as delinquency or drug misuse, most texts discuss family therapy as a multi-purpose therapy for a range of problems. This reflects the single common denominator that we discussed at the outset of this chapter, namely that it is difficult to understand or intervene in a range of personal, interpersonal and social problems without looking at the contexts in which they occur. These contexts embrace biological systems (as in mental illness or child temperament), family systems, peer systems, neighbourhoods and wider society.

The evidence base

> Over time, the practical nature of marriage and family therapy (MFT) has changed in terms of models, modalities, emphases, and, for some, philosophy of science. The field has developed widely disparate models of therapy ranging from prescriptive and formulaic sets of interventions to postmodern philosophies that view change as 'emerging' through conversation.
>
> (Nelson and Smock, 2005: 355)

There is growing evidence of the importance of incorporating a systemic approach into assessment and the structuring of interventions (see below). When it comes to assessing the effectiveness of family therapy per se this diversity of approaches makes the task very difficult, and this is further complicated by the eclectic nature of the approaches and techniques used irrespective of the particular 'school' of therapy to which they belong – a long-standing matter, much discussed, but never to be settled, it seems, unless we get a grip on it.

This means that, except where an evaluation concerns a 'manualized treatment' (where the intervention is stipulated and monitored), one is more often looking at the effectiveness of family therapists or working with the family as a whole (compared with groups or individual sessions) rather than anything more clearly differentiated. Second, there is only a small number of controlled trials of family therapy, particularly if one excludes couples therapy and behavioural family therapy. Those systematic reviews and meta-analyses that are available usually combine very different theoretical approaches, many of which are dominated by behavioural family therapy, or forms of family therapy that make substantial use of behavioural techniques (see overleaf).

These issues are aptly illustrated in two overviews of the evidence produced by Carr (2000a, 2000b), drawing on 'important review papers' and meta-analyses where they exist, and controlled group trials where they do not. In the first paper on children's problems he concludes that there is evidence for the effectiveness of family therapy for: the management of child behaviour problems; conduct disorder such as oppositional defiant disorder; hyperactivity and attentional problems; antisocial behaviour and substance misuse in adolescence; anxiety; depression, eating disorders; psychosomatic problems, and child abuse and neglect. In the companion paper on adults' problems Carr presents evidence for family therapy's effectiveness regarding relationship problems, anxiety and depression, mood disorders, psychoses, substance misuse and chronic pain (Carr, 2000b).

One could therefore be tempted to conclude that family therapy is clearly effective in helping to ameliorate or resolve many of the problems that bring people to the attention of mental health agencies, youth justice, counselling and social services. That would be somewhat misleading though, and although Carr sometimes talks about 'family therapy' he most often uses the language of 'family-based interventions' – a somewhat different thing based on formats rather interventions.

Table 8.1 provides an overview of the evidence reviewed by Carr in relation to child-focused problems. One might argue that it suggests that Carr overplays the role of structural or strategic psychotherapeutic traditions, and underplays the cognitive behavioural elements already shown to be effective. Overall, the evidence points to the importance of family-focused assessment and intervention in a wide range of problems. Beyond that there is evidence to suggest that for some problems, family-based interventions – broadly defined – outperform 'treatment as usual' or 'other treatments' and do better than no treatment at all. Here is a summary.

- *Conduct disorders and delinquency.* Behavioural parent training is clearly the treatment of choice for conduct-disordered children, in conjunction with behavioural couples therapy or social support where necessary (see e.g., Serketich and Dumas, 1996). Although inconclusive, there is *some* evidence that multisystemic therapy may be effective in helping adolescents avoid out-of-home or more restrictive placements, may help attenuate offending, and may improve family functioning (see Curtis *et al.*, 2004; Littell *et al.*, 2005; Chapter 12, this volume).
- *Drug misuse.* In relation to drug abuse, Stanton and Shadish (1997) conclude that the evidence 'favors family therapy over (a) individual counselling or therapy; (b) peer group therapy, and (c) family psychoeducation'. They go on to say that family therapy did better at retaining people in treatment, did equally well for both adults and adolescents, and appeared to be a cost-effective adjunct to methadone maintenance. There were insufficient studies to examine the differential effects of particular kinds of family therapy, but the authors point out (1) that only two studies specifically compared interventions, and (2) that 13 of the 15 studies shared similarities, including an emphasis on behavioural tasks (p.183).

Table 8.1 Summary of Carr's overview of evidence for child-focused problems

Problem	Approach	Evidence base
Oppositional defiant disorder	Behavioural parent training	Serkevitch and Dumas, 1996
ADHD	Multimodal: drugs plus behavioural parent training or structural family therapy	Hinshaw *et al.*, 1998 Barklay, 1990
Pervasive conduct problems in adolescents	Functional family therapy and multisystemic therapy	Kazdin, 1998 Chamberlain and Rosicky, 1995
Adolescent drug use	Family therapy and multisystemic therapy Family-based therapy	Liddle and Dakof, 1995 Waldron, 1996 Stanton and Shadish, 1997
Anxiety	Cognitive behavioural interventions Behavioural family therapy	Range of single studies
Depression	Conjoint family therapy and concurrent group-based cognitive-behavioural parent and child training	Brent *et al.*, 1997 Harringon *et al.*, 1998 Lewinsohn *et al.*, 1990, 1996
Common psychosomatic complaints	Behavioural, family-based behavioural and a narrative therapy externalizing (cognitive) behaviour Family therapy	Houts *et al.*, 1994 Thapar *et al.*, 1992 White and Epston, 1989 (single study) Gustaffson *et al*, 1986
Anorexia	Family therapy and combined individual therapy and parent counselling with or without initial hospital-based feeding	Wilson and Fairburn, 1998
Child abuse and neglect	Family-focused casework, multisystemic family therapy	A number of controlled studies

- *Relationship problems.* Behavioural couples therapy has been shown to be more effective than no treatment (Shadish and Baldwin, 2005) though there have been fewer investigations of its effectiveness relative to other forms of treatment, and in an earlier systematic review of family and marital therapies Shadish and his colleagues concluded that it was generally *not* possible to differentiate the relative effectiveness of different therapeutic schools, primarily due to the eclectic and integrative nature of the therapies (Shadish *et al.*, 1993). A long-standing problem.
- *Schizophrenia.* Pilling and colleagues undertook two systematic reviews of the effects of psychological treatments in schizophrenia (see also Chapter 13). One looked at social skills training and cognitive remediation (Pilling *et al.*, 2002a)

and the other at family interventions and cognitive-behavioural therapy (Pilling *et al.*, 2002b). Family intervention was defined as a supportive, family-based intervention lasting for at least six weeks and comprising at least one of the following: psycho-educational intervention; problem-solving/crisis management work; or intervention with the identified patient. Sometimes intervention took place in groups of families (usually without the patient) and sometimes with single families. Family therapy, thus defined, had 'clear preventative effects on the outcomes of psychotic relapse and readmission, in addition to benefits in medication compliance'.

- *Eating disorders.* Guidelines on treatment choice in the deployment of psychological therapies (DoH, 2001) identify evidence that family therapy may be effective for the early onset of adolescent anorexia, though broadly based individual therapy may be more appropriate for later onset (Russell *et al.*, 1987). The evidence, however, is mixed, and there is limited evidence to support the use of systemic therapies for bulimia nervosa, though they are regularly provided (Asen, 2002; see also Chapter 13, this volume)

Compromise conclusions

With some exceptions, the evidence base for family-based interventions is promising but slender, and requires a careful unpacking of what exactly is being evaluated. In his review of psychotherapy for children and adolescents, Kazdin reminds us that of some 550 treatments available and in common use, only a handful have been empirically evaluated (2003: 258). Family-based interventions in general, and systemic approaches in particular, are promising approaches, but one's enthusiasm should reflect the strength of the evidence currently available. In research terms, these approaches do well until they meet the full face of RCT methodologies and systematic reviews of these approaches (see Littell *et al.*, 2005), which suggests that the jury, though smiling at the defendants, is still out on these approaches regarding any *distinct* impact.

9 Social work and community work

> It seems that whenever our policy-makers reach an intellectual impasse they cover their embarrassment with the fig leaf of community.
>
> Pinker, 1982: 242

Perhaps; but there was a time (see Chapter 1) when virtually all social work was a form of community work. Indeed, until quite recently, most qualifying courses had a community work element, but only in Northern Ireland is competence in community development a requirement of the professional qualification. The question arises however: to what extent are social workers now generally involved in such pursuits? Certainly the adjective is everywhere: we have community mental health teams; community support teams, even 'community punishments' (which remind one a little of the stocks), but is this, as Pinker thought, so much heart-warming, sepia-toned sentimentality? We shall try to answer this question, but first we will conduct a short survey of the literature, in which the following themes are present:

1   Some books, and many more articles, celebrate the idea that the onerous responsibilities with which social work is charged (e.g. community care in mental health, community care to enable frail, elderly people to live at home, Sure Start) envisage a community organization element to the work. That is, the planned involvement of extended families, neighbours, voluntary groups and volunteers. The problem, and it is very evident, is that this is often supposed to happen via some catalytic process, without allowing professionals the time to get involved in a supportive capacity.

   Further, some writers devote considerable space to the question of whether communities still exist beyond what is implied above (i.e. is this just the *place* where governmental initiatives are carried out?). They have a point, for are we not more atomized as citizens than ever before: staying in for hours watching TV or reviewing our e-mails, taking what R&R there is time for after increasingly long hours in increasingly demanding jobs? In 1966, the sociologist Veblin warned us that we would soon have leisure to burn and had better adapt quickly to this fact, but it turned out not to be quite the case. But perhaps other expressions of community spirit exist in the 'communities of interest' which spring up when local environments are threatened, or in the growth in the health field of amazingly well-informed interest and support groups for people with physical and mental conditions. Certainly the *idea* of community has not gone away, because we miss the benefits, but are we prepared to go outside and join in any more?

2   Some authors, in somewhat 'dialectical' fashion, see so many 'contradictions' (coded Marxist terms) in the way society is developing, that a (Newton's Third Law type) reaction is bound to occur; for example:

> Even if public-agency social work becomes completely absorbed in assess-ments for social assistance payments, care packages, training programmes and treatment regimes, the original principle and values of social work will not disappear. They will be kept alive in many unofficial activities and small-scale organisations, and in the everyday practices of ordinary people. In this way they will remain available to collective decision-makers when – at some future date – all semblances of voluntarism and co-operative engagement has drained out of public-sector agencies, and the costs of enforcement have come to threaten economic efficiency itself. Then the historical wheel will have to come full circle, and social work may start again from roughly its late nineteenth century beginnings.
>
> (Jordan, 1997: 2)

Or not, of course.

However, although wary of the idea of historical 'inevitabilities', we do find some of these arguments persuasive, wishing only that they could be incor-porated into a view of the broader ills with which social work – the resolution of some of which lie in necessarily more individual interventions. For these and community-based work could reasonably be seen as elements of a *continuum* of provision. The problems which regularly come our way are indeed diverse, and so, logically, must the attempted solutions be. Subdisciplinary tunnel vision is a self-imposed handicap in these matters, or as Sigmund Freud called it (and he would have known), 'the narcissism of small differences'. Nowhere is this more self-affirming the case than in the family therapy approaches discussed in Chapter 8.

3   Much of the literature on community work is getting on a bit, not a sin in itself, except where the social conditions being addressed have changed markedly. The publications making the largest claims come from community work's 'golden age' in the 1960s and 1970s, but these ambitious projects also tended to employ the weakest evaluation methods, on the dubious principle that if the cause was right, then the results would be obvious to everyone except those determined to disregard them for right-wing political reasons. These players also suspected that 'spurious' scientific arguments were being used to constrain radicalism. Therefore, the money quickly ran out, because existing civic arrangements – the very ones that many in this field are now trying to get back to – were being damaged by the 'free radicals' (as it were). And then another type of radical, Margaret Thatcher, put an end to most of this.

4   What we have left is a cluster of publications from more pluralist community workers and academics whose approach is (although they may dislike the term) more professional. These concentrate on *how* to harness non-state-directed cooperation and goodwill for local purposes, so that the genuine concerns of people with common interests get a hearing, and that other than official

definitions of what is wrong and right in a particular area can be taken forward from within it (see Ghake and Hazel, 2004; Sutton, 1994).

Jordan's subtitle to his intriguing book (2004) is *The Transformation of Collective Life*, and here he quotes the sociologist Thomas Scheff's (1997) ethological ideas to support his view that the stickiness of the 'social glue' needs regularly to be checked up on from time to time:

> My model of the Social bond is based on the concept of *attachment*, mutual identification and understanding. A secure social bond means that the individuals involved identify with each other and understand each other, rather than misunderstand and reject each other. I assume that in all human contact, if bonds are not being built, maintained, or repaired, then they are being damaged.
>
> (from Jordan, 2004: 76)

Consequently sociologists today are much concerned with the concept of 'social capital' – actually an old idea; here is the coiner of the term's original definition:

> In the use of the phrase *social capital* I make no reference to the usual acceptation of the term *capital*, except in a figurative sense. I do not refer to real estate, or to personal property or to cold cash, but rather to that in life which tends to make these tangible substances count for most in the daily lives of a people, namely, goodwill, fellowship, mutual sympathy and social intercourse among a group of individuals and families who make up a social unit, the rural community, whose logical center is the school.
>
> (Hanifen, 1916: 130)

Hanifen, an active educational reformer observed, 'It is not what [professionals] did for the people that counts for most in what was achieved; it was what they led the people to do for themselves that was really important' (p. 138).

5   The feature that this body of work still lacks, however, is not ever more refined conceptual analysis, or ever changing 'buzz-words', but robust, routine, empirical research on the practical effectiveness of these ideas when implemented, and on what works best in what circumstances. There are many opportunities for comparisons in community work projects, where services are provided/developed in one area but not in another area with similar problems. There do exist a few American evaluations (see Campbell at www.campbellcollaboration.org) but one has the sense in these later 'task-centred' projects that the community is a backdrop as much as a central resource.

6   This said, there is a large empirical literature on the sociological origins of social problems. These routinely implicate a breakdown in community among the main causes: run-down estates with little social cohesion where most of the burglaries are done neighbour upon neighbour; places where near-feral children intimidate neighbours and force them indoors; problems of isolated elderly people, or those with mental health problems, and so on. This naturally leads on to (for us) the most interesting branch of the literature, one which examines what happens when any sense of community has broken down or was stifled at birth by planners and architects; the 'you don't know what you've got till it's gone' research. The

best of these deliver a robust critique of the effectiveness of current arrangements within the social and other services for providing credible, practical help (see Holman, 1987, 1992, 1995, 1999). The main obstacle to recovery aided by statutory involvement, to which such writing turns again and again, is the tyranny of 'the case' as the unit of accountability for the costs versus benefits of any potential good being attempted. This is an old preoccupation:

> Present institutions train several kinds of persons – such as judges and social workers – to think in terms of situations. In their activities and world outlook and in their professional work, they tend to show an occupational incapacity to rise above 'cases'.
>
> (Wright Mills, 1943: 165)

An example follows in support of this argument.

Case example

There was once, on the outskirts of a city, a run-down council estate, which had at its edge a hostel for refugees left over from World War II. They were all then elderly men who had escaped from Nazi occupation and had never gone home because there was nothing much to go back to. They were housed in concrete blocks surrounded by a fence, and so the conditions, though clean(ish) and orderly, were nevertheless reminders of the much worse conditions they had fled to avoid. The men were predominantly Poles, plus a few Estonians and Lithuanians. The hostel was run by the Housing Department and had a superintendent who saw social welfare as nothing much to do with him. No staff member spoke a word of the languages of the residents, who had only limited English. Across the road was a Social Services Department Tardis (Portakabin) which, *contrariwise*, didn't really 'do' housing. However, it did aspire to 'patch-based' social work. This agency also contained a student unit comprising six undergraduates from three different courses. One of these was required to conduct a 'community audit', and noticed that older Polish men being seen by duty social workers were highly over-represented on the agency case load. There was also another consistent pattern of problems: few GPs were willing to take the refugees as patients, so if they fell ill they had to go to Casualty; few translation services were available; many found the various forms they had to fill in to obtain top-up benefits an impossible task; there was no support for writing to enquire about lost relatives; and depression was a common problem; forms of jovial cultural expression (aided by the local off-licence) were frowned upon, and in passing, they heartily disliked the 'traditional English' food they were fed. One deceased resident's death certificate had 'malnutrition' on it – still a problem in our hospitals. The student also noticed later that few of the clients had the remotest notion of a longer term future (Poland, Estonia and Lithuania having been occupied by Soviet Russia) and some of these men having 'previous' with that regime.

The group of students proposed a small community project with the following aims: (1) that since most of the problems reported either arose from *inside* the hostel or were due to casual discrimination against residents by public services, therefore, the main targets of influence had to be the Social Services and Housing Department – which, awkwardly, were the employers and hosts of those concerned; (2) that there ought to be open access by social workers/ students to the hostel rather than the prevailing visit by appointment/'Yes, can I help you?' system, and that all residents had a legal entitlement to a local GP, though this right had never been insisted upon; (3) that the citizen status of these men should be clarified with their consulates, and that they should be invited to take an interest in their welfare and their futures; (4) that ways should be found to improve cultural contacts, via organizations within travelling distance, and through a supply of books and magazines in their own languages.

By far the hardest part of the project was to get the Housing Department and Social Services to talk to each other. Neither wanted to take on new responsibilities, having enough already; the hostel manager fought hard for the retention of his control over these refugees' lives, and was intimidatory towards residents who supported the initiative; open access was granted only after a meeting between the Director of Social Services and the Director of Housing Services (this took three months of hard advocacy to set up); the consulates were helpful and financed a library of books and other relevant materials; the local GP practices had to be forced by the NHS to enrol these 'new' patients; the benefits review system involving the Citizens Advice Bureau resulted in an increase in income for many residents. The interpreters' service was difficult to set up since the nearest available sources were 20 miles away – but interestingly, when they came, they would spend 20 minutes on practical problems and half an hour 'just talking'.

Throughout the project the main opposition from both within and without the Social Services Department, and indeed in the students' universities, was that (*à la* C. Wright Mills) these groups of people were not official 'cases' and therefore did not really count for case study purposes. This would not happen today of course, unless you visit a Polish fruit-pickers' hostel or a disused RAF base used to house asylum seekers.

What is community?

Social scientists who study the concept of community have a rather self-defeating habit of rolling their eyes, either metaphorically on the page, or literally at conferences, when asked for simple definitions. It *is* a complex idea, but then so are many others in fields where conceptual constipation seems less of a problem. For example, Daniel Barenboim (the 2006 Reith lecturer) who had the task of defining music – now there's a challenge – came up with 'Sonorus air' but then spent five hours on examples of the mysteries. Hence we should define community social work as 'helping people in their locales to live better, more socially integrated aspirational and more fulfilled lives, where informal support is routinely given and received', and then write the footnotes.

Here is the *OED* definition of community:

> Joint ownership, as of goods; identity of character; fellowship; organized political, municipal, or social body; body of people living in the same locality.

Social-scientific definitions (which vary greatly) contain the following themes:

1   A defined geographical location (village, town, area of a city, neighbourhood) where there is a customary pattern of social exchange, reciprocity and altruism over and above the obligations of law or regulation: *communtitas* not *polis*. But then there are some areas of towns and cities where mere geographical closeness is no predictor of reciprocity or altruism, rather of fear and alienation.

2   A sense of belonging to a social space as a symbolic entity reinforced by routine interaction, mutuality and custom. But then there are more scattered communities based on ethnicity or religion which transcend local environments. Thus, the Sikh community in the whole of the city of Leicester probably has more contact and fellow feeling than any single, geographically closer, mixed neighbourhood within it.

3   The concept of community has to encompass the idea of moral goods, of natural altruism and mutual aid. Refer back to p. 6 for an argument that these attributes have become as hard-wired into us as the basic reflexes for aggression and self-protection, yet they are by no means free of environmental contingencies. Thus, we can speak easily of the 'wider Muslim community', recognizing patterns of its common values and its provision of mutual aid under pressure, but never of the 'paedophile community', which is *highly* organized in support of perverted aspirations. If we speak of 'the criminal fraternity' we do so ironically.

   Therefore, inescapably, definitions of community must encompass the idea of positive, intendedly helpful, moral interactions, at least semi-independent of state control. This is the 'gluon force' that holds a decent society together independently of governmental supply drops.

   The current switch-off of interest in politics in Britain (about 30 per cent of electoral voters exercise this hard-won right – compared with Iraq where the turn-out was 80 per cent, defying threats of bombings and beheadings) is because it's all been 'fixed' in Whitehall, and because 'consultations' which are not affirmatory tend not to make it through to the policy stage. A mistake. Many definitions (e.g. Putnam, 2000) measure levels of community spirit by the existence, or absence, of informal, self-run organizations, clubs and pressure groups; neighbourhood and civic societies; youth facilities; parent/teacher groups, which are widely, and in our view rightly, seen as the 'glue' (interestingly, this word is hardly ever absent from a text on the subject) which binds democracy and civil society together. These institutions represent, in Jordan's (2004) terms, 'communities of choice' rather than 'communities of fate'.

4   The idea that seeding these troubled communities with professional helpers who might well know better than to try to impose their views, but who can support local aspirations, is, as we have seen, an old one. But governmental funders especially tend to impose daunting targets upon them and require levels of evaluation that their own departments hardly ever achieve. Without losing

sight of the need for methodological rigour, surely something more sympathetic could be put together given the complexity of this field? After all, the primary aims of community work, the NHS and Social Services should not be to make the government of the day look re-electable. We are directly or indirectly their servants, but they are also ours.

The skills of community-based work

There is an overlap between the skills of community work and social work, though there are some differences. What follows is a discussion of these differences. Note, though, that no 'free-range' community worker would be very effective without the communication skills described in Chapter 6, however good his or her knowledge of community assets, but conversely, no 'battery' social worker who did not know where to go to and who to talk to would be likely to gather support for a project or for the wider aims of a complicated case. Here are our views on the additional factors.

Assessment

There are several well-designed scales for measuring social deprivation, and for auditing social assets which go beyond the subjective (e.g. the Social Deprivation Index; Hudson's scales are also very reliable; free school meals take-up a reliable indicator, and so on). In our work in Cornwall (see Lovering *et al.*, 2006) the problem of securing funding for community projects, often from London-based civil servants or voluntary groups, is that people associate this English county with holidays. The people who actually live there all year round are among the most disadvantaged outside the inner cities. The travelling distances also complicate any notions of 'outreach' services. Thus, without objective evidence of deprivation and social exclusion, the case for funding could easily have fallen for sentimental reasons. Therefore, as in the rest of social work, the schemes which produce the most convincing results are those that incorporate the need for the equivalent of a public health review of troubling local conditions, and of promising community responses to these. However, this is one of the last things funders wish to hear about, because review and evaluation plans usually use up a quarter of the available money.

The ecological model has some attractions here. It proposes not just 'hanging around' problems until they are better understood, but analysing systemic interconnections (see Jack, 1997; Jack and Jack, 2000), thereby recognizing the complexity and the socio-economic embeddedness of problems with which the personal Social Services are involved. It takes a telescope to community deficits and assets, the only problem being that microscopy is the fashion of the time. But there *could* always be both.

A thorough assessment of community deficits and assets is thus effectual, but, awkwardly, it requires time spent on the ground getting to know about these things and building up trust. In the case example (p. 182) variations of 'everybody thinks we're shit because we live here' about sum up the opinions of residents.

Networking

Alan Twelvetrees (2002: 14) has this to say about the labour-intensive process of initiating, maintaining, renewing and making use of contacts with potentially influential individuals, voluntary groups and local politicians:

> Because community workers control almost nothing, we need the support and goodwill of as many other people as possible if we want to get anything done. Unless we take care to cultivate this goodwill and mutual understanding widely, and to develop a sense of ownership in others about what we want to achieve, we may find that the natural conservatism and resistance to change of most people will turn into opposition.

The ubiquitous finding of public consultations about policing in Britain is that we greatly miss (and not just romantically) a routine, reassuring police presence on the streets to prevent trouble, rather than relying upon high-speed, blue light responses to what has already happened. Yet this clear and persistent message seems almost impossible to implement. In social care the analogy holds up well: clients in receipt of 'community care' also want to get to know *someone*, not just in dire circumstances, but in a preventive role. The elderly, infirm, housebound, somewhat deaf and myopic mother of one of us regularly received postcards through the door from her 'mobile community support worker' saying, 'Sorry you were out when I called . . .'[tick]. Real community workers get to know the individual circumstances of people on their case loads (the milkman and a neighbour were better at it in the latter case), but all concerned should follow Alan Twelvetrees' wise advice: *'Walk, don't ride!'*

Community-level interventions

The greater part of the literature of social work is concerned with single clients, or perhaps families closeted in interview rooms. Community work is different in the sense that most of the targets of influence will be large groups of people with similar problems or who are members of other organizations who either hold the keys to the releasing or locking up of resources. Community workers need therefore to be persuasive people.

Here are some findings on the nature of persuasive communications as investigated by comparison trials where various factors are held constant and differences introduced one at a time (see Cohen, 1964; Sheldon, 1978).

1   Reputation is a powerful factor, worryingly so perhaps; nevertheless, it usually trumps the fine detail of arguments. However, reputations for trustworthiness and reliability have to be *built*.
2   There are *order effects* in persuasive communications. Those which summarize the main arguments and/or goals of what is being argued for and then explore them are more persuasive. Two-sided arguments are better than determined preaching in the medium and longer term.
3   Non-defensiveness about aims and means, sometimes signalled by a little humour, also convinces more than the 'total commitment to mission statements'.

4   Would-be persuaders who pre-raise possible objections to their ideas and either deal with them as best they can, or publicly scratch their heads and ask for help, are more than likely to win influence.

5   Anxiety-reduction techniques prefigure that in some situations, organizations and community groups are not anxious *enough* to collaborate, and may need to be made more so. We have seen skilled community workers gently doing just this kind of thing: 'What will happen if we ignore "out-of-control" children until they get big enough to do some real harm around here?'; 'Immediate costs aside, what will the press make of our failure to act on this?' Proposals based on licensed, reasonable radicalism, as well as good evidence, with properly costed, well-evaluated projects that might just make a difference, are more persuasive.

Community-based projects

Workers on community-based projects require levels of persistence and benign assertion which transcend the ordinary social training of most of us. Assertiveness is a much misunderstood concept and is normally, in our culture, associated with aggressiveness, yet it equates more to calm directions.

The problem then is how to teach communication and influence skills. Some efforts have been made before using closed-circuit television, but these are now a rarity given the numbers of students on courses. All we can say is that if medical students were denied access to laboratories because there were too many of them to accommodate, it might cause a stir. We have both seen good results from role-play work involving real funding representatives, real senior managers, real councillors and real service users, to whom students must make a case for cooperation and learn from the feedback they receive.

Case example

There was once a left-over, scruffy council estate on the outskirts of a large city. Left over, one suspects, because the residents had always voted against transferring their tenancies to a private housing company, a plan dear to the hearts of the cash-strapped local authority. It had no outpost of the Social Services Department on it although many of the residents were clients. Social disadvantage measures showed the area to be very poor, with free school meal rates approaching 80 per cent. It had one, steel-shuttered convenience store which charged high prices; no bank; no community centre; no post office; no health centre, and the churches seemed not to be interested in the lives of the people who lived nearby. The bus service into town was infrequent and expensive.

The population profile was of young single mothers and children and elderly people, with few working couples in the middle. Debt levels, utility arrears and threatened eviction rates were high. Unemployment rates were nearly three times the city's average, so much so that to give this postcode on an application for credit produced a near automatic refusal. When families from elsewhere

---

were evicted for rent arrears, they were relocated to this estate. Social and Health Services were deployed by car from outside; in and out quick. Tallymen, drug dealers and 'loan sharks' were the most reliable visitors.

Into this bleak picture came a voluntary organization which had secured a medium-sized government grant for an urban regeneration project. A community worker (plus a part-time assistant) was appointed. She asked for a year to get to know local people and to establish their needs. Not surprisingly this was refused, and only three months were set aside for the exercise – good by modern standards.

Alan Twelvetrees has brought the problems of this 'task-centred community work' approach to our attention, so an academic interlude here:

> Many of the community work projects that do exist are often short-term: three years at the most. It will be six months, at least, before the project is 'up and running'. It will be at least another six months before much of value is delivered, probably longer. And after another year and a half the staff will be looking around for new jobs. Much of any good may well be unsustainable, as a result of which the community-run initiatives supported by the staff run down, leaving a very disillusioned community . . . For these reasons, community work needs to become strategic, long-term and integrated to the organisations which seek to deliver it.
>
> (Twelvetrees, 2002: 11)

Amen; but such expert commentaries are unlikely to change the current managerial culture, which is better suited to the efficient semi-commercial production of 'things' rather than acknowledging that services for human beings require tailored solutions based on stable and continuing acquaintance.

What was done?

- The first problem was insufficient numbers of staff on the ground. The grant had been given to a voluntary organization with no great presence in this locale, on the optimistic grounds (only the brave challenge unfounded optimism from grant providers at the outset of a project and risk early exclusion) that they might come up with something new.

  The solution to this problem for the single (heroic) community worker in this case was: (1) to draw students on practical work placements in by contacting courses. They came, and were useful well beyond being extra pairs of hands; they were keen and they had evaluative projects to complete in order to qualify; (2) there were many city, statutory and voluntary organizations (e.g. CAB, Social Services, public health projects) with declared responsibilities throughout the area, though they were rarely visible on the estate.

  Two approaches were taken. First, there were attempts to engage with front-line Social Services and other staff to try to involve them in the project. This typically produced heart-warming offers of general support but led to little in the way of practical resources. Second, it was decided to adopt an 'up-and-over' approach by contacting senior managers, and reminding them of their own declared responsibilities for outreach work. Next came an attempt to get a few, somewhat disaffected, councillors on side; they were surprised to be asked, but did rally round.

- The next problem that emerged was a lack of premises in which to hold meetings. The project workers had been allowed to rent a house on the estate and lived there, turning the ground floor into a base for operations. The area contained a number of publicly owned facilities, but gaining access to these facilities required determined work.

- So far, so routine, but what was done next, though it might sound banal, contained deeper purposes. A committee was put together to organize a summer fête (there had never been anything like this since the Coronation in 1953). The idea came from a student who had read about the theory of 'cognitive dissonance'. Thus, although the idea was to encourage the local community to come together and have a good time, the subtext was to incite city organizations to participate. The city police; an army motorcycle team; the fire brigade; the scouts and guides; the Air Training Corps, and the Lady Mayoress all turned up, and therefore, so did the local press. There were food stalls, cooking competitions and so on. At the end of the day, which, according to police officers, passed without incident, the Chair of the residents' committee duly handed over a cheque to the Lady Mayoress for a city children's charity. The local newspaper headlines next day ran: 'Those who have little give to the even worse off.' The sense of pride, the fact that the day went well; the fact that the community worker and the students took a back seat and acted as 'fixers'; the contradiction of the prevailing stereotype of residents as 'spongers', were all palpable in the air, as was the sense of empowerment – they did it again the following year and it became a fixed event.

An integrated model of social work and community work?

William Schwartz (1969), in his article 'Private troubles and public issues: one social work job or two?', raised the question as to whether social workers are to be both individual and family practitioners *and* forensic, community development workers. The answer was, sensibly, a little of both, if a way could be found to integrate these skills and services. However, the situation is now more complicated, particularly at a management and organizational level, because it is now quite routine to be communicating to 'Housing and Social Services', or to 'Libraries, Education and Children's Services', and this constant merging and reorganizing is the price of not presenting to local and national politicians a clear idea of who exactly we are.

However, there is a clear case for a (re) merger between social work, community work and community development, since community work is to social work what public health is to general practice in medicine. The novelist A. J. Cronin (1932) (who was himself a chief officer for public health) portrayed two young, idealistic doctors, keen to do their best for their patients in the dire conditions of a South Wales mining community in the 1920s. The most common request from patients was for 'the usual bottle of pink medicine'. The conditions of which they complained, however, ranged from pneumoicosiasis, to TB, to malnutrition, to worse diseases caused by leakages of sewerage into the water supply. Cronin's characters were persuaded on the evidence to stop going along with this palliative approach, and instead got their miner patients to demolish the old sewers with dynamite, forcing the authorities to build new ones. (A valid analogy, but probably you shouldn't try this at work.)

So, the question before us (we are far from the first to raise it) is: Could social workers bring these wider 'public health equivalent' factors, not just into their understanding of the origins of the social and personal problems (we are quite good at this), but into their routine practice? We are quite bad at the latter because we belong to organizations that are best thought of as large-scale behaviour modification schemes, increasingly designed to constrict professional imagination wherever it might embarrass politicians and thus the security of employment of managers – who, from close acquaintance, we know would dearly like to do a broader, more meaningful job, but are discouraged from doing so.

This brings us back to the question as to whether social workers, in their daily practice, should/could try to harness contributions from the community in ameliorating the problems of individuals and families. There have been several attempts, most notably those of Goldstein (1973), Pincus and Minahan (1973), and more recently Gordon Jack, Bill Jordan and colleagues. Concentrating on the first authors for now, they were foolhardy enough to offer a definition of 'integrated social work' in the following terms; it was to:

- Help people to enhance and more effectively use their own problem-solving and coping capacities.
- Establish linkages between people and resource systems.
- Facilitate interaction and modify and build relationships between people and societal resource systems.
- Facilitate interaction and modify and build relationships between people within resource systems.
- Contribute to the development and modification of social policy.
- Dispense material resources.
- Serve as agents of social control.

(Pincus and Minahan, 1973)

They add that, 'in practice, a given activity might be performed to achieve several of these functions at the same time' (no point in hanging about, but imagine a weekly work diary with several of these functions listed).

But this volume contains enduringly interesting ideas – indeed we are proposing a revival of it in modified form. The problem is that it is a product of American cultural optimism (don't knock it), but it shies away from questions of raw political power and bureaucratic inertia, and it assumes widespread rationality and as yet unreleased goodwill. It was also a reaction against a failure of individualized casework (i.e. of quasi-psychotherapeutic methods) to solve society's ills. This list of proposed social work functions is derived from systems theory (see Chapter 8) and is worth discussing further:

1   Previous texts on social work, though they paid lip-service to familial and social factors, sought mainly to teach the skills of one-to-one engagement – all the rest was context.

2   The next useful idea was to restore *advocacy* as a social work skill worth teaching. At present we have hundreds of initiatives to help 'lift people out of poverty and social exclusion', with millions in the pot, but then financial accountability requires tight eligibility criteria; otherwise 'parasitism' occurs, as it has done in the incapacity benefits system. Therefore the entry criteria for such otherwise creditable schemes tend to verge on the labyrinthine. Social workers and community workers have a key role here as 'street-level bureaucrats'.

3   The two illustrations contained in this chapter are examples of projects with better than prima facie claims to effectiveness. But beneath the plans, the consultations and the sub-projects lies a steady buildup of skills in influencing and coordinating contributions from staff residents and volunteers who are not always really convinced at the outset.

4   Pincus and Minahan remind us that it is not unusual to see clients struggling with their own lives and circumstances in the midst of what, on paper at least, look like considerable reserves of unrealized social capital, friends, neighbours and so on. Social workers should aim to realize these resources.

5   As for the aim of influencing social policy, we know from our research on the history of the profession (see Chapter 1) that this has long been a reasonable aspiration. The only problem is that we are not very good at it. Voluntary organizations devote considerable resources to this. Barnardo's, MIND and Help the Aged are good at it. The Association of Directors of Social Services in Britain have a go, but are fearful about seeming 'off-message' in volatile political climates. Individual social workers and community workers feel that they cannot do this; only report back, observe patterns in their case loads and pass on the concerns of local people. Influencing social policies requires alliances of organizations which represent service users and professionals but which are free to operate outside the confines of the protocols of grant-funded projects or employment regulations.

There is thus a Royal Collage of Nursing, a College of Occupational Therapists and a Royal College of Surgeons. There has also long been a British Association of Social Workers (visit www.BASW.org), but its political influence is minimal, since few people join it – a mistake. Distancing oneself from the compromised world of politics does of course give a sense of ideological purity, but little sway. So, join something is the advice, or soon you will have all the occupational influence of a call centre employee, and it will serve you right.

There are two major contributions within Pincus and Minahan's model. First, they propose that there are 'Four basic systems in social work practice':

1 *The change agent system.* This notion focuses our attention on the internal politics of social work agencies, since often ineffective approaches to social needs are more a product of bureaucratic inertia, or perverse incentives and disincentives, than the tractability or otherwise of the problems coming through the front door. Therefore, social workers need to use their skills to put their own house in order. It is an interesting exercise when invited to conduct an audit of who comes where for help, with what problems. More often than not no one has a clue, because no data are problem-based and are squeezed into the department's own preferred frame of reference.

2 *The client system.* This denomination reminds us that however convenient it is to have a single name on a manila folder, or a single reference number on a database, there are usually social entanglements which might either impede progress or, if harnessed, might have a good influence.

3 *The target system.* An unfortunate phrase perhaps, but this term simply reminds us of where, on the basis of our assessments of clients' troubles, we should focus our influence. There are a couple of examples below which will serve to illustrate this point.

4 *The action system.* This spin-off from task-centred casework (see Chapter 6) reminds us that social workers achieve most of their results when working in organized collaboration with other people. Often, particularly where there is a community element either to the causes of problems or to their potential improvement, we regard such people as friendly allies. Pincus and Minahan counsel us that at least as much effort should be put into collaboration as into direct work with clients.

The second important contribution from these authors is the idea of thinking about cases and community projects as having common stages, namely:

1 *Collecting data.* Gained by asking questions such as: How typical or unusual is this case? What do we know about similar problems in the literature? What is the typical route to referral for such cases? What do we know about the effectiveness of our usual measures?

2 *Making initial contacts.* Taking testimony about problems from the referred clients is typically an automatic reflex, but beyond this, contacts, say, with the school or the GP or members of the local community, can sometimes be just afterthoughts or are triggered by a crisis. Our assessments and our attempted solutions are the poorer for this.

3 *Negotiating contacts.* Over many years of professional experience we have yet to meet a client, or a collection of people who might be able to aid that client, who did not value the idea of writing down who is willing to do what for what purpose. Things can get very fuzzy, very quickly without this precaution.

4 *Forming and maintaining action systems.* This is the essential feature of community-based work, and reminds us of the issue of just who can be persuaded to join in a campaign to improve something with specific, achievable limits. Our experience is that if potential collaborators know that they are not having problems dumped on them, but that there is a sense of continuing project or case 'ownership' by the agencies making the request, then collaboration is likely to be better.

5   *Exercising influence.* Social workers have long been wary of the idea of *direct* influence (should the opportunity even arise) since it raises ethical problems, but not wary enough of the ethical consequences of limper forms of intervention or mere 'containment' (see Chapter 6). What shots do we have in the locker? Well, knowledge and expertise about how social and personal problems typically arise in the first place; knowledge of what – one hopes from the evidence-based literature – seems to work; knowledge of, and established working relationships with, other organizations in the community who might provide additional support; information; advocacy skills; relationship skills, and an ability to focus and coordinate the efforts of well-wishers on to the needs of either a case or community project.

6   *Termination.* This stage should have included the word 'evaluation' in its title, but we have written enough about this in other chapters. Suffice it to say that there is ample evidence that if potential collaborators know what they are signing up for, and for how long, that the scheme is being monitored and the interim results fed back to them, then they are more likely to stay involved.

This model has, in our experience, provided a good structure for the design of a social work training curriculum. The stages are similar, and one can always move sideways to particular implications, say, in mental health, childcare or the care of older people. The alternative is to go specialist in each of these fields and repeat the sequence of stages over and over again, which is inefficient.

What is wrong with this formulation as presented is not its structure but the *language* in which it is presented, which is pretty techno-awful. Systems-theory-based projects have done tolerably well in the empirical literature so that isn't the issue; it is rather that just adding the word 'systems' to the back of a description – though it rightly signals the often unattended-to complexity of arrangements in our field – does little else of practical value. 'Tailgunner Parkinson', of *Social Work Today* fame, once lampooned all this via a nursery rhyme parody:

> As I was going to St Ives
> I met a man with seven wife-systems;
> Every wife had seven catsystems, and
> Each subsystem had seven cat-systems . . .

However, having based a couple of curricula on Pincus and Minahan's model, we did see practical results. Here are some examples:

• A group of students noticed that elderly clients with chronic debt problems were over-represented in the agency caseload. These clients typically came from a large council-owned block where electricity bills were cripplingly high and there were constant problems with damp. Rather than continuing to see these clients individually, they gathered in the bills and organized a (well-attended) public meeting. Several of those present had written to the council complaining about the bills and the fungal growths on their inside walls, and had received individual replies recommending that they should all turn *up* their underfloor electrical heating and then open the windows to allow a flow of air (so using even more energy and producing even bigger bills). The students brought in 'Friends of the Earth' (who worked for nothing, incidentally) to solve the condensation versus structurally induced damp, and the inefficient heating system dilemma. With the aid of a few meters they pronounced for the latter cause. A report was prepared and sent to the Director of Housing, whose first response was to contact the Director of Social Services to ask who (the hell) these students were and what were they doing 'inciting' local people to complain. Much flack was taken, but thanks to a good Social Services team leader, the outdated electrical heating systems were eventually replaced.

- It was noticed by a group of community social workers that the 'meals on wheels' service for the frail elderly people living at home reported that, although grateful for the service, they often did not eat the food provided. Attempts were made to ask clients what kind of food they most enjoyed, but the responses contained a sub-text about how it felt to eat alone from a tin-foil box. The social workers piloted a scheme whereby a small fleet of buses provided by community transport would bring people to a centre to eat together, watch a film afterwards or just sit and talk to each other. An evaluation of this simple scheme showed that overwhelmingly the clients preferred it.
- A group of social workers concerned with the welfare of learning-disabled children and adolescents noticed that many of the problems coming their way – adverse attitudes at school, problems with peer relationships – were experienced in common. Rather than visiting each family individually, they organized meetings with families at the local community centre. The result, with the help of MENCAP, was a concerted as opposed to an individual approach by parents to pressure schools into something more inclusive.

The main message for social workers in this outline is: Look carefully at the case in front of you; where did it come from? How many others like this are there? What does the literature suggest you should do? If you are allegedly 'not allowed' to do that, how can you get it changed? The message for community workers is that beneath the commonalities of socio-economic position and neighbourhood conditions lie individuals with different, not always common, needs; the message for social workers is that 'liaison', collaboration and advocacy are not forgoable luxuries.

Part III

Client groups: common problems and what helps

10 Social work with children and families

Maxima debetur puero reverentia, sispuid turpe paras, nec tu pueri contempseris annos.

[A child deserves the maximum respect; if you ever have something disgraceful in mind, don't ignore your child's tender years.]

Juvenal (AD *c*.60–*c*.130) XIV: 47

Introduction

A scan of the legislation underpinning the involvement of the State in family life indicates that it is primarily structured around children's welfare. This reflects the dominant focus of social work policy and practice with families. It is true both with regard to helping families care for their children (family support) and the more interventionist area of child protection. As described in Chapter 1, the state has generally been reluctant to intervene in family life beyond a need to offset risks to the most vulnerable. Child abuse and neglect constitute such risks. In relation to family support, there have been political concerns since the Poor Law days that the more help one affords families the less responsible they become ('take responsibility away from people and they become irresponsible': Keith Joseph, 1974). While such concerns centre largely on the provision of financial aid, they have also coloured the ways in which family support has been conceptualized, namely addressing parental inadequacy and preventing undesirable outcomes. Delinquency, child abuse and neglect, and the costly alternative of removing children from the care of their parents, feature large in the list of 'undesirable outcomes'. Only with the introduction of the Children Act 1989 did policy and practice recognize the need for a more collaborative approach, based on a recognition that *all* families need support at some time.

The shift towards a more positive approach to family support is informed by a growing awareness of the part families play in promoting a range of important outcomes for children. The quality of children's experiences within the family can impact upon their educational achievement, their employment, their psychological and emotional adjustment, their physical and mental health and the extent to which they feel part of their community and society as a whole. For the state then, family support is an investment in securing a range of policy goals such as an effective labour force, good citizenship and in preventing spiralling costs in public services.

The organization of services

Parenting is a challenging task. For some, the everyday tasks of bringing up children are more difficult because they have other things to contend with. Domestic violence, substance misuse, serious mental health problems, problems with housing, immigration status and debt are serious enough challenges when they come as single issues. In some families these challenges come in bundles, and although the labels used are the same, the detail and meaning of such things as 'domestic violence' or 'mental health problems' are as varied as the families concerned. Having a particular problem does not mean someone is unable to be a good-enough parent. It does mean that some parents need additional support to provide adequate care. Unless effectively addressed, adults' problems can undermine the well-being of children, directly or indirectly, and in the short and long term. In a minority of cases, such difficulties can contribute to the neglect of children's physical, emotional and psychological well-being and adversely effect their development in a range of ways.

Research confirms the close relationship between parental problems and families coming to the attention of child protection services (see Hayden, 2004; James, 2004; Statham and Holtermann, 2004). It is not only childcare social workers, therefore, who have a role in family support, but social workers and other professionals working in education, health, mental health, substance misuse, housing and disability services. The need for cooperation is recognized in guidance to councils on the eligibility criteria they should operate with regard to adult services. This stresses the importance of them being 'prepared to address their responsibilities under the Children Act 1989' (DoH, 2002) and the importance of all those working with people who are parents to be alert to the support they may be need to carry out their parenting role. The *Framework for the Assessment of Children in Need and their Families* makes clear that the needs of parents form an important feature of a good-quality assessment and that other professionals with relevant expertise have a contribution to make to that assessment (DoH, 2000).

Unfortunately, the organizational separation of services has proved one of the most persistent obstacles to providing timely and appropriate support to families (see Darlington *et al.*, 2005). This exacerbates the resource constraints under which all agencies operate, driving up the thresholds of eligibility criteria. Not only are thresholds in both adults' and children's services high, but they tend to be 'independent' of one another – unlike the experience of families. Family 'B' may be eligible for help from *children's* services owing to worries about the impact of low intellectual ability and parental depression on a parent's capacity to provide care, but the same parent may fail the eligibility threshold for help from either the council's learning disability services or mental health community services (see CSCI, 2006).

Following the death of Victoria Climbié, Lord Laming conducted an inquiry whose report resulted in significant organizational and philosophical changes in England and Wales. The importance of inter-agency working, good-quality assessment, case planning and engaging with the child were all highlighted, as in previous inquiries. Laming, however, advocated additional changes in relation to organizational accountability and leadership that he hoped would bring about more effective practice and inter-agency collaboration (Laming, 2003). The government's response was encapsulated in the Green Paper *Every Child Matters* (Great Britain Cm 5860) and the Children Act 2004. *Every Child Matters* reinforced the importance of prevention and early intervention, and the Children Act 2004 introduced a range of measures designed to improve overall outcomes for children as well as strengthen the organizational arrangements underpinning child protection (see below).

Improving outcomes for children

In the Green Paper *Every Child Matters* (DfES, 2005a) the government set out policies aimed to reduce the number of children who experience educational failure, suffer ill-health, become pregnant as teenagers, are the victims of abuse and neglect, or become involved in offending and antisocial behaviour. In line with the views of those who were consulted, including parents and children, ministers 'wanted an approach that was less about crisis or failure, and more about helping every child to achieve his or her potential . . . an approach that involved children, families, communities and public services working to a shared set of goals, rather than narrow or contradictory objectives' (p. 14). The following five outcomes were identified as those that 'really matter for children and young people's well-being':

- Being healthy: enjoying good physical and mental health and living a healthy lifestyle.
- Staying safe: being protected from harm and neglect and growing up able to look after themselves.
- Enjoying and achieving: getting the most out of life and developing broad skills for adulthood.
- Making a positive contribution: to the community and to society and not engaging in antisocial or offending behaviour.
- Achieving economic well-being: overcoming socio-economic disadvantages to achieve their full potential in life.

In addition to the perceived benefits for children and future generations, the Green Paper notes that society as a whole benefits from reduced spending on avoidable problems and maximizing the contribution to society of all citizens. It notes that a child with a conduct disorder at age 10 will cost the public purse around £70,000 by age 28 – up to ten times more than a child with no behavioural problems (Scott, 2001). The overall cost of providing foster and residential care placements for 60,000 children is £2.2 billion per year.

The Children Act 2004 provides the statutory basis for the changes required to deliver these policy objectives, namely:

- *The integration of children's services.* The Act required the appointments of Directors of Children's Services and a Lead Member to assume responsibility for ensuring the integration of education and children's Social Services (DfES, 2005b).
- *New governance arrangements.* Leading local public bodies must work together under a new duty of cooperation in new children's trust arrangements (DfES, 2005c). In addition, children's services were required to set up new Local Safeguarding Children Boards and a range of partners to cooperate in establishing them (DfES, 2007).

- *An integrated strategy.* Local partners in the children's trust should develop a Children and Young People's Plan (DfES, 2005d) that sets out their shared priorities for improving outcomes for children and young people, and their plan for delivering the local Change for Children programme.
- *Integrated processes.* To support these changes, partners should introduce common assessments (DfES, 2005e), better arrangements for sharing information DFES, 2006), and processes and procedures to support integrated responses to children's needs.
- *Integrated front-line delivery.* Partners are expected to work together to refocus local children's services around the needs of children, young people and families, rather than professionals or organizations (DfES, 2005f).

The Act and the Green Paper make it clear that all those working with children, young people and families need to change how they work to achieve improved outcomes.

Children in need

Some services, such as health care and education, are available to all children. Others are only provided on the basis of particular eligibility criteria. For example, income support is only available to those whose income falls below a certain threshold. In England and Wales councils have a 'general duty':

- to 'safeguard and promote the welfare of children within their area who are in need';
- so far as is consistent with that duty, to promote the upbringing of such children by their families,

by providing a range and level of services appropriate to those children's needs (Children Act 1989, Section 17 (1)). Similar legislation governs the work of agencies and social workers in Northern Ireland and Scotland. Being a 'child in need' is the basic eligibility criterion operated in the allocation of family support services.

The Children Act 1989 (section 17(10)) defines a child in need in the following terms:

- he is unlikely to achieve or maintain, or to have the opportunity of achieving or maintaining, a reasonable standard of health or development without the provision for him of services by a local authority under this Part;
- his health or development is likely to be significantly impaired, or further impaired, without the provision for him of such services;
- he is disabled.

The Act is clear that 'development' refers to physical, intellectual, emotional, social or behavioural development; 'health' means physical or mental health and 'family' includes 'any person who has parental responsibility for the child and any other person with whom he has been living'. What the Act is less clear about is how to identify 'significant harm' or what 'a reasonable standard' means. It states: 'whether harm suffered by a child is significant turns on the child's health or development, his health or development shall be compared with that which could reasonably be expected of a similar child' (31(10)), and that priority should be given to the most vulnerable children. This suggests ambiguity and considerable scope for variation in how the Act is interpreted and implemented, and several studies confirm that this is indeed the reality. Colton *et al.* (1995a, 1995b) examined how childcare social workers and their senior colleagues defined need. The study revealed little consensus with regard to how need should be defined, about available guidance, and about what such guidance said.

Social workers tended to see 'reasonable care' and 'significant impairment' as opposite sides of the same coin. That is to say, a child who does not meet reasonable standards of development is, by definition, significantly impaired. Second, such children were believed, almost by definition, to be in need of protection. Colton and his colleagues are of the view that the dearth of guidance then available on how to assess need left a vacuum that social workers were filling by 'stretching' guidance on child protection to fit circumstances for which it was not designed. Colton *et al.*'s study also highlights the unintended consequence of finite budgets and growing demands (see also Aldgate and Tunstill, 1996). Despite wishing to be proactive in the help they offered families, managers were unable to do so for financial reasons. Finite budgets mean that the primary focus of agencies has typically been on children in need of protection 'now', leaving few resources available to families whose difficulties are at a relatively early stage. Families whose children are deemed to be in need of safeguarding continue to include substantial numbers of families who were unable to access appropriate help earlier (CSCI, 2006).

Safeguarding

Language shapes perception and behaviour, and itself is shaped by the ideologies of the day. The tendency to see family support and protection as separate and, with respect to resources, competing activities is partly attributable to the way that statutory duties and responsibilities are set out in the Children Act 1989, partly due to the way that services were organized, and the political and economic climate in which it was introduced (see Tunstill, 1997). The Children Act 2004 has introduced a change in terminology that it is hoped will change the way agencies and professional staff operate. It is specifically designed to bridge the artificial divide between 'prevention' or 'family support' and child protection. The language is the language of 'safeguarding' and was anticipated in two important overview reports produced by those Inspectorates responsible for children's services (SSI, 2002; CSCI, 2005).

The new organizational arrangements introduced in England and Wales by the Children Act 2004 are designed to improve the well-being of children and to safeguard their welfare. Sections 10 and 25(2) outline the duty of cooperation as follows:

(2) The arrangements are to be made with a view to improving the well-being of children in the authority's area so far as relating to –

    (a) physical and mental health and emotional well-being;

(b) protection from harm and neglect;
(c) education, training and recreation;
(d) the contribution made by them to society;
(e) social and economic well-being.

'Well-being' now has a legal status based on the five outcomes outlined in *Every Child Matters* (see above). The Act goes on to state that arrangements to safeguard and promote welfare 'must have regard to the importance of parents and other persons caring for children in improving the well-being of children' (10(3) and 25(3)). These arrangements include the setting up of Local Safeguarding Children Boards and the abolition of child protection registers that will be replaced by electronic records of children in need of protection. They also include the establishment of Children's Commissioners in each country within the UK.

As indicated earlier, there has been a growing appreciation of the range of factors that influence children's development and the outcomes and life chances they can expect. In the next section we consider the model that affords the most helpful way of making sense of these many types of influences, and that informs the assessment framework which most social workers now follow.

Ecological-transactional models

The reciprocal or interactive nature of factors influencing child development is well recognized, as is the importance of sensitive periods in which children are particularly susceptible to particular kinds of stress or adversity (see Glaser, 2000; Rutter and Sroufe, 2000). A number of models have been put forward better to understand the interplay between factors often operating at different levels (e.g. Sameroff and Chandler, 1975; Bronfenbrenner, 1979; Cicchetti and Rizley, 1981). They emphasize:

- the dynamic contribution of genetic, biological, psychological, environmental and sociological influences, and their cumulative impact over time;
- the fact that some factors increase vulnerability, while others exert a protective or insulating effect;
- that some factors can have an enduring impact on development, while others can vary or have a transient effect.

The ecological model provides a means of synthesizing research in a number of areas, including developmental psychology and developmental psychopathology. Most versions of this model identify the following interacting systems that impact upon development. The language leaves something to be desired, but here it is:

1   *The microsystem* refers to those systems in which an individual lives their day-to-day lives. For the child, this is his or her family. Infancy is usually spent with one or two adults in relatively simple activities: feeding, bathing, cuddling, sleeping, playing. As the child grows, the complexity of the activities in the home increase, as does the number of people with whom the child interacts. Exposure to a growing range of people and systems provides the basis of social development,

through the experience of relationships, as well as observation and new experiences. In this sense, the microsystem refers to the closeness or directness of influence on an individual.

2   *The mesosystem* refers to the relationships among microsystems and particularly between the family and other microsystems. It is sometimes represented as a part of the exosystem (see below). The stronger the relationships between the attitude to education that is present in the home and the school the stronger the influence of school.

3   *The exosystem* encompasses the social structures in which people live, including local councils, schools, churches and work groups. It includes informal as well as formal networks, the availability of services, of employment, of good housing and so on. The socio-economic climate of a community is part of the exosystem. They are systems in which the child does not play a direct role, but whose welfare is affected by the decisions and actions of those who do play a direct role within them. There is a wealth of research testifying to the impact of these factors on the experiences and life chances of individuals. If you live in a violent community you are more likely to be exposed to violence and to be the victim of violence. If the planning committee decides to build houses on the only green spaces in the neighbourhood, then a child's opportunities for sport, leisure and possibly friendship networks are influenced. Parents whose employment is regimented and oppressive may be more rigid in their styles of upbringing than those who are able to exercise influence over some choices.

4   *The macrosystem* is the term used to refer to the wider social milieu in which families and communities exist. It signals those aspects of cultural values and beliefs that foster societal attitudes, including law and policy, as these mediate the kinds of support and resources made available to citizens and communities. So, for example, societies that legislate against domestic violence and that take clear and decisive action to prevent it are likely to differ in significant ways from those that do not, with concomitant affects on the experiences of women and children. Cultural variation from the majority cultural group is seen as the legitimate adaptation to the contextual demands of that majority macrosystem, and valuable in their own right. The advantages of this approach include the reframing of cultural variation away from deficit or pathological models (see Garcia Coll *et al.*, 2000).

Within these interrelated systems the child is not a passive recipient of the actions of others, but – particularly in the early stages of development – can be adversely effected in ways that have long-term consequences. Maltreatment at a very early age can adversely effect a child's ability to negotiate the central tasks of that and subsequent developmental periods. For example, children need to learn how best to regulate their emotions in the face of a range of arousing and emotionally challenging situations. Early parent–child interactions play an important role in this 'developmental com-petency' (Cicchetti and Schneider-Rosen, 1986). Maltreated children present with a range of problems in their emotional self-regulation. Many express excessive amounts of negative affect, while others appear unable to express positive or negative affect ('blunted affect'). They have difficulties processing emotional stimuli and go on to have considerable difficulties coping with emotionally stressful situations, unable to make rational assessments of their experiences. Physically abused infants as young as 3 to 4 months old show early manifestations of these problems, including fear which, in non-abused children, do not usually emerge until months 8 to 9. Researchers hypothesize that maltreatment speeds up the development of fear, which in turn brings about corresponding neurobiological changes in the negative affect pathways of the brain. At this age, children do not have the cognitive capacity to process fear-inducing stimuli. This, in conjunction with distorted affective relationships with care-givers, may lead to serious problems in their ability to regulate and organize their emotional experiences (see Cicchetti and Toth, 1997; Cicchetti and Valentino, 2006). Thus, in terms of safeguarding, children with very poor attachments to care-givers may not be in 'imminent harm', but may be undergoing hard-to-observe changes that will seriously undermine their future well-being.

In short it seems that (1) a range of factors can play a causal role in child physical abuse; (2) some factors are 'proximal' (i.e. they operate in the 'here and now' or are of recent origin), while others are 'distal' and/or have a more cumulative effect (e.g. early childhood separation); (3) some factors may exert a protective influence and act as 'buffers' against the deleterious effects of adverse events (e.g. a supportive adult partnership or social network); and (4) the dynamic interplay of all factors means that the significance of one set of variables depends, to some extent, on the presence or absence of others.

In relation to child abuse and neglect, econological models emphasize four important factors:

- First, they emphasize that in order to understand how the care that some adults provide their children falls short of 'reasonable' or can lead to maltreatment, one needs to look beyond neat singleton factors to the range of influences which research suggests shape and trigger abusive behaviour.

- Second, they highlight the importance of *process*, that is, how factors interact. Checklists of so-called risk factors do not lend themselves to summative interpretation (i.e. the more factors, the more risk). Risk factors, particularly those from different 'categories' (e.g. environmental, interpersonal), interact in a range of ways, with some factors acquiring force over time, and others having more the characteristics of straws breaking the backs of already over-burdened camels.

- Third, they direct our attention to the strengths and strategies which appear to protect some individuals from engaging in abusive behaviour despite sharing many of the circumstantial and personal characteristics (or 'risks') that seem to precipitate it in others, and protect some individuals who are mistreated from the deleterious consequences which beset many others.

- Fourth, they signal the centrality of assessment to effective work. The principles of a good assessment are outlined in Chapter 5. The guiding principle should be that assessors consider the wide range of factors which research suggests may be contributing to family difficulties, and how these interact in a particular family.

In light of the above, we look first at an area that is gaining more significance in both policy and practice, namely primary prevention strategies. We then turn to the evidence of what interventions appear to be most effective in dealing with high-risk situations (secondary prevention) and situations where issues have already impinged upon children's well-being and safety (tertiary prevention).

What works in safeguarding children and promoting well-being?

Because we are concerned with the particular role of social workers, this chapter inevitably focuses on those issues within the family that, if not addressed, are thought adversely to effect children's well-being.

Decisions about when to intervene in people's lives is a complex business. Timely help may be critical in securing good outcomes, but it is not always clear when something is 'timely'. Despite the general consensus that early intervention is crucial, the evidence does not always bear this out (see below). For some problems, the evidence points to the cost-effectiveness of targeting interventions at those with already established problems. One of the factors that should influence policy decisions about what interventions should be undertaken is the evidence base for their effectiveness.

In this chapter we draw on terminology more commonly found (though not originating) in health, to distinguish three levels of intervention:

1 *Primary prevention* strategies are those used to prevent the occurrence of problems. They are usually aimed at whole communities or populations. Vaccinations are primary prevention health care interventions. Medico-social interventions such as health visiting fall into this category. Primary prevention interventions targeting social problems are known as 'early interventions'. Examples include parent education and day care. Primary prevention interventions may address a range of desiderata, some proximal (near in time) and others distal (longer term objectives). Some primary prevention strategies have explicitly targeted child abuse and neglect (see below) but most address more immediate concerns that may later have an impact upon the likelihood of maltreatment, such as parenting, school attendance, literacy and so on.

2 *Secondary prevention* approaches are those aimed at individuals or groups of individuals who are identified as being at high risk for a certain problem. Such groups would include those that research indicates may be at high risk of poor outcomes (e.g. children of disadvantaged teenage mothers, disabled children and their families).

3 *Tertiary prevention* refers to interventions aimed to ensure that problems that have already occurred do not occur again, or their adverse consequences are minimized. This includes work with families, the provision of services to children who may need to be removed from the care of their parents (either temporarily or permanently) and therapeutic work with children who have experienced these and other traumas.

Primary prevention

Economic and social interventions

Despite differing views about the magnitude of the impact of poverty and inequality upon children's health and development, and the mechanisms whereby poverty has its effect, there is little disagreement that it is a key factor in bringing about poor outcomes in the health and development of children (see Davey-Smith and Egger, 1986; Gelles, 1992; Roberts, 1997). Spencer (2000) observes, 'there is a consistent positive correlation between low socio-economic status and adverse . . . child health outcomes' (p.170). Roberts (1997) points to the 'long shadow forward' (p.1123) cast over physical and emotional health that can result from the experience of living in poverty during childhood. Children from these groups are less likely to fulfil their potential in education and are more likely to be unemployed or working in unskilled and poorly paid jobs in adult life. It is not surprising, therefore, that a serious contender for primary prevention is a series of changes aimed at redressing inequality, or, minimally, improving the socio-economic circumstances in which some children are raised. Where the aims have been explicitly to improve the conditions of children living in poverty, there have, typically, been four approaches used in the UK and USA (see Goodson *et al.*, 2000):

1   Enhancing children's educational experience: schemes designed to provide compensatory experiences by exposing children to experiences designed to optimise their intellectual, social, and emotional development.
2   Improving knowledge and skills in regards to the difficult task of parenting.
3   Improving economic resources.
4   Broad-based programmes of family support.

Early education

There is evidence that good-quality day care and pre-school education can help promote a range of good outcomes for children (see Sylva, 1994; Barnett, 1995). This evidence comes from a series of experimental evaluations of the impact of pre-school educational programmes upon disadvantaged children in America. It suggests that not 'any educational experience' will produce good outcomes for disadvantaged children. Rather, it is the *active-learning component* of particular pre-school programmes (e.g. plan/do/review) that appears to account for their effectiveness in providing children with long-lasting academic, cognitive and social gains. Here is Sylva's description of the curriculum:

> In the High/Scope curriculum children learn to be self-critical, without shame, to set high goals while seeking objective feedback. There is a deliberate encouragement to reflect on efforts and agency, encouragement to develop persistence in the face of failure and calm acceptance of errors.
>
> (Sylva, 1994: 142)

The positive experience of school which these programmes seem to engender appears to reduce the likelihood of early school failure and placement in special education, both key turning points in the lives of many children. Further, this positive attitude to school may be protective against later risk of maladjustment, delinquency and maltreatment. Evidence for the potential impact of these programmes on abuse and neglect is summarized in the following quote from two reviewers of early childhood programmes:

> Parents made positive changes in their own educational and employment levels and showed reductions in *Child Abuse and Neglect*. Early childhood programs clearly do help overcome the barriers imposed by impoverishment.
>
> (Campbell and Taylor, 1996: 78)

So, as a primary prevention strategy, early education may take a generation to make its mark on child protection, but it is not surprising that increasing a person's life chances appears to impact on their later ability to be a good parent.

These are important gains in an area where it has proved very difficult to make inroads. However, we need to be careful not to go beyond the evidence. With the exception of some flagship programmes such as the Perry Preschool project (Sweinhart *et al.*, 1993), the evidence about the impact of these programmes reliably to lift children out of poverty is all too slight. Even in the Perry Preschool programme a large number of participants remained living at, or just above, the poverty line some 30 years on. Generally, it seems that broader based, more intensive and longer term programmes that start early are what are needed.

Improving parental knowledge and skills

Expecting to bring about improvements in children's outcomes by enhancing parental knowledge and skills presumes that socio-economically disadvantaged parents know less and act differently from their financially secure counterparts. Research does indeed indicate that differences exist, but these may be attributable to other factors. Clarke-Stewart (1983) argues that once we take into account race, ethnicity, religion and family structure, these apparent differences disappear. Others have argued that socio-economic status is associated with differences in parenting styles owing to differences in exposure to the range of acute and chronic stressors that go hand in glove with poverty.

Improving economic well-being

That is, addressing the issue of lack of money through financial assistance is one way of seeking to improve family circumstances. Those reviewing the evidence note that while the mechanism for the impact of income on child health is not clear, it appears likely that household income in itself is important over and above access to resources. A systematic review of nine trials including more than 25,000 participants indicates that providing additional income to families may have a positive effect on children's emotional health, school achievement and their cognitive development (Lucas *et al.*, 2007).

Broad-based family support programmes

Partly due to the disappointing results of more 'focused' interventions (such as parenting education) and because of the recognition of the importance of the family in children's development, there have been a number of broader based interventions aimed at supporting parents and helping children. Among many such programmes in the USA, the Comprehensive Child Development Program (CCDP) was one of the most tightly designed and rigorously evaluated. These 22 successful projects that bid for funding were mandated to serve 'infants and young children from families who have incomes below the poverty line and who, because of environmental, health, or other factors, need intensive and comprehensive supportive services to enhance their development' (Public Law 100–297, Part E, Section 2502 – see Goodson *et al.*, 2000). The services these projects were required to provide included:

- Case management – based on the assumption that low-income families needed help to access and to use existing services, and might also require tailor-made resources. Case managers (lay professionals) conducted biweekly 30- to 90-minute home visits to each family for a number of years (families were enrolled in the programme for five years, though not all families remained for the duration). They undertook regular need assessments arranged for appropriate services, including specialist help.
- Early childhood education – projects had to ensure that all children received developmentally appropriate early childhood education. Up until age 3 this was generally provided in the home, often by the case manager, and usually worked via offering training to the parent. At age 3 children were enrolled in centre-based programmes.
- Developmental screening – leading to early referral to specialists if problems were identified.
- Referral to other services – including adult literacy education, child health services, prenatal care for women, mental health services for children and adults, substance-abuse education, parental education in child development, health and nutrition and vocational training.

The project organizers had to agree to participate in the evaluation – which was a randomized controlled trial. Four and a half thousand families were followed up for five years. To say the results were disappointing would be an understatement. Families in the experimental group (that received this intensive, multifaceted and long-term support) improved on a range of measures, including: improvements in vocabulary and achievement scores for children; a reduction of reliance on benefits (AFDC and food stamps); a reduction in the number of mothers experiencing depression; an increase in the number of parents gaining employment and/or continuing their education, and so on. But so did those in the control group, who had access to local services only, without the support of a case manager. In reflecting on the possible reasons for this 'draw' result, the researchers concluded that it was 'a fair test of this key policy alternative' (St Pierre *et al.*, 1999: 31). Their main conclusions? That the intervention did not work and that it demonstrated that 'the case management approach does not lead to improved outcomes for parents or children' (see also St Pierre *et al.*, 1999: 32). Importantly, the researchers note that had they not conducted an experimental evaluation they might have been misled into thinking that the intervention was effective, when in fact whatever was responsible for the observed changes was happening in the control group as well.

What of the UK? We have tended to look to the USA for examples of what might work, not least of all because of their better track record at funding demonstration projects with tight evaluations. Unfortunately, in the UK we have a habit of adopting promising approaches before the evaluation data are in.

Broad-based interventions of the type described above have received considerable attention and investment in the UK in recent years with initiatives such as SureStart. This £21-billion initiative was established with the aim of eliminating child poverty and social exclusion (Tunstill *et al.*, 2005). It is a universal programme, delivered on an area basis. This, it was hoped, would tackle the problem of stigma that may otherwise become attached to those who took up such services. The areas targeted were those marked by a high degree of deprivation, though as Rutter has pointed out, this meant that there was considerable variation among families, as most areas in the UK are heterogeneous in their make-up. While the initiative was based on previous research about what appeared to be effective, it was left entirely up to each community to decide what they wished to do and how they wished to do it ('flexibility'), although they did have to provide five core services: (1) outreach and home visiting; (2) support for families and parents; (3) good-quality play, learning and childcare; (4) primary and community health care, including advice about child and family health, and (5) support for children and parents with specialized needs. Like the CCDP, SureStart aimed to coordinate, streamline and 'add value' to existing services (cf. case management functions) and to augment and develop early years facilities (the childhood education function).

Unfortunately, the evaluation of SureStart was not constructed in such a way that the evaluators could easily disinter the effects of the SureStart intervention(s). In the circumstances the evaluators have been described as doing what they could to ensure that the results were 'unlikely to be due to either social selection or chance association' (Rutter, 2006: 3). The results of this expensive 'flagship' policy initiative are disappointing. The initiative was rushed, the interventions neither sufficiently well described, controlled nor implemented (unlike the CCDPs above), and rolled out nationally before the results of even the first pilot projects were available. Family and child functioning after three years for those 150 areas with SureStart, compared with those without, showed 'very few significant differences, with some indications of adverse effects in the most disadvantaged families', i.e. those families with teenage mothers, lone parents and workless households. Those who benefited most were the least needy.

SureStart is one of a number of major changes introduced into early years provision in the UK since 1997. In addition to SureStart there is now (1) an official early childhood curriculum (Foundation Stage of the National Curriculum); (2) free nursery education for 3-year-olds, and (3) the introduction of the Every Child Matters policy initiative (relatively new at the time of writing). In addition, the most deprived communities now have neighbourhood nurseries, and a national network of children's centres was launched in 2003 (Merrell *et al.*, 2007). Researchers at Durham examined the performance at school entry of some 35,000 children and found that their vocabulary, ability to count and name shapes were no better than that of children some six years ago (Merrell *et al.*, 2007). While it is argued that it is too early to draw firm conclusions (Hughes, 2007), Merrell and her colleagues reasonably contend that after five years one might have expected to see some return on this £51-billion investment.

The simplest conclusion from the evidence on early years intervention to date is that, while this is clearly the optimum point at which to intervene, it is very difficult objectively to demonstrate changes at the level of primary prevention. The evidence continues to suggest that (1) broad-brush approaches are a good bet and that (2) in seeking to improve intellectual capacity, work needs to be focused directly with children, rather than through their parents. The evaluations of the CCDP programmes suggest that if they are to be effective, services need to be relevant to families, of high quality, and sufficiently intensive and long term to bring about meaningful changes.

Primary prevention of the sexual abuse of children

Primary prevention interventions are key tools aimed at protecting children from the risk of sexual abuse. A number of carefully considered reviews exist (Carroll *et al.*, 1992; Finkelhor and Strapko, 1992; MacMillan *et al.*, 1994b), two of which have included meta-analysis (i.e. they have combined the results of single studies to ascertain a more secure estimate of effectiveness) (see Rispens *et al.*, 1997).

MacMillan and her colleagues identified 19 controlled studies published in English-language journals between January 1979 and May 1993 (MacMillan *et al.*, 1994b). All the studies took an educational approach, and compared verbal instruction alone or with one or more of the following: behavioural training, film, video or play. The effectiveness of the programmes was generally measured in relation to children's knowledge (via questionnaires) or skills thought to relate to prevention (assessed by verbal response to vignettes or to simulated conditions (e.g. stranger approach)). Only two studies included data on child disclosure of sexual abuse. Rispens *et al.*'s later review (1997) produced similar conclusions, although somewhat different inclusion criteria were used, as did a Cochrane review of school-based interventions (see Zwi *et al.*, 2007).

The Cochrane review identified 15 trials that measured knowledge and behaviour changes as a result of child sexual abuse intervention programmes. Children who participated in these interventions demonstrated statistically significant increases in knowledge of child sexual abuse and reported self-protective behaviours (12 studies). Two studies measured safe behaviours (in simulated situations). Children in these studies showed an increased likelihood of protective behaviours. Retention of knowledge was demonstrated in most studies at two to three months after the intervention but few studies looked beyond this time. Harms were not formally measured in most studies, but some reported increased negative outcomes (Zwi *et al.*, 2007). The overall conclusions in this area are as follows:

- All studies yielded positive results at the end of the programme. Children of all ages benefited and showed improved knowledge and, where measured, self-protection skills.
- At follow-up these improvements are not maintained at their original, post-intervention level, but still reveal significant changes.

- Programmes that include specific behavioural training in self-protection skills are more effective than those that do not.
- Longer/more intensive programmes achieve better results.
- Younger children generally demonstrate greater gains immediately following a programme, but these 'fade' at follow-up, adding weight to the argument that there should be more opportunities for repeated learning.
- Studies which provided data on socio-economic status (50 per cent) suggest that children from lower socio-economic groups benefit most from preventive programmes. However, there is also evidence of a 'fading' of effects over time, suggesting that socio-economic status may also be associated with poor retention of knowledge and skills.
- There is no evidence on the transferability of knowledge and 'proxy' skills to real-life situations in which children are at risk of sexual abuse.

The findings of one study suggest that behavioural skills training may be less confusing for pre-school children than 'feelings-based' programmes (see Wurtele *et al.*, 1989). More attention needs to be paid to developing programmes which are tailored to the developmental age of children, particularly their cognitive ability. Note, however, that adverse effects were reported in three of the studies included in the Cochrane review.

Secondary prevention

As with primary prevention, most promising interventions in secondary prevention are multifaceted, seeking to address a range of factors associated with enhanced risk (see Barth, 1989). Although there are emerging trends, all too few interventions have been rigorously evaluated. Those that have are directed at factors thought to be associated with inadequate parenting. This includes those factors believed to place children at risk of maltreatment, although studies rarely collect data on abusive behaviour per se. In this section we begin with a consideration of interventions based on attachment theory before moving on to some broader based interventions. We conclude with a consideration of other factors that impact on parenting.

Attachment-based interventions

Attachment is an important concept for social workers. Prior and Glaser (2006) have published an excellent overview of research in this area, covering the origins and development of attachment theory, research on prevalence and incidence, and the evidence about what works in helping parents whose infants have experienced attachment difficulties.

Attachment is often described as an emotional bond between two people. It does not indicate *any* attachment between *any* two people. Rather, it signifies the tie between an infant and his or her care-giver, based on the infant's need for safety, security and protection. Small children do not have the wherewithal to meet their own needs or to protect themselves from threats to their well-being. They therefore need to stay close to someone who can do this for them. This attachment behaviour is a set of behaviours essential to survival and adaptation.

Our early experiences of care-giving impact upon the nature and security of our attachments. In turn these shape the people we become (see above). Howe (1995: 24) has summarized this as follows:

> In our development, what is on the social outside eventually establishes itself on the psychological inside. In this sense, relationships with others become internalised. It is in our relationships with others that our self forms, the personality takes on many of its characteristics.

In attachment theory, the concept of 'internal working models' is used to signify the mental representations children develop of the relationship between the self and the care-givers to whom they are attached, irrespective of the nature of that attachment. The theory also talks of the defences children develop when the care-giving they experience is not adequate. These can include the denial of feelings.

For most infants, the development of attachment follows a predictable course, although the phases are not tightly defined:

- *Phase 1*: From birth to not less than 8 weeks, the infant uses those behaviours available to him or her to attract attention from, or respond to, his care-giver(s). Even in this 'initial pre-attachment' phase (Bowlby, 1969) the infant is learning to discriminate between adults.
- *Phase 2*: From 8 weeks to around 6 months of age, the infant becomes more adept at distinguishing familiar from unfamiliar adults and becomes especially responsive to his or her main carer.
- *Phase 3*: From 6 or 7 months the infant's behaviour becomes more organized. Bowlby writes: 'Thenceforward, it seems, he discovers what the conditions are that terminate his distress and make him feel secure, and from that phase onward he begins to be able to plan his behaviour so that these conditions are achieved' (Bowlby, 1969: 351). This phase continues until well into the child's third year. Because he or she can now walk and communicate, the child actively uses the carer (usually a mother-figure) as a base from which to explore (secure base) and a place of safety when threatened ('secure haven' – Ainsworth *et al.*, 1978).
- *Phase 4*: For some children this phase might start in the second year, though for many it will be much later – in or after the third year. When children reach ages 3 to 4 they can begin to understand the reasons underlying separations, and can make appropriate adjustments. In this phase the child begins to recognize the carer as an independent person.

The majority of children establish effective attachments, particularly with their mothers, but also with other adults responsible for their care, though attachments usually have a recognizable order of importance for the child. For some children, however, their attachment behaviours do not develop securely. For a variety of reasons some carers are unable to provide the sensitive and kindly protection that their child's attachment behaviours are designed to trigger.

Through a series of carefully controlled experiments Ainsworth identified a number of types of attachment. Her experiments are known as the 'stranger situation' experiments. Infants (12–18 months) were brought into a laboratory setting with their mother and subjected to varying forms of stress involving a number of two- to three minute separations. A stranger is sometimes present. The infant's behaviour was observed before, during and after separation. Ainsworth identified three kinds of attachment behaviour, to which a fourth was later added. She used a system of letters to denote each category. These are as follows:

Secure	B	Uses care-giver as a secure base. Misses parent on separation. Greets on reunions. Goes to when upset.
Insecure/avoidant	A	Explores, but little display of secure base. Little distress when left. Avoids parent on reunion, stiffens or looks away.
Insecure/ambivalent	C	Distressed on entering the laboratory. Little exploration. Distress on separation. Passive or angry on reunion. Hard to comfort.
Disorganized	D	Incomplete, interrupted movements. Freezing. Fear of parent. Main feature is lack of coherent attachment strategy.

In general, certain patterns of attachment are associated with particular kinds of parenting style (Table 10.1).

Table 10.1 Types of parenting style

Parenting	*Attachment*
Consistently responsive	Secure B
Consistently unresponsive	Avoidant A
Inconsistently responsive	Ambivalent C
Dangerous/frightening	Disorganized D

There is a large literature on attachment and the problems associated with insecure attachments (see Howe, 2006; Prior and Glaser, 2006). In essence, we may conclude that:

1 We all need relationships that provide a safe haven for emotional support and a sense of safety and a secure base for 'exploration'.
2 These relationships are *selective* and are indicated by a desire for proximity and distress at forced separation.
3 Insecure or disorganized attachment behaviours in infancy and early childhood carry risks for later relationships and of subsequent psychosocial problems.
4 Marked disturbances in early care-giving (such as abuse, neglect, multiple carers) frequently lead to problems in developing secure attachments to new carers.
5 The longer the poor experiences have lasted, the greater the likelihood of problems. Problems are not specific to 'attachment' relationships but tend to generalize to all relationships.
6 These problems are often very difficult to deal with and challenge new carers' normal care-giving capacities to the limit. Affection and stability often seem insufficient on their own – ask any foster carer.

Children experiencing neglect, children whose mothers are psychologically and emotionally 'unavailable' (due to mental illness, for example), and children who have experienced physical and/or emotional abuse are likely to develop wary and insecure attachments. This tendency can have long-term consequences. Sometimes, it appears that some mothers have difficulty in responding appropriately to certain of their children. It is this latter group that we are considering in this section.

Attachment theory-based interventions

As will be evident from our brief summary of attachment theory, the quality and sensitivity of a child's primary care-giver is essential to the development of secure attachments. When a parent or other carer is insensitive to their child's needs they are also likely to be neglectful of them, posing further risks to the child.

In a meta-analysis of interventions designed to enhance carer sensitivity and promote attachment, Bakermans-Kranenburg *et al.* (2003) identified 81 studies that met their inclusion criteria, 51 of which were randomized controlled trials. The measures used included assessments of care-giver sensitivity and ratings of attachment security. Interventions were categorized according to whether they were designed to improve sensitivity (see Black and Teti, 1997), to bring about changes in carers' mental representations (see Cicchetti *et al.*, 2000) or to provide social support and practical help in changing behaviour (Barnett *et al.*, 1987), or a combination of these. The reviewers sought to answer a number of questions, but of particular interest is what were the most effective interventions.

Maternal sensitivity

Overall the authors concluded that interventions targeting maternal sensitivity produced a significant, albeit moderate effect when measured statistically. Based on the randomized controlled trials, they concluded that interventions focusing only on sensitive maternal behaviour (compared with those also providing 'support') appear 'rather successful' in improving sensitive parenting as well as infant attachment insecurity. The most effective interventions:

- Incorporated video feedback.
- Start after the child is 6 months old.
- Were short. Interventions with fewer than five sessions were as effective as those with 5 to 16 sessions and more effective than those longer than 16 sessions.
- Were provided by non-professionals.
- Involved fathers (though they note that this association should be viewed with caution as there were few studies and these were not randomized controlled trials).

Infant attachment

When looking at the impact of interventions on infant attachment, a similar pattern of findings emerged from the 23 randomized controlled trials that measured this outcome:

- The impact on attachment security was statistically small but significant.
- Interventions aimed only at enhancing sensitivity were the only interventions that indicated a statistically significant effect on attachment security.
- By and large, these improvements were achieved irrespective of socio-economic status.

High-risk families

The authors went on to examine the effectiveness of interventions with families with multiple risks. They hypothesized that these families would need more intensive and multifaceted interventions. In fact, from the 15 relevant studies, the findings echoed those reported above. The most effective interventions were those that focused on sensitivity, started at age 6 months, used video feedback and were behaviourally based.

Relationship between sensitivity and infant attachment security

The authors also concluded that the only intervention studies that yielded a significant effect size on attachment security were those that also brought about significant shifts in sensitivity.

As may be seen from a perusal of the studies included in the review by Bakermans-Kranenburg and her colleagues, attachment interventions vary considerably in design, their conceptual assumptions, and the goals of therapy. Most entail providing a safe and supportive environment, helping the carer to 'tune' into her child; to be physically accessible (perhaps by sitting on the floor with him or her) and to be emotionally responsive (perhaps via play). There is often an element of information sharing or education, but this is only one small element in the most effective interventions. As indicated above, one of the most powerful mechanisms for change appears to be the chance to learn by doing, to receive feedback (via video) and to have an opportunity to reflect on that feedback with a supportive person.

Home visiting

Home visiting programmes occupy the same space as attachment interventions insofar as many schemes are directed towards mothers whose circumstances place them at risk of less than optimal parenting. Home visiting programmes vary enormously, but most focus on helping (1) to shape parenting skills, (2) to enhance the parent–child relationship, and (3) to improve relationships with informal and formal networks. Visitors may be trained nurses, laypeople or para-professionals. There have been a number of reviews of the effectiveness of these interventions (Olds and Kitzman, 1990; MacMillan *et al.*, 1994a; Clémant and Tourginy, 1997).

MacMillan and her colleagues undertook a systematic review of home visiting programmes that included a specific focus on abuse and neglect. It is important to note that of the 11 studies reviewed, only two reported outcomes directly relevant to child abuse (i.e. reports of abuse), and of these, one was a primary prevention study as defined in this chapter (Hardy and Street, 1989). The other (Olds *et al.*, 1994) was a fairly long-term programme of visiting by trained nurses, begun *during* pregnancy and designed to address a number of aspects of maternal and child functioning, namely:

- outcomes of pregnancy for mother and child;
- the qualities of care-giving (including associated child health and developmental problems);
- maternal life-course development (helping mothers return to education or work, and to plan future pregnancies);
- the prevention of child maltreatment.

(Olds, 1997: 133)

Versions of the Olds programme have been widely adopted and held up as a model in the UK. The programme is grounded in an ecological framework (see p. 198) and conceptualizes the adequacy of care provided by parents as a function of other relationships, and the wider social context. Home visitors therefore focus attention on the social and material environment of families. They seek to promote informal networks of friends and family members who can provide reliable sources of material and emotional support. In the course of its development the programme has gradually paid more attention to theories of human attachment, and to the perceived importance of self-efficacy theory (i.e. that human behaviour is partly a function of how effective people perceive themselves to be). The latter have resulted in an emphasis on behaviour rehearsal, reinforcement and problem-solving. This has had particular relevance to the process of helping, stressing the importance of:

- establishing an empathic relationship between mother and home visitor;
- reviewing with care-givers their own child-rearing histories;
- the development of an explicit focus on promoting a sensitive, responsive and engaged care-giving in the early years of a child's life.

Mothers received an average of nine visits during their pregnancy and 23 visits (SD = 15) from birth through the second year of the child's life. The results showed that of those who received home visiting, only 4 per cent abused or neglected their children, compared with 19 per cent of those who did not receive this service. Between their 24th and 48th month of life, children of home-visited women were 40 per cent less likely to visit a physician for an injury or ingestion (poisoning) than those in the comparison group, and they lived in homes with fewer safety hazards, and which were deemed more conducive to their intellectual and emotional needs (Olds *et al.*, 1995). However, there were no differences noted in referrals for child maltreatment during this period. The authors point out that child maltreatment in the comparison group is likely to be under-detected, and over-detected in the experimental group due to the increased surveillance. The reality is that subsequent replications of the programme have had less striking results.

The *Child Development Programme* is a UK-based programme (Barker, 1988, 1994). Essentially it makes available a source of social support for first-time mothers, and encourages them in the task of parenting. This support was provided originally by specially trained health visitors, known as 'first parent visitors', but has subsequently been provided by experienced mothers who receive support and training. The programme seeks to empower parents, and to give them a sense of control over their lives and their children's upbringing. The visitors focus on all areas of a child's development, health and nutrition, and use semi-structured methods to foster parents' development. Parents are encouraged to set themselves developmental, dietary, health or other tasks to carry out with their children in the coming months. As with the Olds' programme, there is an emphasis on the health and well-being of the mother, in her role as a woman with her own interests and future, and not merely the mother of her children. Some of the work is done in groups in order to promote social support. Finally, enhancing the role of the father/partner is taken seriously.

Two randomized controlled trials have been conducted into the effectiveness of this programme. The first focused on trained health visitors (Barker, 1988), the second examined the effectiveness of the programme using specially trained community mothers (Johnson *et al.*, 1993). Other evidence comes from the analyses of longitudinal data gathered on the very large numbers of families served by the programme over a number of years. Results indicate improvement on a variety of home environment factors, such as language and cognitive development, and the nutrition of 'intervention' children, as well as reductions in child abuse and neglect. Barker attributes the success of the project to the involvement of laypeople, 'community mothers' whom he believes are more acceptable to new parents, and are more likely to be able to understand and assist. This is a complex debate, with more opinions than data.

Parenting programmes

A variety of circumstances can undermine a parent's capacity adequately to care for a child. If substance misuse or depression are major causes for concern, then staff need to take into account what is known about the relative effectiveness of different treatments. In this section we consider other factors that make parenting particularly challenging and that are now generally addressed through some form of parenting programme. These difficulties take the form of problems in understanding, perception, knowledge and skills, or combinations of these. Problems might arise from not having had a good experience of parenting oneself, so being short of 'know-how', or having a child who is temperamentally difficult and/or behaviourally demanding (see Chapter 7). High levels of negative emotion can distort a parent's judgements about their children's behaviour, increasing their negative expectations. Negative emotions, psychological or mental distress can also disrupt parents' ability to monitor and attend to their children's behaviour, and disrupt their ability to problem-solve and think clearly about child-rearing conflicts (Patterson, 1982; Dix, 1991). Broadly speaking, parent training programmes endeavour to address these problems areas. Fundamentally, they aim to enhance parents' abilities to manage their children's behaviour, to reduce conflict and confrontation while increasing compliance, cooperation and pleasant interaction, and generally to alter the balance of reward and punishment in favour of the former. This may entail any combination of the following:

- providing information about child development, health, hygiene, safety and so on;

- helping parents reconsider and reframe 'age-inappropriate' expectations and misattributions;
- enhancing the quality of child–parent relationships by, for example, teaching play skills, structuring the day so that they set aside some time for them and their child(ren);
- developing parents' ability to monitor and track their children's behaviour and respond appropriately, including the management of challenging behaviour;
- building up support networks.

However, there is great variation in the 'recipes' to be found in the literature (see Polster *et al.*, 1987; Smith, 1996) and few programmes of any formula have been subjected to rigorous scrutiny (see Barlow and Parsons, 2003). Of these, only a handful involve work with parents deemed to be at 'high risk'.

In their systematic review, Barlow and Parsons demonstrated the effectiveness of parent-training programmes in improving behaviour problems in children aged 3 to 10 years. Overall, group-based programmes produced superior results to individual programmes, and behavioural programmes produced superior results to either Adlerian or Parent Effectiveness Training (PET) programmes. Cognitive-behavioural programmes enjoy considerable support in helping parents at risk of abusing or neglecting their children, and the evidence for this is discussed in relation to tertiary prevention, as studies often combine parents known to have maltreated their children with those considered to be at risk of doing so. The results are, for the most part, encouraging. However, the evidence suggests that effective interventions for such families need a broader focus than purely child management, and need to be provided on a longer term basis (Patterson *et al.*, 1982). What is also important is a more considered approach to the recruitment and retention of families who most need this kind of help and support.

Evidence from studies conducted by Webster-Stratton and Herbert (1993, 1994) reinforce the importance of attending to the *process* of helping as well as to the content. Working collaboratively with parents, helping them to develop their self-esteem and self-efficacy are key components of success in these interventions. Before moving on to consider one particular cognitive-behavioural intervention – anger management – it is worth noting a further promising use of cognitive-behavioural approaches relevant to secondary prevention.

Work with learning-disabled parents

Learning-disabled parents face particular problems in parenting which can contribute to problems of neglect, developmental delay and behaviour problems in their children (Tymchuk and Feldman, 1991; Feldman and Walton-Allen, 1997). Learning-disabled parents are more likely to have their children removed from their care than other parents. This reflects prejudice and discrimination, but also indicates the parenting difficulties that learning-disabled people encounter in the absence of appropriate support from informal and formal networks (Feldman, 1998). Some studies have indicated that learning-disabled parents experience high levels of stress and depression, which may contribute to their parenting difficulties (Feldman *et al.*, 1998) and these may arise, in part, from the adverse social circumstances in which they often live. Children of learning-disabled parents are themselves at risk for developmental delay (Scally, 1957; Reed and Reed, 1965; Feldman and Walter-Allen, 1997) and may need compensatory social and educational experiences, in addition to interventions aimed at improving their general level of care and stimulation.

Feldman describes a home-based parent-training intervention designed to help learning-disabled parents improve their parenting skills, and reduce the risk of child neglect, developmental delays and behaviour problems. Trained parent education therapists visited participants' homes twice weekly (more often if necessary, and for new-borns). In addition to parenting skills training, the staff provided ongoing counselling, stress management, community living and social skills training. The programme was sensitively and carefully structured, and made use of direct observation, modelling, instruction and reinforcement. Training was pitched at the skills required for caring for a child at the age relevant to the family. Trainers saw their work as an essential component of a multi-agency approach.

The results of a number of evaluations testify to the promise of these programmes (see Feldman *et al.*, 1989, 1992a, 1992b, 1993). Feldman and his colleagues do not regard parent training as a panacea, and are aware that other interventions, such as specialized pre-school programmes, may have more to offer some children whose parents are learning disabled. However, they rightly highlight the need for specialized and carefully tailored interventions to help with problems faced by those with learning disabilities. A problem with parent training as a 'one-off' is that the skills necessary to care for a 1-year-old baby will not suffice to meet the needs of a toddler or an 8-year-old. Parents with learning disabilities may need long-term help and support that is shaped by the developmental needs of the child.

Anger management

Anger control training typically involves the following steps:

1   Teaching parents to identify cues that signal potentially uncontrollable anger. These may be physiological: tension, shaking, 'going hot'; or situational: provocative situations such as at bedtimes or at the supermarket, where the parent feels particularly vulnerable.
2   Teaching parents how to relax when these cues are identified and to use various coping strategies. These might include: deep breathing; engaging in an alternative activity; changing the way he or she thinks about the situation.
3   Problem-solving – teaching parents to generate alternative (non-aggressive) responses to situations in which children provoke their ire.

Whiteman *et al.* (1987) compared the relative effectiveness of three components of anger management by allocating participants to one of each of the following:

- cognitive restructuring (aimed at rectifying misattributions of children's behaviour – see Graham, 2004 and Chapter 7);
- problem-solving skills (learning to think of alternative ways of resolving conflicts or dilemmas);
- relaxation (staying calm so that the parent will be less likely to hit out);
- a combination of relaxation, cognitive restructuring *and* problem-solving skills.

The results of this small, randomized controlled trial showed a reduction in anger measures for those in each of three experimental groups, with the composite group doing best. Unfortunately this study relied rather heavily on self-report and role-play measures.

Finally a cautionary note. One of the dangers of résumés of effective strategies is that they tempt practitioners to adopt a 'tool-box' approach to intervention. If there is one thing that the better studies teach us it is that careful assessment is (almost) all. Because the aim of anger-management strategies is to help individuals identify the buildup of aggression from its earliest signs – when they are most likely to be able to intervene successfully – this approach is contraindicated for those whose tempers, coupled with physical violence, is 'instantaneous' and unpredictable.

Tertiary prevention

When children have already experienced significant harm, or where the risk is such that if we do not do something decisive then harm will result (nothing predicts behaviour like behaviour), we find ourselves in the arena of tertiary prevention. At this level there are very few rigorous evaluations of interventions. The studies we have recruit both families who have abused or neglected their children with those thought at serious risk of doing so. This further complicates our evidence base. Do poor results simply mean that seriously maltreating families are masking good outcomes with those families who are 'only at risk' of doing so? Are good results due to the inclusion of high-risk families?. In short, the available evidence base underpinning what therapeutic (as opposed to administrative or legal) interventions are rather slight and not always clear-cut. In the next section we provide an overview of promising trends.

Cognitive-behavioural parent training

One important emerging trend is that behavioural and cognitive-behavioural approaches have much to offer in dealing with the problems which need to be changed if abuse and neglect are to be prevented from recurring (see Gough, 1993; Wolfe *et al.*, 1997). These programmes typically combine parent training with self-management techniques (such as anger control) and problem-solving and are increasingly delivered in contexts which also attend to the broader social conditions in which children and families live. Other sources of evidence of the effectiveness of such approaches may be found in Wolfe and Sandler, 1981; Wolfe *et al.*, 1981, 1982; Egan, 1983; Crimmins *et al.*, 1984.

However, while there are more outcome studies of cognitive-behavioural approaches in tertiary prevention than anything else, controlled *group* studies are still relatively few in number, and most have been conducted in the USA.

A common theme emerging from the research is that long-standing, complex problems generally yield less optimum outcomes, and may well require broader based, long-term, intensive patterns of intervention. This is in contrast to the general trend in psychotherapeutic literature which suggests that if change is to occur it usually does so within the first 12 weeks of an intervention, and that thereafter the gains are marginal (see Rachman and Wilson, 1980). Task-centred or brief approaches, while appropriate for many situations, may need to give way to longer term, more broadly based programmes.

Broader based cognitive-behavioural interventions

As well as encountering problems in child management, families in trouble are likely to need help with relationship problems, problems of depression and/or low self-esteem, substance misuse, as well as the socio-economic troubles which are of such importance. An appreciation of the role played by these other factors in the aetiology and maintenance of family problems, including abuse, has influenced the development of two rather broader based approaches to cognitive-behavioural assessment and intervention. The first is known as behavioural family therapy (see Griest and Wells, 1983; Thyer, 1989). The second is called 'ecobehavioural'.

Behavioural family therapy is an approach based on the premise that many factors conspire to produce abuse and neglect, that a number of these factors are located within the family (or can be intervened with at the level of the family), and that cognitive-behavioural approaches are effective ways of intervening in these difficulties. The substantial evidence base for behavioural family therapy lies predominantly in reports of work directed at specific, relevant aspects of family functioning, such as inter-parental conflict, alcohol misuse or depression (see Chapter 8), but we still lack a sufficiency of studies which clearly explore the use of these techniques (and any other approach) on families where abuse and/or neglect has occurred.

Family-based behavioural approaches have also been evaluated in the context of the broader, multi-systemic approach called ecobehavioural. These programmes target identified problems in a range of settings including, but not restricted to, the family. *Project 12-Ways* is among the best known and best evaluated of these, and derives its name from the 12 core services described in the original programme: parent–child training, stress reduction for parents, basic skills training for the children, money management training, social support, home safety training, multiple-setting behaviour management *in situ*, health and nutrition, problem-solving, couples counselling, alcohol abuse referral, and single mother services (*in situ* in order to help maximize the generalization and maintenance of newly learned skills).

The overall picture is that this is an effective intervention which reduces abuse and neglect. A five-year follow-up of more than 700 families, 352 of which had received services from this project, indictes that families had consistently lower rates of abuse across all years, except one (1981, when the rate was similar to that of the control group: Lutzker and Rice, 1984). In another report, Lutzker makes the case that those families who receive services from *Project 12-Ways* are significantly less likely to be reported again from child abuse and neglect up to four years after services (Lutzker and Rice, 1984), even though – in some of the evaluations – project families had more severe problems than their control counterparts. The authors note, however, that over time the incidence of reported abuse increases for both groups, and the gap between them, while still statistically significant, looks clinically less impressive. In other words, there seems to be what they call a 'wash-out' effect over time, perhaps because some families dropped out of the project, or had not been successfully helped. It may just point to a need for 'booster services' or additional support to these families in order to maintain the early differences between the group.

Social network interventions

Social network interventions are those that explicitly aim to address the problems of abuse and neglect by increasing the amount and quality of social support available to needy and socially isolated parents. Only one controlled study has been conducted to date, but it is methodologically quite secure, and is one of the few studies primarily to target the needs of neglectful parents (Gaudin *et al.*, 1990–1991; Gaudin, 1993).

The intervention begins with an assessment of existing community formal and informal support, and an individual assessment of a family's informal support network, covering size, composition and supportiveness. This is followed by a psychosocial assessment aimed at identifying the range of problems facing a family, across a range of settings (e.g. school, home, housing, substance misuse, debt). Significant material and psychosocial barriers to the development of supportive networks are identified (e.g. lack of telephone, poor verbal and social skills, poor self-esteem, unresolved conflicts with family members or neighbours) and goals for intervention are agreed with the family. Five approaches are used alongside professional casework/ case management activities that include extensive advocacy and brokering of formal services:

- Personal networking. Direct interventions to promote family members' existing or potential relationships with family members, friends, neighbours or work associates.
- Establishing mutual aid groups which focus on teaching parenting and more broadly based social skills, to develop mutual problem-sharing, problem-solving and to enhance self-esteem.
- Recruiting and training volunteers to do tasks akin to 'family aides' in the UK.
- Recruiting neighbours as informal helpers. These people were paid a small sum, and received the support and weekly guidance of the social workers.
- Social skills training.

Given the recognized difficulties in intervening effectively with neglectful families (Daro, 1988), the results of this study are particularly encouraging. Eighty per cent of those who received at least nine months' help improved their parenting from neglectful or severely neglectful to marginally adequate parenting (on the standardized parenting measures used in the study). Almost 60 per cent of cases were closed because of improved parenting. However, the authors point to a number of problems. First, in terms of the study, all the participants were voluntary, so it is unclear whether these results would generalize to reluctant or resistant parents. Second, there was a high drop-out rate due to the extreme mobility of the families involved. One of the major implications for mainstream practice within the UK is that this intervention requires frequent, consistent professional consultation for problem-solving and support, and successful implementation depends on manageable case loads of 20 or fewer, and well-trained social workers with specific knowledge and skills.

Family therapy

We have discussed family therapy in more detail in Chapter 8. Here we highlight one or two interventions that relate particularly to child maltreatment.

Brunk and her colleagues compared the effectiveness of parent training and multi-systemic therapy – systemic family therapy which encompassed attention to the role of cognitive and extrafamilial variables in maintaining problem behaviours, in this case child abuse and neglect. Eighteen abusive and 15 neglectful families were randomly allocated to either parent training (run in groups) or multi-systemic family therapy (conducted in the home). Each programme operated for 1.5 hours per week over eight weeks. In brief, both interventions appeared to bring about statistically significant improvements in the following areas: parental psychiatric symptomatology, overall stress, and the severity of identified problems. Pre-post-test comparisons suggested that parent training was most effective in reducing identified social problems (perhaps because of the group format) and multi-systemic family therapy had the edge on changing parent–child relationships, and facilitated positive change in those behaviour problems that identify maltreating families (see Crittenden, 1981).

In the UK, we have made a considerable investment in the legal and administrative infrastructures aimed at preventing child abuse and neglect. We now need urgently to focus our attention on the *content* of our services for such vulnerable children and their parents. The evidence base regarding *what works* in helping parents to care more adequately for their children is not bewilderingly large or complex, and has some clear messages. The evidence points consistently to a handful of approaches that merit consideration, but which are not routinely used in the UK, although they are gaining ground. Many others that enjoy no such evidence of effectiveness are routinely used none the less. In working with vulnerable children and their parents, we owe a duty of care to deploy those interventions most likely to prove effective.

Addressing the problems of parents

We conclude this chapter with a discussion of some of the problems that can beset adults and which routinely impact upon the welfare of children.

Parents who misuse drugs and/or alcohol

The literature on substance misuse is large, reflecting the complexity of the subject matter, and it is difficult to find unequivocal messages regarding 'what works'. Nowhere is this more so than in relation to women who misuse legal or illegal substances, where researchers have done more to document the failure of professionals to tailor interventions to their particular needs than to develop effective interventions for this group (see Finkelstein, 1994; Howell *et al.*, 1999). To some extent this is reflected in policy guidance, where there is more information available regarding the prevalence and incidence of substance misuse, its impact upon children and how to go about assessing this, than on effective treatment options (see Royal College of Psychiatrists, 2002). Robust outcome studies are few, and often fail to differentiate between different kinds of substance misuse.

Most evaluative work has focused on the use of drugs, such as imipramine or naltrexone. Few psychological interventions have been rigorously evaluated and no good-quality systematic reviews can be identified at the time of writing. A review conducted in Sweden suggests that psycho-social treatment methods with a clear structure and well-defined intervention have favourable effects on alcohol dependence. These include cognitive-behavioural therapy and the 12-step treatment (Berglund *et al.*, 2001). This review also concluded that relearning therapies (cognitive-behavioural therapy) targeted at the behaviour of drug abusers are the most effective among the psycho-social methods for treating heroin and cocaine dependence. The authors conclude that psycho-social therapies used to address other drug addictions have no proven effect or are insufficiently studied. This was not an international systematic review, so the results must be treated with some caution (see also Kownacki and Shadish, 1999 and Chapter 13, this volume).

We urgently need better to understand what factors encourage or inhibit people from entering or remaining in treatment programmes, if we are to provide services that are acceptable as well as effective (Tracey and Farkas, 1994; Nelson-Zlupco *et al.*, 1995; Tsogia *et al.*, 2001). Reviewing the literature on substance abuse treatment for pregnant women, Howell *et al.* conclude there is no clear evidence that one form of provision is better than another (e.g. residential versus outpatient) but that retention within programmes is an essential pre-requisite to good outcomes (Howell *et al.*, 1999; see also Plasse, 2000). Attention to the qualitative aspects of care are therefore crucial. Programmes need to be culturally and ideologically acceptable to potential users; practical obstacles removed (e.g. childcare, financial concerns, transport); anxieties and fears minimized, and other problems addressed. For example, alcohol misuse may be coterminous with, or mask, other deficits in parenting, or other relationship problems. Unless tackled, relapse is likely, even if the programme is initially successful. One review suggests that family- or couples-based treatment may be more effective for drug abuse than other kinds of intervention, both psychosocial and pharmaco-therapeutic (Stanton and Shadish, 1997). Given the role that partners and others can play in relapse, this is likely. Reviewing the evidence from four studies, three of which used experimental methodology (family-based training and home visiting) Barnard and McKeganey (2004) conclude that effective interventions will likely be resource intensive, relatively long term, and need to intervene on a variety of fronts, including extended families and partners with drug problems.

Parents with mental illness

Many parents will suffer from mental illness at some time in their lives, and for most, their children will be protected from any adverse fall-out by the temporary nature of the illness, and the presence of significant others – another parent, extended family, neighbours, friends, schools and so on. For some children, however, serious mental illness in a parent can pose a significant threat to their well-being and, for a few, their safety. Such threatening circumstances include those children whose only carer is seriously depressed and socially isolated, and who perhaps has other problems such as substance misuse. Infants and young children are particularly vulnerable to the adverse effects of carers who are emotionally unavailable to them. It is important when drawing up plans to help such families that due regard is given to providing effective help to the parents, as well as taking steps to safeguard the welfare of the children concerned.

Domestic violence

Domestic violence is a significant child protection issue, though importantly not one that is necessarily best dealt with through child protection procedures (see Humphries and Stanley, 2006). Domestic violence has been defined as typically involving:

> A pattern of physical, sexual and emotional abuse and intimidation which escalates in frequency and severity over time. It can be understood as the misuse of power and exercise of control (Pence and Paymar 1996) by one partner over the other in an intimate relationship, usually by a man over a woman, occasionally by a woman over a man (though without the same pattern of societal collusion) and also occurring amongst same sex couples. It has profound consequences in the lives of individuals, families and communities.
>
> (Mullender and Humphries, 1998)

One in four women are affected by domestic violence, and one in five experience physical assault (Kershaw *et al.*, 2001). The effects on children, who are more often than not aware of the abuse, can be profound and long-lasting. Seeing or hearing domestic violence ('the ill-treatment of another') is now deemed to post a significant risk of harm to children (Adoption and Children Act, 2002). Children may be accidentally injured as a result of living in a household where violence takes place, and many directly experience abuse by the person abusing their mother. Mullender and Humphries point out that the deaths of Kimberley Carlile, Sukina Hammond and Tony Dale all involved domestic violence. These men then went on to kill the child (Mullender and Humpries, 1998). There are particular risks to the unborn children of women subject to domestic violence (see Mezey and Bewley, 1997).

Domestic violence can adversely affect children's behaviour and emotional adjustment (Hester *et al.*, 2007). These may have a detrimental effect on their cognitive abilities and academic achievement, although the evidence is mixed – a minority of children seek solace in education (see Jaffe *et al.*, 1990; Mathias *et al.*, 1995). Clearly, not all children are affected in the same way. Some are more resilient than others, and it is important not to take a 'one-size-fits-all' approach when making decisions about risks of significant harm and when deciding what services are needed:

> This complex interplay of risk and protective factors reinforces the need to shift from blaming women for their 'failure to protect', to exploring strengths, the potential to create places of safety and support for survivors and challenges to domestic violence offenders.
>
> (Mullender and Humphries, 1998: 17–18)

These authors identify the potential of education interventions to help raise awareness of domestic violence among children, particularly boys (whose attitudes differ markedly from those of girls from age 13 and who are much more likely to excuse the perpetrator). They also discuss the opportunities provided within shelters and group work with children to affect children's ability to come to terms with their experiences, to feel less responsible for what has happened, and to learn how to stay safe and to seek help safely in the future.

The importance of a coherent, multi-agency approach to intervening in domestic violence is now recognized (see Crime and Disorder Act, 1998; Home Office, 2004). However, the effectiveness of local partnerships continues to be limited by (1) a lack of services available for women and children, (2) a reluctance to use legal powers to remove the perpetrator (rather than requiring that the woman leave to ensure her safety and that of her children), and (3) reliance on, and inappropriate use of, child protection procedures (see Hague, 2001). Insufficient attention is given to the issue of securing women's safety, which continues to undermine many of the interventions offered to them and their children.

Ramsay *et al.* (2005) produced a systematic review of controlled evaluations of interventions designed to promote the phsycial and psycho-social well-being of women who experience partner violence. They concluded that advocacy can be an effective means of reducing abuse, increasing social support and improving the quality of women's lives. It can also enhance safety and the use of community resources. Only one support group has been subjected to rigorous evaluation but it too found a reduction in abuse and improved psychological outcomes for participants. The evidence from the 11 studies of counselling was not sufficiently robust to permit conclusions about the effectivness of this approach over and above the passage of time and other influences. Nevertheless, Ramsey *et al.* recommend that counselling be available to women who have left an abusive partner (and good-quality studies conducted regarding counselling effectiveness) but should take a back seat to advocacy for those women currently in abusive relationships.

In terms of addressing violence, most research has focused on violent men, since these account for the large majority of perpetrators. Two approaches dominate, both in service delivery and evaluation, namely the Duluth model and cognitive-behavioural approaches. The Duluth model is a psycho-educational approach anchored in feminism which seeks to raise participants' awareness of the ways in which violence is part of a pattern of behaviour that includes intimidation, isolation, emotional and economic – as well as – physical abuse, underpinned by patriarchal ideology. The aim is to move participants away from a 'power and control' approach to resolutions to one of equality. Cognitive-behavioural approaches take as their starting point the proposition that violence – like other behaviour – is learned. That is to say, it is aquired via modelling and reinforcement (violence 'pays'), and maintained because it serves a range of purposes, however 'dysfunctional' (i.e. it reduces tension, secures compliance, provides resolution and leaves the perpetrator with a sense of control). As learned behaviour, violence can also be unlearned and more appropriate modes of relating put in place. This typically involves an educational component (about the components of violence; problem-solving), anger-management skills (identifying the triggers for aggression and ways of handling it), modelling and behaviour rehearsal, to acquire new skills.

In a systematic review of treatment efficacy, Babcok *et al.* (2004) note that in fact both approaches incorporate features of the other (i.e. cognitive-behavioural approaches include a focus on attitudes to violence and to women); the Duluth model looks at the way violence is learned and transmitted. Evaluations of these approaches in a 'pure' form are therefore non-existent. It is primarily a question of emphasis. The 22 studies included in their review suffered from a range of methodological weaknesses and the reviewers suggest 'caution in interpreting these results is warranted. Meta-analyses are only as robust as the individual studies taken into account' (p. 1047). Against this warning, here are their conclusions:

1   Claims for the superiority of one intervention over another is not defensible on the available data.
2   There is no discernible difference in the effectiveness of either method, possibly owing to the degree of overlap between them in the detail of content and delivery. The average effect sizes between the two interventions were the same for both police records and victim reports.
3   Estimates of the size of effect for both interventions are small. Based on partner reports, men who have participated in a treatment programme have a 40 per cent chance of being successfully non-violent, compared with 35 per cent for untreated men. In other words, we are only talking about a 5 per cent increase in success rate that may be attributed to treatment. Although statistically small, this may be a 'clinically significant' effect (i.e. a 5 per cent decrease in violence among those participating in violence programmes in the USA would equate to around 42,000 women per annum being free from physical abuse).
4   The review should not be used as a reason for abandoning these programmes. They argue that the present evidence base should be used for tailoring future programmes to particular groups of perpetrators (rather than a 'one-size-fits-all' approach) and then undertaking careful evaluations of these to learn what works best, with whom.

Domestic violence is a significant social problem. Those working in mental health or in children's services need to be informed about it and clear about their legal and professional responsibilities. Good coverage of the issues may be found in edited volumes by Humphries and Stanley (2006) and Hester *et al.* (2007).

11 Social work with looked-after children

'Looked after' is the term used to describe children in public care (DoH, 1989). They may be placed in the care of a local authority by a court (under an order) or provided with accommodation by Social Services for more than 24 hours. It includes children placed in foster care, in residential care and those who, though living with their parents, are subject to care orders. There may be times when parents are unable to care for their children due to personal circumstances, such as illness or a crisis. In these circumstances children may need to be looked after by others until things get back to normal. Some parents need periodic respite from their caring responsibilities, perhaps because their son or daughter has complex needs. Some children may therefore have to be looked after for short periods of time. Others may need longer term, perhaps permanent, arrangements. This may be because the risks to the children of remaining with their parents are too great, or the reasons why their parents are unable to provide adequate care cannot be resolved in a time frame that meets their developmental needs.

At any one time there are around 60,000 children looked after in England. Comparable figures for Wales, Scotland and Northern Ireland are 5,000, 13,000 and 2,500 respectively (Scottish Executive, 2006; DfES, 2007; DHSSPS, 2008). During 2005 to 2006, some 90,000 children entered the care system in England, with almost half returning home within six months, and most within 12 months. The majority of children coming into care are at least 10 years of age.

Children in long-term care are among the most vulnerable in society. The majority have suffered abuse or neglect and children leaving care have notably poorer outcomes than other children in terms of physical, emotional and mental health, education, and economic well-being. These poorer outcomes are not just a function of children's experiences before coming into care, they also reflect inadequacies in the care system. Many children experience unplanned endings to their placements ('placement breakdown'), with some moving several times in one year. For example, between April 2004 and March 2005, 13 per cent of all looked-after children in England experienced three or more placements. Of those under age 16 who had been looked after for two and a half years or more, only 65 per cent were living in the same placement for the past two years or had been placed for adoption. The remaining 35 per cent experienced more than one placement in the previous two years. Each placement breakdown is likely to add to a child's difficulties. There is therefore considerable room for improvement in experiences of children in public care. It is also important that those providing for children who cannot be cared for within their birth family are familiar with what works for children in these settings, and how to maximize their life chances within them.

This is a large field, and readers are recommended to use other sources that discuss these specialist aspects of childcare practice, including children's participation in decision-making (e.g. Thomas and O'Kane, 1998; Aldgate and Statham, 2001; Thomas, 2005; Cocker and Allain, 2007). In this chapter we focus on the evidence concerning those key factors that appear to be essential to successful fostering and residential care.

Children in foster care

The majority of children who become looked after are placed in foster care. Most are placed with strangers, often in places they don't know, some way away from their families of origin. This can be difficult for well-attached, well-loved and well-adjusted children (remember – or imagine – what that first visit to a new family on an 'exchange visit' was like). In addition to the inherent trauma that such a placement can represent, children who become looked after often have to cope with this on top of very traumatic experiences within their own families, for which they may feel responsible, most probably won't fully understand and will have difficulty processing emotionally. Some children's histories may be such that they come into care with a range of challenging emotional and behaviour problems, with ambivalence about the move (and possibly downright opposition), and with little trust in adults. To return to attachment theory, different children may seek to cope with their experiences in different ways, some of which can be extremely challenging to foster carers:

> Those who have experienced consistent patterns of rejection may have learned to deactivate their proximity-seeking attachment behaviours and demonstrate avoidant attachment patterns. Those who had insensitive, unpredictable care may have learned to hyperactivate their attachment behaviours and demonstrate an ambivalent/resistant attachment pattern. Many maltreated children who have experienced particular kinds of frightening and unpredictable environments will have developed representations of caregivers as dangerous or neglectful and will have found it impossible to organise a strategy for coping. They may demonstrate a disorganised attachment.
>
> (Schofield, 2003: 8)

Those caring for such children need considerable understanding, patience, skill and support if they are to help children to settle and develop new, good-enough attachments with them. It is important that children in care experience stability in their care arrangements. Placement stability is really a shorthand term for the continuity and security children need in their relationships with adults if they are to flourish and realize their potential. Children, particularly older children, may need time to become attached to new carers. They may struggle to do this, and to maintain contact and optimal relationships with their own parents. Foster carers need to be able to manage these tensions and potential conflicts, and social workers need to be able to support them to do so.

There have been growing concerns about the experiences of children looked after who are all too often not well served by the care system. They frequently leave care with few or no qualifications, and have little support when they do so. Many experience frequent moves which effectively prevents them from forming strong attachments or working through their difficulties in ways that help them secure good outcomes. When children in care were asked about their experiences, many acknowledged the support and care they were given. They liked being part of a family and valued the opportunities this provided. What they did not like included:

- The lack of choice they had about their foster placement;
- The lack of information given to them about their foster family prior to their move;
- The loss of contact with their parents;
- Missing their friends and family.

(Morgan, 2005)

In 2003 the government provided increased funding to improve placement services. A key objective was to develop the range of placements available so that the needs of looked-after children could be appropriately met. The policy, known as *Choice Protects*, also sought to improve the support and training to foster carers, develop new services to meet specific needs, and provide specialist services that would help foster carers improve outcomes for children in their care, particularly in relation to their health and educational achievements (see DoH, 2003). There has been a significant body of research looking at some of these areas, and fostering agencies and the local authorities who commission their services have been inspected against a set of national standards for several years. Of particular relevance is the overview of 16 research projects in the UK published since 1998 that was conducted by Sinclair (Sinclair, 2006). In addition, the Social Care Institute for Excellence also conducted a 'knowledge review' of what works in fostering (SCIE, 2006) and the Commission for Social Care Inspection produced a bulletin aimed at helping fostering agencies improve the quality of their services (CSCI, 2006). What emerges from this work is a set of good practice measures that fostering agencies, commissioning bodies and individual social workers should seek to achieve. These include the following.

Effective recruitment and retention of foster carers

Placement choice depends upon the availability of a range of foster carers. There are a number of ways of securing this, most of which need to start with an analysis of what obstacles are responsible for any shortages. Things that have helped include: promoting a positive image of foster care, working with experienced foster carers; social workers and local managers; paying foster carers for introducing another carer; dealing promptly with enquiries; innovative approaches to marketing, including the local media; targeted recruitment, for example, of black and minority ethnic carers; ensuring that carers receive what they regard as adequate remuneration and support; prompt payments to carers (see Triseliotis *et al.*, 1999). Some fostering agencies, particularly in the independent sector, pay enhanced remuneration to carers and provide enhanced levels of support from professionals.

Matching children and carers

Getting the right 'match' between child and foster carer has long been a good practice mantra in social work. It clearly makes sense to place children in families where they are likely to be at ease and with people best able to meet their needs. There is, however, evidence that too often placement decisions are made using 'rigid rules of thumb' on what works, with professionals relying too much on matching children and carers on the basis of their backgrounds and experiences (see Sinclair, 2006). It is certainly important to consider whether or not foster carers have their own or other children, what the age gaps are between the child to be placed and other children already there, and whether to place a child with or without their siblings. As well as minimizing the trauma inherent in a move, factors such as ethnicity and religion may be important to a child's identity and approach to life. However, one can match children and carers on all of these dimensions and fail to secure a good placement. As with other relationships it is important that children and carers 'get on' and the stock matching criteria will not guarantee this. As children themselves indicate, they want choice, and a chance to size up carers before committing themselves. Best practice means giving a child the chance to say 'no'.

Providing information to children and carers

This issue comes up in many areas of social work. Adults need to put themselves more often in the shoes of the children they are seeking to place, giving more thought to the experiences of children who get to the point of needing foster care, any worries they may have, any self-blame they may harbour, their confusion about what is happening and their sense of loss. It is with these worries that children are transported into the homes of strangers. Sometimes we cannot avoid this, particularly when true emergencies arise, but these are perhaps rarer than they are recorded as being the case. Children need to know exactly why they have been placed in foster care. As well as reassuring them that it is not 'their fault' it helps them construct an answer to the questions about their circumstances that will inevitably come their way and which children have said often preoccupies them (Cleaver, 2000). Carers who are well informed about the children they are being asked to look after are less likely to report feeling misled and being ill-prepared (Farmer *et al.*, 2004). The same applies to adoptive parents.

Maintaining important relationships

It is generally thought that children who come into care should continue to maintain contact with their parents and other significant family members, if only via the telephone or mail, including email. The evidence is not straightforward (see Quinton *et al.*, 1997; Ryburn, 1999). Current best evidence suggests that effective contact arrangements are those that are underpinned by a realistic assessment of the attachment between a child and his or her parent(s); a risk assessment of the potential risks and benefits of contact with a wide range of relatives; clarity about the purpose of contact, its desired frequency and who should be involved; discussions with children, parents and carers about contact arrangements; and agreement about the venue and a risk assessment of the practical and other barriers to successful contact and arrangements (Sinclair, 2006).

Effective training and support for carers

There is currently no blueprint for the effective training of foster carers. We know what carers need to be able to do, and what they might need to know, but it is much less clear how to achieve this. Sinclair's overview (2006) summarizes the kinds of things that appear to be important. These include how to manage contact, attachment problems and challenging behaviour – not just at home but at school. Carers also need to understand the importance of identity, and how to validate and nurture this. They need to be able to respond to a child's emotional age (rather than his or her chronological age), to be able to help children develop age-appropriate skills and to monitor the activities of adolescents (Sinclair, 2006: 116). Where possible, carers and social workers should be working to the same understanding of the nature of problems and how best to handle them. However, the latter are often available only at times of crises.

Foster carers are increasingly caring for children with complex needs, and in order to do this effectively they need good-quality, reliable support that is available in a timely manner. The eligibility thresholds for child and adolescent mental health services are often so high that children have to wait for assistance, and even then they cannot be guaranteed an evidence-based approach. As indicated above, some independent fostering agencies use their fees to employ therapists or support workers to provide children and carers with the help they need, or commission dedicated services for looked-after children from relevant agencies.

Promoting educational achievement

This is a major concern of government owing to the impact this has on a range of other outcomes in adult life. Placement stability supports good educational progress, and children who are settled in school are also more likely to be settled in the foster home. Research and inspections have highlighted the confusion that often exists about the role of foster carers in relation to school. Carers need clarity. From the child's point of view, foster carers provide the most 'normal' point of contact with the school, and it is foster carers who are best placed to advocate for the child at school, to support their learning at home and to ensure that they attend school and are happy there. If a child is reluctant to attend it is important to find out why this is and to tailor the response accordingly. A child who is being bullied is in a different position from one who is reluctant to go to school because he or she is embarrassed by the taxi journey there. Given children's experiences, their educational achievement may be very low when they first come into care. Foster carers therefore need to invest considerable energy in ensuring that they achieve success, on the grounds that 'success breeds success' (Sinclair, 2006).

Finally, social workers should provide consistent, reliable and sympathetic support to children. One of the most difficult things children say they have to contend with is the continuous turnover of social workers and their unresponsiveness. While there may be little one can do in the short term about the former, there is surely something that can be done about the latter.

Concurrent planning

Before turning to foster care provision, we consider an important development in practice that is intended to reduce the chances of looked-after children 'drifting' in care. Given the consequence of delays in securing permanent placements for children (see below) this is an important issue. Concurrent planning is just what it says on the tin plus a bit more. It means that workers concerned with decisions about a looked-after child's future operate simultaneously on two plans: one to reunite the child with his or her parents by successfully resolving the issues that led to their removal; the other to secure the child's future with another family in a timely fashion should the first plan fail. The 'bit more' is that the child is looked after by foster carers who, should reunification fail, become the adopters. Clearly this approach requires much of foster carers, who need to be able to seek the child's best interests over any desire they may have to adopt a particular child (which grows in some cases). It also requires much of birth parents and of professional staff. The target group for concurrent planning is precisely that group of families where there are substantial problems of parenting and where it is difficult to determine when and where to draw the line in the provision of 'further chances'.

The origins of this approach lie in the USA (Katz *et al.*, 1994; Gambrill, 1997). A number of agencies are currently exploring its effectiveness and to date there is one study that has examined the success of concurrent planning (Monck *et al.*, 2004). The research found that of those birth parents interviewed, most recognized the advantages of the approach, as did carers, although the latter reported high levels of personal anxiety. One aspect of the findings of the study were unexpected, and limit the generalizability of the findings. All but one of the children accepted for concurrent planning were under 12 months of age. This effectively blocked any meaningful comparison of the outcomes of concurrent planning with routine adoption services. The authors conclude that concurrent planning delivered earlier permanence and fewer moves between carers for this particular group. They note that the success of this approach – even for this less complex group of children – is dependent on the support of other professionals involved in decision-making appreciating the detrimental impact of delay. It is fair to say that the study does not provide a robust test of the value of concurrent planning for the majority of children for whom it might be most needed, namely older children. Those interested in this area should read the careful discussion of this and other issues relevant to concurrent planning in the paper by Monck and her colleagues.

Family and friends foster care

Repeated research findings concerning the poor outcomes for children in public care led to the Children Act 1989 prioritizing the goal of placing children needing substitute care with relatives or other members of their social network. Family and friends foster care is also known as kinship care or relative care. It can be arranged in a number of ways, including informal, private or formal arrangements. The last is a legal arrangement in which a child who is subject to a care order is placed in a relative's care by a local authority. Nationally, around 16 per cent of children who are fostered are placed in the care of relatives, although practice varies from local authority to local authority. It makes intuitive sense that if children cannot remain in the care of their parents the best alternative is for them to be cared for by relatives or close friends of the family. The thought is that family and friends care:

> enables children to live with persons whom they know and trust, reduces the trauma children may experience when they are placed with persons who are initially unknown to them, and reinforces children's sense of identity and self esteem which flows from their family history and culture.
>
> (Wilson and Chipungu, 1996: 387)

Such arrangements can mean that children are more likely to stay in the neighbourhoods they know. This means they are more likely to maintain contact with birth parents and siblings; keep their friends; stay at the same school, and be able to continue in any activities or clubs in which they are involved. Kinship care offers one way of overcoming the challenges that may arise when seeking to place minority ethnic children with foster carers of the same ethnic group.

Current evidence about the effectiveness of kinship care is limited, not least of all because of the difficulties in evaluating it. A systematic review by Winokur and colleagues (2007) indicates that kinship care may be effective in enhancing the behavioural development, mental health functioning and placement stability of children. However, the findings from the review do not support implementing kinship care solely to increase permanency rates and the use of supportive services of children in out-of-home care. Most of these outcome studies were conducted in the USA. A number of UK studies have shed some light on a number of important issues when considering family and friends foster care. Of particular importance is Hunt's (2003) scoping review, conducted for the Department of Health. In addition, Sinclair *et al.* included some friends and family carers in their study of foster carers (Sinclair *et al.*, 2004), as did Selwyn *et al.*'s study of the outcome of adoption (2003). The tentative messages from these studies are as follows:

- There is evidence that some children benefit in the ways suggested above.
- Carers who are relatives are more likely to be committed to the child.
- Children in kinship care enjoy more placement stability, although this may be explained by the profile of children in kinship care.
- There may be less tension between the foster-child and other children in the home, compared with placements with previously unknown foster carers.

Hunt points out that few of the benefits identified by those promoting kinship care relate directly to the impact of kinship care on outcomes for children. These tend to be assumed, based on 'proxy outcomes' such as placement stability, contact, and keeping sibling groups together and so on. Noting that the outcomes studies then available were of poor methodological quality, and the evidence 'fragmentary' and in some respects contradictory, she points out that kinship carers are not always operating on an even playing field, partly because of the disadvantages they bring to the situation and partly because of the unequal treatment of kinship carers by Social Services, compared with other foster carers:

- Kinship care *may* have limited resources to manage the challenges of caring for the child(ren).
- Kinship carers are often less well educated than other carers, poorer and less well remunerated by Social Services.
- Kinship carers may receive less training and support from social workers.

Kinship care enjoys growing support. While it does not have to be 'better' than other forms of foster care, there have been some concerns that kinship care can bring particular problems for children, including a lack of protection from those who may have abused them in the past, perhaps because relatives do not believe the allegations made, or because they are themselves intimidated by the birth parents. The conflicts that can arise between kinship carers and birth parents, or others, can have adverse effects on children (Hunt and Macleod, 1999). Social workers therefore need sound knowledge of the particular characteristics of these placements and what does and does not work. They need to use this knowledge when assessing potential placements, and when monitoring and reviewing them. They need to deploy particular care and sensitivity when working with kinship carers, not because they are more difficult to work with, but because they have not sought to be foster carers. Relatives may find the statutory responsibilities that social workers seek to execute unduly intrusive or onerous (e.g. assessment, reviews).

Such placements are different and need to be differently addressed. Hunt identifies actions that need to be taken at the levels of local and national policy, in training and in practice. At the practice level, social workers need different skills and a particular knowledge base. While there are training materials available, these have not been extensively used (Pitcher, 1999a, 1999b; NFCA, 2000a, 2000b) and, in order to extend the use of kinship care in the UK, Hunt argues that a 'strong push is needed to ensure that they are widely circulated and used' (Hunt, 2003: 75). Alongside this a change in professional attitudes to kinship care is needed. Social workers need be trained and supported to recognize and value what relatives, including those from older generations, have to offer children who need alternative care arrangements (see Broad, 2004; also the response of the Kinship Care Alliance to the *Care Matters* Green Paper (Kinship Care Alliance, 2007)).

Family group decision-making

Family group conferencing is an approach to decision-making in which family members assume a central role in discussing the problems that have brought a child to the attention of the state, and identifying the most suitable ways forward. Family group conferences are used in the context of child welfare, child protection and juvenile delinquency. The origins of family group conferencing are found in New Zealand where, in the late 1980s, they were established as a modern-day equivalent of established decision-making practices in the Maori community, and where community elders convened meetings with the extended family, friends and community members to decide how to manage situations in which children were experiencing difficulties.

Since then, family group conferencing has been implemented in a number of places, including Australia, North America and Scandinavia. In the UK the approach has been highlighted as a means of identifying kinship placements at an early stage in decision-making (Cabinet Office, 2000) and of ensuring that plans for children make full use of the potential resources available within the extended family (Nixon, 2001). Although the claims made for its impact on child outcomes often exceed the available evidence, there are persuasive reasons why family group conferencing is an important development, not least of all in relation to children's rights.

> Societies can give children the legal right to participate, but without removing some of the social, economic, and cultural barriers to children's involvement in decision making, this legal right may be worth little in day-to-day practice.
>
> (Nixon, 2007: 20)

The adversarial nature of much child protection practice means that it is all too easy for the needs of children and parents to become polarized. Family group conferences afford an opportunity to reframe difficulties in ways that are solution focused, recognizing the strengths and resources that exist within families and communities, and ensuring that these are used to the full in the endeavour to keep children within their families of origin or, if that is not possible, within their extended family. Family group conferences are typically chaired by an independent person, either within the council with Social Services responsibility or in the agency to which this work is often contracted out. Those concerned about a child's welfare or well-being, including professionals, present their concerns in an open, specific and transparent way, and children and families are invited to share their views about what the problems are and what would help to address these, including safeguarding children's welfare. A key part of the model is giving families a period of 'private time' (i.e. without the presence of professionals or the chair) to consider what they have heard, what they know, and to devise a protection plan.

In New Zealand and in a handful of other jurisdictions, family group conferences are mandatory, but not in the UK. This may account for the patchy development of such schemes, their limited use where schemes exist, and the rather diluted approach to participation (Brown, 2007; Nixon, 2007). Barriers to implementation include concerns that family group conferences exist only as an adjunct to statutory child protection procedures. This places strain on resources and time-scales and provides reluctant professionals with a reason for side-stepping them where such provision exists. Professionals have expressed concerns that families or children may be unable to participate, that it is too risky to leave decision-making to families they perceive to be 'dysfunctional', or that the statutory location for decision-making is care proceedings and associated child protection procedures (e.g. Marsh and Crow, 1998; Morris, 2003). Participation is diluted because too often professionals adopt a 'consultative approach', in which members of the child's network are invited to participate 'in existing professionally led processes, where key decisions have already been taken' (Morris and Burford, 2007: 210). Children are all too often bystanders at events where they should be centre-stage. Children have a legal right to have their views heard and taken into account, but this is rarely realized in any meaningful way. Nixon (2007) has written a particularly helpful paper on the challenges of enabling children to participate in family group decision-making in ways that enable them to have their views heard, and what things help. The paper has wider application than family group conferences. Nixon highlights the importance of:

- Giving children good-quality information and listening to them.
- Using independent advocates where necessary.
- Continually checking that children understand what is being said or what is happening, in a way that is not patronizing.
- Ensuring that children hear positive things about themselves and their future prospects.
- Ensuring that children can chose from a variety of ways to express themselves, including letters, videos, audiotapes or drawings in the event that they do not wish to be present or to speak at the conference.
- Using plain English when developing plans, making clear responsibilities and time-scales.
- Involving children in the arrangements for monitoring and review, since the plan affects them the most. One of the most frequently cited problems in family group decision-making is the lack of follow-through on plans, particularly by professionals.

Residential care

As at 31 March 2007 there were 6,500 children in residential care in England, 5,200 of whom were in community homes for children that were subject to children's homes regulations. The remainder were in secure units (200) or other provision not subject to regulation, such as boarding-schools (SFR-2007). Of a similar number of children in residential care on 31 March 2006, all but 170 were aged 10 years or more at the time of placement (SFR-2006). This section focuses solely on community homes for children (or 'residential care' or 'children's homes'), most of which provide accommodation for between two and six children. In a small proportion of cases young people in residential care have chosen to be there. For most, however, residential placements are placements of last resort, despite a policy stance that residential care should be a positive choice for some children (Utting, 1991). This is perhaps because many children, particularly older children, find themselves in residential care because they cannot be appropriately accommodated elsewhere – either because they cannot cope with the demands of family life, or because their behaviour is too disruptive. For example, the social workers of 223 young people in residential care reported that seven out of ten had been excluded from school or were frequent truants; one-third had engaged in self-harm or attempted suicide; six out of ten had been involved in delinquency, and that significant numbers (at least four out of ten) had been involved in violence to others, including adults and children, had run away from home or from care, or put themselves at risk through sexual behaviour (Sinclair and Gibbs, 1998).

Sinclair provides a memorable categorization of the function of community homes based on his study of homes in the early 1990s, namely:

1 Forming part of tertiary prevention – receiving the walking wounded of family warfare and returning them quickly to the front line.

2 A method of 'career management' – receiving children under emergency situations and enabling them to be assessed and held so that sensible plans could be developed and implemented.

3 As a source of specialized treatment designed to prepare the young people – for reintroduction to family, for a new placement or for independence – and as a long-term shelter in which a minority of residents are brought up.

(Sinclair, 2006: 206)

The shape and texture of residential care has shifted considerably over the past half century. Berridge (2002) has pointed out that the approach to government-sponsored research currently in vogue does little to build a sound picture of current best evidence, focusing as it does on 'themes'. The last time residential care featured as a theme was in the early 1990s, so the results of these studies need to be interpreted cautiously. However, there are some consistent patterns that can help inform decision-making.

Problems in providing effective residential care

For some, the notion of effective residential care is an oxymoron. The shrinkage of the sector reflects a general view that wherever possible children should either remain with their families of origin, or be placed in substitute family care. Bullock argues that this is mistaken, that residential care is neither good nor bad per se. Rather, the appropriate questions concern which residential provisions are appropriate for whom (Bullock, 1999: 267). Unfortunately, there are currently too few places in too few homes to support such choices, with the result that the profile of residents is often such that it presents staff with serious management problems (see Whitaker *et al.*, 1998). Others consider that residential care should be confined to a 'service response to a perceived safety crisis' which, once resolved, should result in young people being moved on to a family placement (Barth, 2005). Here, the dearth of foster placements, particularly specialist foster schemes, means that this is currently not a viable alternative.

Fiscally, it is unlikely that we will ever attain a level of funding that will make placement choice a reality. Residential care is the most costly placement provision, often accounting for one half of social services expenditure on children (see Carr-Hill *et al.*, 1997). Providers cannot afford to run with unfilled beds and commissioners cannot afford to fund empty ones. One positive trend is the growth of specialist residential provision in the independent sector. These homes are better able to ensure a fit between what they have to offer and the children they admit. Further, they typically have a distinct theoretical orientation designed to address particular problems, such as challenging behaviour, substance misuse or the consequences of abuse. Ideology aside, for some children distance from their families of origin may be beneficial, but without studies of the outcomes of these changes in provision, we cannot say whether or not this is so. We return to the question of the effectiveness of residential care later. First, we consider what the children involved want from this form of provision.

Although there have been no representative surveys of young people's views of residential care, there have been a number of studies that have included their views, and some independent surveys by the Children's Rights Director (see Morgan, 2006) and children's organizations such as the Who Cares Trust (1993). Understandably, children value homes where they are not bullied, sexually intimidated or led astray. They also want to be in homes where other residents are friendly (Sinclair and Gibbs, 1998). What they want from staff is not dissimilar from what they want from foster carers. They want staff who afford them respect, who are approachable and can be trusted. Children want staff who 'know what looking after really means'. Some of the most important issues for children are that staff need to be good at coping with problems; to be able to 'talk a situation down' without recourse to physical restraint, and to deal effectively with bullying and abuse without making it more difficult for the victim. They want staff who can listen to children, who are careful to ensure that they find out what the 'quiet children think', that is, those children who are unlikely to speak out in groups (Morgan, 2005). They also said they wanted staff to be able to cope when children speak their minds strongly, perhaps because they are upset or angry, and to understand why that might be the case. Where such things happen, many studies reveal very positive relationships between children and staff in care homes (see Triseliotis *et al.*, 1995; Sinclair and Gibbs, 1998; Anglin, 2004).

Homes that do well

In addition to meeting those things that children themselves value, researchers are generally in broad agreement about the characteristics of children's homes that are well run and provide good-quality care (see Berridge and Brodie, 1998; Sinclair and Gibbs, 1998). This is not necessarily the same as an *effective* home, but it is certainly a necessary prerequisite. The 'active ingredients' are as follows:

- Heads of homes have a clear remit and sufficient autonomy to pursue it.
- They are clear about how the home should be run.
- There is a consensus among the staff and between the staff and the head of the home about how it should be run.

Homes with these characteristics appear to have less staff turnover, less delinquent behaviour among residents and elicit more positive accounts in evaluation from both staff and residents. In a study of children who go missing from residential and foster homes by Wade and Biehal (1998), the researchers found that rates differed from 25 to 71 per cent across the sample. The researchers asked children why they went missing. Among the reasons given were: bullying and intimidation; being unsettled or insecure in the placement, and a general lack of confidence and sense of disempowerment among residential staff (p. 197).

Good leadership and clarity of role are among the things that homes are inspected for (see CSCI, 2005). In addition, national minimum standards for children's homes specify strong management, rigorous recruitment procedures, training for staff and clear procedures, particularly in relation to complaints, care planning, training and development. Aside from the evident importance of preventing unsuitable people from becoming residential care workers, there is limited evidence that training is correlated with good-quality care provision (see Sinclair and Gibbs, 1998). This may be because the training provided is not appropriate, or because the turnover of children and staff is such that homes are unable to put training to best use. In addition to the problems already highlighted, such as absconding, they place children at risk of other associated problems: the strain of having to develop new relationships with a range of people; separation from friends and family; the neglect of those things that families might prioritize such as education, and a loss of 'normality'.

Finally, there are some things that residential settings cannot or do not do well. Bullock (1999) writes as follows:

> The weaknesses of residential settings lie in their inability to give continuing unconditional love, the constraints they place on a child's emotional development, their inability to ensure staff continuity and the peripheral role they often allocate to children's families.
>
> (Bullock, 1999: 262)

Outcomes of residential care

Sadly, we know too little about the outcomes of residential care, however good the quality of it *appears* to be. Whatever improvements occur during placements there is little evidence that they persist after children leave. Sinclair argues that influences that persist probably do so because of the changes they have effected in how young people think about themselves. Similarly, the correlation between residential care that emphasized employment training and success is more likely to be attributable to the impact this had on individuals' sense of responsibility, rather than on their actual employability. Sinclair concludes by saying that the long-term effects of residential care are likely to depend upon the following:

- Control of absconding, offending and other antisocial behaviour.
- Helping young people acquire pro-social skills in education and work.
- Developing a culture that values these things and builds young people's self-esteem.
- Effective work on the relationships between a young person and his or her family.
- After care that enables that young person to use the skills he or she has acquired.

(Sinclair, 2006: 211)

He notes that these are little more than hypotheses. They do, however, chime with the concern with focusing more on outcomes, and reinforce the importance of attending to the maintenance of any positive changes that may have occurred (see below). He does, however, enter a note of caution:

> The case *against* the current homes is strong. They are unstable, and prone to scandal and disorder. They lack a coherent theoretical justification. Their most notable difference from foster care – the existence of a resident group – is commonly seen as a threat rather than an asset. Their outcomes are, if not

demonstrably worse than would be the case for similar young people in foster care, certainly discouraging.

(Sinclair, 2006: 214)

This is the conclusion of someone with very considerable expertise in this field. We might add that residential care can expose young people to risks of involvement in a range of deviant behaviour via their contact with peers, as well as to risks of abuse (see Farmer and Pollock, 1998). Children in residential care are unlikely to receive therapeutic help when needed.

Finally, it is not clear whether, had young people the option of a family placement that provided what they see as the selling points of residential care, they would still choose residential care. These include being able to manage the tensions between their family and current carers (residential workers are not seen as being in competition for their affections) and not feeling able to manage the demands of life within a family.

Leaving care

It should be evident by now that children leaving care are in a very different place to those leaving home in the general population. Although some will have flourished in supportive placements, for many children their time in care – even if helpful – will have done little to compensate for the difficulties they experienced before coming in. For some, their experience will have exacerbated their problems or added to them. These young people are probably among the least well equipped to fend for themselves at the ages of 16 to 18, but are most likely to be doing so. This is in stark contrast to the pattern typically found in mainstream society, where the median age of leaving home is 22.4 years for men and 20.3 years for women (Billari *et al.*, 2001).

Moreover, their move to independent living is often abrupt. For many it is triggered by a placement breakdown and/or or the absence of a suitable placement for them. Since the Children Act 1989 attention has been given to preparing young people for the transition to independent living, but less thought has been given to the support they may subsequently need. Some groups were particularly ill-prepared by Social Services, including disabled young people, young parents and young people from minority ethnic groups (see Stein, 2004).

In addition to leaving care abruptly, poorly prepared and at a younger age than most young people, care leavers have fewer educational qualifications (see Cheung and Heath, 1994). Often they have none. Of the 8,100 children leaving care during 2005 and 2006 aged 16 or over, just 48 per cent had at least one GCSE or GNVQ, and only 6 per cent left with at least five GCSEs at grades A to C. The percentage in the general population stands at 63 per cent. In that year just over half of children in care (54 per cent) were entered for only one GSCE. Not surprisingly, care leavers are also less likely to go on to further or higher education, are more likely to be unemployed, more likely when they obtain work to secure semi- or unskilled manual work and to be living on or near the poverty line (see Biehal *et al.*, 1994; Cheung and Heath, 1994). Young women in care are more likely to become teenage parents than those in the general population (see Biehal *et al.*, 1995). Disabled young people may be further disadvantaged by the lack of sufficiently advanced planning (see Chapter 14).

Stein, a researcher with in-depth knowledge of this area, describes the transition to adulthood for care leavers as too often:

> a final event; there is no option to return in times of difficulty . . . [care leavers] often have to cope with major status changes in their lives at the time of leaving care: leaving foster care or their children's home and setting up a new home, often in a new area, and for some young people starting a new family as well; leaving school and finding their way into further education, training or employment, or coping with unemployment. They are denied the psychological opportunity and space to focus or to deal with issues over time, which is how most young people cope with the challenges of transition.
>
> (Stein, 2006: 274)

This is markedly different from the experience of most young people leaving home. Typically, higher education provides this 'space', and young people can – and do – turn to their parents for all kinds of assistance and increasingly have a tendency to return home for periods of respite and support before finally standing on their own feet (see Mitchell, 2005).

Helping care leavers towards a successful transition

The Children Act 1989 set out a duty to prepare young people in care for adult life. The best preparation begins as soon as a young person starts to be looked after, and is best delivered within a stable and nurturing environment. The accompanying guidance to the 1989 Act set out three key areas to which attention needed to be paid in preparing them for independence: enabling young people to build and maintain relationships, to develop their self-esteem, and to acquire practical and financial skills and knowledge. The *Quality Protects* initiative aimed to maximize the number of looked-after children aged 16 years who were engaged in education, training or employment at age 19. For those who left care after their sixteenth birthday, the aim was to maximize the number still in touch with Social Services or a designated contact person at age 19 and the number who had suitable accommodation at that age.

While there was a growth of specialist schemes set up to address the needs of children leaving care during the 1980s these were somewhat piecemeal, and the evidence suggested that they were not turning the tide of poor outcomes for this group of young people (see Broad, 1998). The Children (Leaving Care) Act 2000 established a new framework for leaving care services (see also the Children (Leaving Care) Act Northern Ireland 2002 Act and the Children (Leaving Care) Act 2000 for Scotland). The Act places a duty on councils with Social Services responsibilities to assess and meet the needs of young people aged 16 and 17; to provide a personal service and to establish a pathway plan for all young people aged 16 to 21 or beyond, for those who qualify for the new arrangements, and to assist those leaving care, including with employment, education and training. The duty to assist with education and training and to provide a personal adviser and pathway plan continues for as long as a young person remains in an agreed programme, even beyond the age of 21. In addition, councils are required to:

- Develop clearly written, comprehensive and accessible policies for those leaving care.
- Develop an appropriate model of service delivery – most established specialist schemes.
- Monitor performance in relation to individual and services outcomes in line with the objectives of *Quality Protects* (DoH, 1998).
- Establish arrangements for consulting young people on service development and evaluations.

Research findings following the introduction of the 2000 Act suggested that these changes were helping to increase the take-up of further education and reducing the numbers of care leavers not in employment or in any form of education or training (see Stein, 2006). These changes appeared to be attributable to improvements in funding for young people; increases in the availability of supported accommodation; better inter-agency working, and clear lines of responsibility and accountability (see Dixon *et al.*, 2004).

Improving outcomes for care leavers

Given the importance of effective transitions for children previously in care, government concerns about social inclusion and exclusion, and the drive to improve outcomes for children, it is striking that there has been little investment in research studies following the introduction of the Children (Leaving Care) Act 2000 (see Broad (2004) for an exception). It is likely that, having taken steps to address the problems identified in earlier research, the assumption is that the rest will take care of itself. This is, frankly, naive.

Evaluations of schemes prior to the 2000 Act provide evidence that leaving care services can bring about significant improvements in the lives of these young people. They can help to equip young people with the skills they need to live independently and to help them find and maintain accommodation. These factors are important in securing good results and are not wholly dependent upon children's previous experiences (see Wade and Dixon, 2006). They can support and help children develop relationships and do well in education, but generally these things depend upon children's experiences while in care.

However, the evidence is that, some seven years after the introduction of the 2000 Act in England, Wales and Scotland, we have a long way to go reliably to improve the transitions of young care leavers. In a consultation with care leavers using a variety of methods, the Children's Rights Director reported:

> A common, recurring theme from what young people told us was that there appeared to be little middle ground in the quality of support and preparation that young people leaving care receive. In most cases help was either excellent or poor and, in some cases, non-existent. What each young person got was not

dependent upon their legal entitlement to leaving care and aftercare support, but most often upon the commitment of individual councils, and their staff.

(Morgan, 2006: 3)

Stein argues that to improve outcomes for care leavers requires four changes. The first is early intervention and family support. Second, better quality care that will compensate for the damaging experiences to which children in care have been exposed. Third, opportunities for more gradual transitions that more closely resemble those experienced by the majority of young people. Finally, ongoing support to those who need it, particularly those who have complex needs, or mental, emotional and behavioural problems (see Stein, 2006).

In their responses to the survey conducted by the Children's Rights Director, young people identified the following as the things that most worried them:

1   Being on your own (loneliness): 'The worst thing for me was moving out of area away from friends.'
2   Not being able to cope.
3   Not being able to get help when you most need it: 'Not being offered guidance and worried about getting lonely.'
4   Not having enough money to get by on: 'Not being able to pay bills.'
5   Cleaning up after yourself.
6   Leaving before being ready to do so: 'Should have a say in when to leave care.'
7   Having nowhere/no one to come back to.
8   Being put in some 'dodgy' places.
9   Becoming homeless: 'Having nowhere to live.'
10   Having to keep moving around: 'Not being able to settle anywhere.'

(Morgan, 2006)

Adoption

For many children unable to live with their own families, adoption is likely to be the first placement choice. As part of the *Quality Protects* programme, the UK government is aspiring to increase the number of children in care in England and Wales placed for adoption by 40 per cent, from 5 per cent in 2000 (DoH, 1998). In the year ending 31 March 2007, the percentage was 5.5 per cent (numbering 3,300). The Adoption and Children Act 2002 was designed to support this, aiming to reduce delay, to strengthen adoption support and bring adoption law in line with the Children Act 1989. As well as providing councils with Social Services responsibilities with additional funding to meet this target, the government has set up a number of support services such as the 'Adoption and Permanence Project' – to provide advice and assistance (www.everychildmatters.gov.uk/adoption); and the National Adoption Register – to speed placement and improve matching. In addition, it has published National Adoption Standards for England and established specialist adoption centres to hear adoption cases.

Who is adopted?

Adoption severs all legal ties between a child and his or her birth family. The adopted person is treated in law as if born to the adoptive parents. Adoptions now appear to be happening more quickly and the average age of children being adopted is going down. This suggests that adoption is being considered earlier on in the planning process, in keeping with the requirement in the National Standards that (1) a permanency plan should be in place within four months of a child becoming looked after, and (2) that adoption should always be considered if returning the child home is not an option. Only 4.5 per cent of children adopted are under 12 months of age; 64 per cent are between 1 and 4 years old, and 27 per cent between 10 and 15. Most are white, have spent between one and three years in care, and became looked-after children owing to abuse or neglect (SSDA903).

How effective are adoptions?

Answering this question is not straightforward. As Quinton and Selwyn point out (2006) it depends on what you mean. Should we be assessing the outcomes of children in relation to children in the general population, with those with similar problems but placed in different settings, or in terms of the changes we bring about for individuals or groups of individuals? Most studies address the issue simply in relation to placement disruptions. This is an important, but limited, indicator of good outcomes. Different researchers measure it differently and at different times, making it hard to synthesize the findings from such studies (see Quinton and Selwyn, 2006). Placements that do not actually break down may not be working well. Some may be unhappy or problematic for children and/or parents (see Rushton and Dance, 2004). The following summary draws on studies and overviews prepared by Alan Rushton (2003, 2004).

Disruption in adoption

Studies of the adoption of children placed under 2 years of age, and with fewer and less adverse pre-adoption experiences, consistently demonstrate that this is a placement in which children can flourish (see Bohman and Sigvardsson, 1990). These children do better than children from similar socio-economic backgrounds on a variety of psycho-social measures, including improvements in self-esteem and mental health, less substance misuse, better stability in relationships, and better educational achievement. More strikingly, they compare favourably with children in the general population (see Collinshaw *et al.*, 1998; Maughan *et al.*, 1998).

As we have seen, most children placed for adoption are now considerably older then they used to be. The majority have troubled pasts, resulting in one or more of a range of problems with which adoptive parents will have to deal, both at the time of placement and beyond. To date, there have been around a dozen outcome studies of adoption of such children with non-relatives. The evidence suggests that adoption works well, with reported rates of disruption similar to those of infant adoptions, ranging from 10 to 50 per cent depending on the sample, and rising with the child's age at placement. Children placed in middle years also do well, though as Rushton observes, 'the picture is much less positive for adolescents and the full story is much more complex' (Rushton, 2004: Rushton and Dance, 2004).

Children's experiences and difficulties

Studies indicate that the factors associated with placement instability are: older age at placement (see Sharma *et al.*, 1995); adverse pre-placement experiences (see Howe, 1995); the child's psycho-social adjustment at the time of placement (see Quinton *et al.*, 1997), and being placed in an established family with a resident child of similar age (see Parker, 1996). In combination these factors can have a cumulative effect. The older a child is, the greater his or her exposure to the adverse circumstances that resulted in their coming into care in the first place. Children may therefore have more and more complex problems of a long-standing nature. They may well have had several moves already. The combination of all of these factors can make it very difficult for children to settle, to take the risk of becoming attached to new people, and to succeed in establishing new relationships. They may feel more torn between their loyalties to their families of origin and their desire for security and stability with their adoptive parents. For some, contact with their birth families will contribute to these difficulties, though for others it may help.

Quinton and Selwyn (2006) note that, while adoption is most likely to be successful when children are placed early, it is also possible successfully to place older children, given careful assessment, careful matching and appropriate support (see below). A factor that raises the age at which children are placed is the time it takes to make and execute decisions to adopt. A delay of one year for a pre-school child amounts to one-fifth of their life experience, and the odds against being adopted increase 1.8-fold for every year of delay (Quinton and Selwyn, 2006). This has implications for all those involved in decision-making, including courts, and many of the changes introduced in adoption law are designed to speed these processes up. Given that most adoptions of older children are contested, it seems that there is a ceiling on the extent to which the length of time cases take through court can be reduced.

Disability, gender and race have no known association with increased risk of placement instability, but the problems that children bring to the placement, as a result of early traumas, do. Three groups of problems place particular strain on adoptive placements and increase the risk of disruption: relationship problems, behavioural and emotional problems, and educational problems (see Rushton, 2004). Children who have been maltreated and who have experienced several changes of caretaker often find it hard to make new attachments. As Schofield's quote above suggests, the way such children cope with such adversity can make it difficult to parent them. They may be withdrawn, unable or unwilling to respond warmly or to show affection. Research indicates that these problems can last for many years (see Rushton and Dance, 2004). Adoptive parents need to be immunized against the expectation of 'quick fixes' based on a stable family environment, and provided with appropriate support. While attachment theory offers a way of thinking about these problems and constructing ways of helping, Rushton cautions that practitioners should not jump to the conclusion that 'attachment theory explains all and that attachment-related therapy is necessary in all such cases' (p. 97).

Non-compliance, tantrums, aggression, lying and stealing are commonplace in samples of older adopted children, as are a range of emotional difficulties such as anxiety. All are challenging to deal with, some particularly so. The challenge to adoptive parents who take on sibling groups, all of whom may present with similar problems, is considerable (Rushton *et al.*, 1998). Many school-age children placed for adoption will bring a range of learning problems with them, and one study suggests the significance of these problems can increase as the placement progresses (Rushton *et al.*, 1998). Many adopters will need to be staunch advocates on behalf of their children if they are to secure educational continuity, to get the help that the child needs and to deal with the behavioural and relationship problems that surface in school. This is an area where there has been little focused research but an area it would seem important to address.

Characteristics of the adoptive family

Rather tellingly, the literature typically talks of the characteristics of children and the risk of disruption and those of adoptive parents, and the likelihood of success. In fact, relatively little is known about the latter. This is partly because 'To date, no studies have collected data at the point of assessment and related it to placement outcome' (Rushton, 2004). There may be a link between the following aspects of parenting style and good outcomes: with warmth, positive regard, sensitivity to the child, the ability to set clear boundaries and the use of authoritative (rather than authoritarian) discipline delivered in a way that helps children to learn to control their own behaviour (see Quinton, 2004). Rushton's view is that given the dearth of knowledge in this area, what is most important is the quality of the relationship between the adoptive parent and the child. He goes on to argue that, therefore, the investment of our energies should be less in detailed assessment of parenting styles and more in ensuring that adoption workers are able to detect the first signs of relationship problems post-placement and to provide speedy, effective help.

Other outcomes

Considerable work is in progress to improve the assessment of outcomes in adoption research and other forms of placement. The tools now available to practitioners in assessing and monitoring children form part of this and will provide much richer sources of data about the well-being and adjustment of children prior to placement. Rushton cautions, however, that this varied and disparate activity may lead to a situation in which it becomes even more difficult to draw together the findings from research because each research team will have opted for a different approach to measuring outcomes. He argues for the importance of longitudinal studies of children placed for adoption and in other placements, since these can enable us to follow children into adulthood, and also to disinter the differential influences of children's pre-placement experiences (for example, of maltreatment), their emotional, psychological and behavioural adjustment and so on.

Rushton observes that an important area of research relevant to adoption which has been underexplored is that concerning the impact of prenatal and early experiences, and the consequences of maltreatment on development, and in particular attachment (Rushton, 2004). We need studies that address these questions and others – such as the success or failure of children placed in adolescence, and the support services needed. Currently, we have little data of this kind on which an assessment of adoption generally, or current adoption policy, could be evaluated.

A follow-up study of 130 children aged 3–8 years, for whom a decision was made that it was in their best interest to be placed for adoption and for whom some important pre-placement data were available, was conducted by Selwyn and colleagues (Selwyn *et al.*, 2006). Not all of the children were adopted. Sixteen placements were disrupted and 34 of the 130 children spent time in long-term foster care or other permanent placements. This important study provides a detailed account of the services provided to children in foster care or adoptive placements, and of the quality and timeliness of decision-making. It also reports on the children's outcomes, but unfortunately the study is limited in its ability to shine a spotlight on the relationships between these and adoption owing to the differences between the groups of children studied. The authors conclude that children in adoptive homes had better stability than those in foster care, but where the latter placements had lasted, these children were also doing well in terms of their emotional and behavioural development (p. 573). They go on to say:

> One of the key differences, however, between these two types of permanent placement was in the adopters' and carers' reports of closeness and confiding behaviours. In comparison with the adopters, foster carers reported that the children confided less and were less close to them.

Where adopted children did much better was at age 16 and over, largely due to the factors discussed in relation to children leaving care, where the adopted child finds him or herself in a very different situation, with different prospects. The young people that fared very poorly at this stage were those who had unstable care careers.

Comparisons with long-term foster care

The problems faced by Selwyn and her colleagues in disinterring the relative contribution of adoption from other factors, such as the early histories and characteristics of the children (even though the study was designed to minimize these), generally bedevils attempts to compare the outcomes of children fostered with those adopted (see Triseliotis, 2002). Children are not randomly assigned to adoption or long-term fostering and those adopted are likely systematically to differ from those who are not. Further, long-term fostering is rarely planned, making it difficult to identify an appropriate comparison group (Quinton and Selwyn, 2006). We do know that long-term foster care placements have, historically, been very vulnerable to breakdown, perhaps owing to the lack of certainty and forward planning that underpins them. Further, the fact that there is no legal change of status may reflect, or possibly result in, less commitment on the part of parents and the child to the placement, rendering it more precarious. Commitment is something that appears to enable adopters to weather difficult times with challenging children (Quinton *et al.*, 1997). In concluding his appraisal of the evidence relating to outcomes in adoption and long-term fostering, Triseliotis makes the important point that when deciding between alternative forms of substitute parenting it is essential to take into account the needs and circumstances of individual children, those of available carers and the range of available placements: 'In the same way that the same shoe will not fit every foot, adoption is not the answer for every child who cannot return to their families.' In this respect, the question 'what works for looked-after children' is very different from the same question applied to something like depression or behavioural problems.

We conclude this section with a consideration of the factors that current best evidence *suggests* might be important in securing successful placements for those who are placed for adoption.

Contact

Since the introduction of 'open adoption', in which the adoptive family has continuing contact with the child's birth family, there has been a tendency to assume that contact is generally a good thing. In fact the evidence base for the benefits of contact on outcomes, particularly children's psychosocial adjustment, is just not available. There are some data from America (see Grotevant and McRoy, 1998) and from a UK study of infant adoptions (Neil, 2000), but neither study addressed the outcomes of contact for the typical UK adoptee (i.e. a child over 4 years of age with a history of adverse experiences and a range of problems). For a critical appraisal of the current evidence on contact and outcomes, see papers by Quinton and colleagues (1997, 1999). For a discussion of the challenges of conducting robust research in this area, and of the importance of doing so, see Rushton, 2004. What we do have are studies that have examined how professionals make decisions about contact (see Harris and Lindsay, 2002); the impact of face-to-face contact on various stake-holders and their relationships, and what factors facilitate or hinder contact (see Logan and Smith, 1999), and what kinds of support help to make contact manageable (see Mackaskill, 2002). Taken as a whole, these studies indicate that contact can be managed in ways that everyone can accommodate, but much depends on how it is introduced and managed by adoption workers. Ensuring that arrangements leave adopters with some sense of control seems to be a key factor.

Post-adoption support

Given the challenges faced by adopters, it is not surprising that research studies, inspection reports and adopters themselves have identified the need for effective support post-adoption. Post-adoption support refers specifically to help with the issues arising from adoption, and perhaps from the steep learning curve with which adopters find themselves confronted. Adopters may need help with managing the kinds of problems described earlier; they may simply want reassurance until they feel their feet. They may want to know that there is someone to turn to as and when problems arise, for example, with school. Support services are very unevenly spread across the country. Even when available, there may be challenges in persuading adopters to have the confidence to take advantage of them. Among the deterrents to seeking help are concerns that they might be blamed for the problems they are struggling with or will be perceived as not succeeding as adoptive parents. Unsympathetic or ineffective help may deter adopters from seeking help in the future.

Finally, adoptive families may sometimes need the same kinds of services that other families need.

Helping children who have been affected by maltreatment

Not all maltreated children become looked after, but most looked after children have been maltreated. We therefore conclude this chapter with a review of research studies seeking to address the question: 'What helps such children?'

It appears that programmes which provide a safe, structured, nurturing environment, which are intentionally geared towards addressing the specific consequences of abuse, and which combine group-based work with individual therapy, are most successful.

Case example

In a study of a therapeutic pre-school for physically abused and sexually abused children, 24 children described as having sufficiently serious developmental delays and problematic behaviour to be judged unsuitable to enter mainstream schooling were enrolled in Project KEEPSAFE (Kempe Early Education Project Serving Abused Families) (Oates *et al.*, 1995). This project aimed to provide a physically and psychologically safe environment, and each child with the knowledge and pre-academic skills required for entry into mainstream school. The rationale for this is that success at school is a major protective factor to offset childhood disadvantage (see Macdonald and Roberts, 1995). In addition to a carefully structured routine and a curriculum designed to meet these aims, the project includes a case-management system whereby one teacher is responsible for each child, including home visits to carer, to provide support and to improve the quality of interaction between the child and the care-giver.

Of the 22 children old enough for school at the end of 12 months, 79 per cent were enrolled at mainstream schools (33 per cent in regular classrooms and 46 per cent into special education). Only 12 per cent required residential placements. Results from a range of standardized developmental tests showed that the majority of the children made developmental gains at a faster rate than would normally be expected. In the absence of a control or comparison groups these results should be treated cautiously, but they mirror the trends of group comparison studies such as those by Culp *et al.* (1987, 1991). What is different about this programme is the addition of home visiting in an attempt to influence and integrate factors in both the major contexts of children's lives.

Helping children who have suffered neglect

Apathy, passivity and social withdrawal are among the documented effects of child physical neglect, along with behaviour problems and academic delay (see Crittenden,

1981; Egeland *et al.*, 1983; Wodarski *et al.*, 1990). Providing compensatory experiences is probably fairly straightforward, but when seeking to deal with the cumulative impact of neglect, the evidence base is limited.

Some of the work discussed in the previous chapter included interventions aimed at helping neglected children (see *Project 12-Ways*). Otherwise, very few studies have focused specifically on the needs of neglected children, or identified neglected children as a subsample of those for whom services were provided. A series of studies by Fantuzzo and colleagues (see Fantuzzo *et al.*, 1987, 1988; Fantuzzo, 1990) evaluated a range of interventions designed to develop social interaction skills in withdrawn, maltreated pre-school children.

Case example

Fantuzzo and colleagues randomly allocated 46 socially withdrawn Head Start children, of whom 22 had been physically abused or neglected, to two groups. In the experimental group, children were paired with 'resilient' peers who, under the supervision of the classroom teacher, initiated play. Results show that these children demonstrated significant increases in positive interaction peer play, and a decrease in solitary play, both among those who had been maltreated, and those who had not. These improvements were maintained at two-month follow-up (see Fantuzzo *et al.*, 1996).

Sadly, in 2007, the picture was much the same as it has long been (see Gershater-Molko *et al.*, 2002). The message therefore is that we should be very cautious in our dealings with children who have suffered neglect, particularly neglect over a long period, and that we should seek to remedy this most serious gap in our knowledge base.

Sexual abuse

Sexual abuse is an event rather than a disorder. The possible consequences of sexual abuse are many and not easily predictable. They may not appear for many years. They may not even exist. The fact that someone has been sexually abused is minimally helpful as an indicator that they might need professional help. A range of factors such as parental support (see Everson *et al.*, 1989), maternal upset (see Newberger *et al.*, 1993) and family functioning (see Conte and Schuerman, 1987) are good predictors of the extent to which sexual abuse results in adverse consequences, and the speed with which children and family members recover. Once again, careful assessment of the impact of the abuse on the child and family is essential. Swenson and Hanson (1997) recommend that this should:

- be comprehensive;
- be multifaceted (i.e. including multiple methods of data collection across different settings, and using multiple respondents);
- cover not just the abusive incident(s) but a complete social history, including a child's history of trauma and of mental health and behaviour problems;

- draw on a range of standardized instruments, including those specifically designed to identify the sequelae of sexual abuse.

This advice is clear and evidence based; its implementation is more rare.

Current best evidence suggests that cognitive-behavioural interventions (see Chapter 7) outperform other therapeutic interventions such as play therapy (see Macdonald, 2001; Corcoran, 2006; Macdonald *et al.*, 2007). In particular they are effective in addressing 'externalizing' behaviours (e.g. aggression, acting out); sexualized behaviour, and the trauma-related (PTSD) symptoms than can affect some children. Interventions that address these abuse-specific consequences have the following components:

- provide information about the nature of sexual abuse and the range of likely consequences;
- facilitate the expression of a range of abuse-related feelings;
- identify and correct distorted or maladaptive cognitions;
- teach anxiety management skills;
- equip children with self-protection skills;
- directly address the management of problematic behaviour associated with the abuse.

Case example

Deblinger *et al.* (1996) randomly allocated 100 children to one of four conditions:

1   Community control. Parents received information about their children's symptom patterns and were strongly encouraged to seek help within the community.

2   Child-only intervention in which children received 12 individual sessions of cognitive-behavioural therapy. One of the reasons why anxieties and phobias are resistant to change is because we avoid those things that trigger them. In the attempt to protect children who have been sexually abused, parents often shield them from abuse-related stimuli or discussion. In doing so they prevent children from processing their abusive experiences. Gradual exposure was therefore used as the cornerstone of this approach. Parents received occasional updates on their child's progress and the workers answered any questions or concerns they had.

3   Non-offending parent intervention. Twelve weekly group sessions in which parents were taught the therapeutic skills deployed by the therapists in the child-only group. They also learned to analyse their interactions with their children, identifying situations in which they might inadvertently have shaped or maintained problems associated with the abuse. Child management skills were then taught to help parents change these unhelpful patterns of interaction.

4   Combined parent and child intervention. A combination of (2) and (3).

Mothers who were involved in this programme described significantly greater decreases in their children's externalizing behaviours (e.g. aggression, acting out), and reported greater use of effective own parenting skills than those assigned to the community or child-only conditions. Their children reported significantly less depression than those children assigned to the community or child-only conditions. Children assigned to both experimental treatments exhibited significantly fewer PTSD symptoms than children not involved in treatment. Children in the control group who received help within the community did no better than those who did not, suggesting that general treatment strategies which are not 'abuse-focused' are not effective for this group (see Goodman *et al.*, 1992; Oates *et al.*, 1994). This study is one of a number that indicate programmes which offer help to parents and to children simultaneously are more beneficial than those with a focus on either parents or children alone.

Conclusions

Sticks and stones may break my bones but words will never hurt me.

Nonsense. Given the psychological traumas that looked-after children have experienced and the precarious service that many receive while in care, it is nothing short of shameful that we have such a weak evidence base concerning how best to help them. In particular we know little about what helps children deal with psychological maltreatment. This permeates all forms of abuse and is thought to be an important factor in accounting for the adverse developmental outcomes of other forms of abuse (see Becker *et al.*, 1995). Rather, as a society, we have concentrated our attention on the forensically more detectable and dramatic forms of physical abuse. This is a mistake.

12 Social work with young offenders

Nemo repente duit turpissimus
(No one ever suddenly became depraved)
Juvenal

Introduction

The first point to note in relation to young people and offending is that the two terms are not synonymous. It is easy to buy into the moral panic that has grown up around 'youth' in many countries. As Muncie observes, 'youth' and 'adolescence', unlike 'child' or 'adult', are not neutral terms. Rather, they conjure up a range of 'emotional and troubling images' which themselves influence the ways in which society responds to them (Muncie, 2004). Given that those working in criminal justice typically encounter young people who have been apprehended for criminal acts and some whose, strictly speaking, non-criminal activity has none the less brought them into the criminal justice system through antisocial behaviour orders, it is important to be aware of how atypical these young people are.

Unless otherwise indicated, the term 'offending' is used here to denote criminal activity, irrespective of whether or not the young person concerned is apprehended, appears in court or is found guilty. The terms 'delinquency', 'crime' and 'offender' imply apprehension and conviction, but then research consistently indicates that most crime is not captured in official crime statistics (see Muncie, 2004; Maguire, 2007). Further, official statistics reflect the age of criminal responsibility, which varies across countries and offences and changes over time (10 in England, Wales and Northern Ireland; 8 in Scotland). The term 'young people' is used in preference to 'adolescents' for two reasons. First, it more accurately reflects the extended social transition from childhood to adulthood (e.g. the 'peak' age for male offending has risen from 14 in 1971 to 18 since 1990) and the continued development of young people beyond the age of legal adulthood (18 in the UK; see Rutter *et al.*, 1998).

Compared with their peers, young people who offend are likely to differ from their non-offending peers in a number of ways. In order to make sound assessments of how and why a young person finds him or herself at risk of entering the juvenile justice system and to decide how best to help them, those working in the field need to understand what factors in young people's lives have contributed to their offending and how. They need also to understand how social and environmental influences shape and maintain behaviour; why some groups are more at risk than others of finding themselves labelled as offenders or receiving harsher treatment within the justice system, and how it is that certain behaviours come to be seen as problematic.

After considering what we know about the prevalence and incidence of youth offending we examine those factors that are associated with an increased risk of criminal behaviour in young people. We then review what we know about effective interventions and the extent to which this evidence has been incorporated into UK sentencing and disposals. After a discussion of substance use, misuse and offending, and what works in helping those so affected, we conclude the chapter with a brief consideration of the overall effectiveness of the juvenile justice system in England and Wales.

The scope of youth offending

Surveys have come to occupy an increasingly important place in our endeavour to capture the extent and nature of criminal activity. This is because of the well-documented limitations of most official data sources. Some surveys, such as the British Crime Survey (BCS), focus on people's experiences of crime. Others, such as the Offending, Crime and Justice Survey (OCJS), focus on self-reported criminal activity. Both testify to the 'tip-of-the-iceberg' nature of official crime statistics and help to build a more accurate picture of the extent and nature of criminal activity. Surveys also assist with the complex task of interpreting the meaning of data collected and, when repeated over time, can identify trends – though not always the absolute causes.

The OCJS has now been conducted over three consecutive years. It focuses primarily on 20 core offences covering property-related offences (e.g. burglary, theft, including vehicle theft, and criminal damage), violent offences (robbery and assault) and drug selling. It does not cover homicide and sexual offences. The 2005 sample comprised 4,980 respondents aged 10 to 25 at the time of the interview. All but 816 had been interviewed in either 2003 or 2004 (the additional 816 respondents represent a 70 per cent response rate of those approached). OCJS samples are drawn from those living in the general household population of England and Wales only, and do not include people living in institutions or those who are homeless. The surveys therefore cover few 'serious' offenders (for further detail see Wilson *et al.*, 2006, Appendix B). Here are some key findings about the extent of youth offending in the 12 months preceding the 2005 survey interviews:

1   Twenty-five per cent of young people aged 10 to 25 said they had committed at least one core offence. Half of these (13 per cent) had committed at least one serious offence (assault with injury, theft from a person, theft of a vehicle, burglary, selling Class A drugs, robbery). This equates to 13 per cent of all 10- to 15-year-olds.
2   The most commonly reported offence categories were assault (committed by 16 per cent) and other thefts (11 per cent). 'Other thefts' included thefts from school or workplace (most common), from shops, from the person and 'miscellaneous'.
3   Criminal damage, drug-selling offences and vehicle-related thefts were less common (4 per cent, 4 per cent and 2 per cent respectively) with only 1 per cent

of young people saying they had committed burglary or robbery in the past 12 months.

4   Males were more likely to have offended than females (30 per cent compared to 21 per cent respectively). For males, the prevalence of offending peaked among 16- to 19-year-olds, while for females the prevalence peaked earlier at age 14 to 15.

5   Seven per cent of young people were classified as *frequent* offenders. That is, they had offended six or more times in the preceding 12 months. This group was responsible for 83 per cent of all offences measured in the survey.

6   One per cent of all 10- to 25-year-olds had committed six or more *serious* offences and were classified as frequent serious offenders.

7   Four per cent of all respondents reported carrying a knife, with males being significantly more likely to have done so than females (5 per cent versus 2 per cent). Eight in ten respondents who carried a knife said they did so for protection.

8   Twenty per cent of 12- to 25-year-olds had handled (bought or sold) stolen goods, a figure that remained stable between 2004 and 2005.

It is instructive to set against these reports of activity the much lower reported rates of apprehension:

9   Four per cent of 10- to 25-year-olds had been arrested, 2 per cent had been to court accused of committing a criminal offence and 1 per cent had received a community or custodial sentence or a fine.

10   Thirteen per cent of those who had offended said the police had spoken to them about at least one of the offences they had committed, although this had not necessarily resulted in arrest. Violent offences were those most likely to bring young people into contact with the police.

The data reported in the three OCJ Surveys indicate a remarkably stable and consistent pattern with regard to the proportion of young people who report committing an offence, the proportion of males and females and of young people from the age groups 10 to 17 and 18 to 25 years who report criminal activity, and the proportion who fall into the 'serious' or 'frequent' offender categories. Although the proportions are substantial, they counter popular notions that 'most' young people are involved in criminal activity and, while reflecting gender differences in criminal activity, they suggest that these may not be as stark as portrayed in other data. There may be several reasons for this. When considering offenders, we should note that young people who offend are at greater risk of themselves becoming a victim. In their survey of 14- to 15-year-olds in Peterborough, Wikström and Butterworth (2006) found that the mean rate of victimization was highest for high-frequency offenders, and the strongest relationship was between committing an act of violence and being a victim of violence.

Age and gender

The 'peak age' phenomenon has generally been taken to mean that most young people who become involved in offending eventually 'grow out of it'. While there is undoubtedly evidence to support this interpretation, there has been little research into precisely why this might be, and which young people are likely to desist (see Laub and Sampson, 2001). Data from the Youth Lifestyles Surveys (YLS) suggest the need for a more fine-grained analysis. The first survey (1992/3) suggested variation in the ages at which young men and women engaged in certain kinds of offending. For example, for 'expressive property offences' the peak age of offending for males was 14, but for violent offences it was 16. For serious offences and drug offences it was 17 and 20 years respectively (Graham and Bowling, 1995). The second survey (1998/9) also found that the rate of property offending remained stable between the ages of 18 and 25, although it tailed off after that (see Flood-Page *et al.*, 2000). The peak age for both young male and young female offences of violence is 14 to 15; and although male offenders commit more violent offences, both are more likely to commit a violent offence than a property offence (Budd *et al.*, 2005a).

Social class and ethnicity

Although the OCJS does not report social class for respondents, there is evidence from other sources that young people who commit offences are disproportionately drawn from social classes IV and V (i.e. the working class) (see Flood-Page *et al.*, 2000). Self-report data indicate that black and white youth generally share an equal likelihood of being involved in crime, with those of Asian origin being much less likely (see Sharp and Budd, 2005; Wikström and Butterworth, 2006). In contrast, police arrest data, victimization surveys and witness descriptions all suggest that black people are more likely than their white peers to commit certain kinds of crime (e.g. robbery, gun crime) and to be the victims of crime. They are also more likely to be treated differently, and more harshly, at various points of the criminal justice process – in terms of being stopped and searched, arrested, remanded in custody and awarded custodial sentences (see Phillips and Bowling, 2007). Evidence from a study by Feltzer and Hood suggests that mixed-race youths are more likely to be prosecuted (rather than being dealt with pre-court) than their case characteristics would indicate. Together with black youths, they are significantly more likely to be remanded in custody and then not convicted. Although neither group is more likely to receive a custodial sentence than white youth, they are more likely to receive a *longer* sentence, both custodial and community. Finally, Asian youths are more likely to be sentenced to custody than white youths with the same characteristics, despite their under-representation in offending statistics, including self-report data (Feilzer and Hood, 2004). It is difficult to resist the proposition that racism contributes to these patterns of differential treatment (Bowling and Phillips, 2002; Audit Commission, 2004).

Drugs

The use of illegal substances is itself an offence, and there is evidence that it can be implicated in other forms of offending, either by dint of its impact on mood, behaviour and judgement, or because offences are committed as a means of funding these habits. Young people aged 16 to 24 show the highest prevalence of drug use in the UK, with vulnerable young people reporting higher levels than their non-vulnerable peers (NICE, 2007a; see also Information Centre, 2005). The vulnerable group includes looked-after children, children with conduct and emotional disorders, and those known to Youth Offending Teams. The British Crime Survey (Roe and Man, 2006) reported that 45 per cent of 16- to 24-year-olds had used one or more illicit drugs in their lifetime; 25 per cent in the last year, and 15 per cent in the last month (see Roe and Man, 2006).

The second YLS reported that 75 per cent of 'persistent offenders' (committing three or more minor offences, and/or at least one serious offence, in the past year) aged 12 to 17 reported lifetime use of drugs, and 57 per cent had used drugs in the previous year (Flood-Page *et al.*, 2000). Serious and persistent male offenders were four times more likely to be using Class A drugs on at least a monthly basis than their female counterparts, though they note these levels are low compared with those reported by offenders who are apprehended by the police or incarcerated (Goulden and Sondhi, 2001; see also Wikström and Butterworth, 2006). This picture comes from a survey of nearly 300 offenders aged 15 to 16 known to Youth Offending Teams (YOTs) (Hammersley *et al.*, 2003). Most of these young people, mainly boys, had committed at least six different types of offence and more than 20 per cent reported shoplifting, selling stolen goods and taking cars without consent at least 20 times in the previous 12 months (p. viii). They were therefore at the serious end of the spectrum of young people known to YOTs. Reported substance use in this group was considerably higher than that reported in either the Youth Lifestyles Survey or the British Crime Survey 2000. Over 20 per cent of these young people had used a Class A drug, and over 20 per cent reported that they had committed drug-dealing-type offences at least 20 times during the year. Substance use, particularly of socially tolerated substances (alcohol, cannabis and tobacco), predicted offending. Substance misuse in this sample was more prevalent than among the 'serious' offenders in the Youth Lifestyles Survey and even more so than among the 16 to 30 subsample of the British Crime Survey. Forty per cent of the cohort interviewed felt there was some relationship between their substance use and their offending.

The relationship between drug use and offending is, however, complex. To put the preceding data in perspective it is worth reviewing the wider picture of drug use by children and young people, most of whom will not be in trouble. In a survey of school-age children in England (Information Centre, 2007), 17 per cent of pupils aged 11 to 15 reported taking drugs in the past year and 9 per cent in the past month (data for the 'ever used drugs' category are not available for respondents in the 2006 *Smoking, Drinking and Drug Use* survey). While the numbers of boys and girls reporting drug use were similar, boys were more likely to have taken drugs in the past month. The prevalence of drug-taking increased with age, from 6 per cent of 11-year-olds to 29 per cent of 15-year-olds reporting drug use in the past year (Home Office, 2007). The annual surveys on smoking, drinking and drug use among pupils in England between 2003 and 2005 provide some information on drug use and ethnicity. Pupils of mixed parentage were more likely than other groups to have taken drugs in the month and year prior to interview (15 per cent and 24 per cent respectively). Figures for other groups ranged from 8 per cent (Asian pupils) to 11 per cent (white pupils) in the past month, and 12 per cent (Asian pupils) to 20 per cent (white pupils) in the previous year. Among pupils from black ethnic groups, girls were more likely than boys to have taken drugs in the past year, but this was not the case for white pupils.

Cannabis continues to be the drug used most by young people, and although reclassified as a Class C drug (thereby attracting a lesser penalty for illegal possession) the increased strength of the cannabis now in circulation is a cause of concern. The BCS in 2005 estimated that 21 per cent of 16- to 24-year-olds used cannabis in the previous year. This is followed by cocaine (6 per cent) and ecstasy (4 per cent) (Roe and Man, 2006; see also Budd *et al.*, 2005b). The 2006 survey of school-children in England reported that 10 per cent of pupils had used cannabis in the year prior to the interview. Volatile substances (glues and solvents) were the next most frequently cited drugs. Just over 4 per cent of pupils reported using any Class A drugs (Information Centre, 2007).

Data on *frequency* of drug use were asked for the first time in the 2002/3 BCS. Cannabis is the drug most likely to be used frequently by young people (defined as more than once a month during the previous year), with 41 per cent of cannabis users saying they used the drug with this frequency (see Roe and Man, 2006).

Until the mid-1990s, surveys tracked a steady rise over 20 years in the use of illicit drugs among young people, including polydrug use (see Parker *et al.*, 1995). Since the late 1990s all surveys indicate reductions in most illicit drug use. For example, the BCS reports an overall (but not statistically significant) decrease in illicit drug use since 1998, attributable primarily to a gradual decline in cannabis use over that period from 28 per cent to 21 per cent. The use of other non-Class A drugs has remained stable, though there has been an increase in cocaine powder use between 1998 and 2000 from 3 per cent of young people aged 16 to 24 reporting use to 6 per cent where it has stabilized.

Alcohol

Alcohol use and misuse (both of which increase with age – see Goddard, 1996; Harrington, 2000) by young people has become a major concern since the late 1990s. So-called 'binge drinking' is of particular concern, and the data from the YLS indicate a general association between this and offending, particularly violent offending (see Richardson *et al.*, 2003). Other research confirms that increasing alcohol use is associated with significant increases in rates of both violent and property crime, even controlling for the effects of confounding influences such as age and deviant peer affiliations (see Fergusson and Horwood, 2000; Department of Health *et al.*, 2007).

Understanding youth crime

Knowing who commits what sort of crime, at what ages and in what circumstances is important information. It can help to provide a basis for determining changes in patterns of offending and, indirectly, the impact of steps taken to prevent or reduce trouble. Such information, in and of itself, tells us relatively little about why some children, and not others, commit offences, and how they differ from their non-offending peers. In and of itself it sheds no light on why some young people continue to offend into adulthood while most desist. Knowing that there is a strong correlation between drug and alcohol misuse and offending does not tell us what the relationship is between the two, whether they are simply highly correlated or whether one influences the other, and if so in which direction.

In order to intervene effectively in the lives of young people we need to understand how patterns of offending develop (from 'initiation', through continued offending and – for most – eventual desistance), how the nature and frequency of offending changes, what factors are influential and how. Recent years have seen a burgeoning of studies that seek to address these general questions. Important sources of data are prospective longitudinal studies that track groups of children and young people through time. A key example in the UK is the Cambridge Study in Delinquent Development. This is a prospective longitudinal survey of the development of antisocial and offending behaviour in a sample of 411 South London boys, born mostly in 1953 (West and Farrington, 1973; Piquero *et al.*, 2007). The survey has tracked participants from age 8 to 48. This survey sits alongside a number of other longitudinal studies conducted in various countries (including the USA, New Zealand and Scandinavian countries), and there is considerable consistency in the findings reported (see Farrington and Welsh, 2007). As in other areas of criminology, we find a pooling of ideas and data from a range of disciplines, including psychology, sociology, biology and genetics. To date we have a number of potential pieces of the offending jigsaw, but how they fit together and what final picture will emerge is, as yet, uncertain.

West and Farrington (1973) suggested (some time ago – but the trends are still present) that there are currently ten widely accepted conclusions about the development of offending:

1   Age of onset of offending is typically between 8 and 14. Self-report data indicate earlier onset than official records. People typically desist from offending between 20 and 29 years of age, though a small group continue well into adulthood.
2   In general, levels of offending peak between ages 15 and 19.
3   An early onset predicts a relatively long duration of criminal activity and more offences.
4   There is a marked continuity in offending and antisocial behaviour throughout a person's life. There is a high probability that people who commit a high number of offences at one stage in their lives, relative to others, will commit a high number of offences, relative to others, at a later age.
5   A small number of people commit a large proportion of all crime. These 'chronic offenders' have generally engaged in crime at an early stage, and have committed offences with high frequency and over a long period of time. These are sometimes referred to as 'early onset' offenders (see Moffitt, 1993).
6   Offending is generally not specialized. That is to say, offenders (particularly violent offenders) commit a range of offences – but see the qualification in (10) below.
7   Offences appear to be one element of a larger syndrome of antisocial behaviour that includes behaviours such as heavy drinking, reckless driving and promiscuous sex.
8   While most offences committed in adolescence tend to be done in the company of others, those over age 20 appear to move from group to lone offending.
9   Adolescent offenders account for their offending in terms of excitement,

boredom and/or emotional or utilitarian reasons. After age 20 the major reasons given are utilitarian.

10   Different kinds of offences are first committed at different ages, and there appears to be some progression such that, for example, shoplifting precedes burglary, which precedes robbery. Offences committed after age 20 appear to be more specialized.

A range of factors have been identified that appear to increase the risk that a young person will engage in criminal behaviour, and that shape the frequency, duration and persistence of offending. The following summary draws on analyses of longitudinal data from a range of studies from within psychology, sociology, criminology and genetics.

Individual risk factors

Genetic influences

Having a convicted parent or older delinquent sibling was one of the best predictors of later offending and antisocial behaviour for boys aged 8 to 10 in the Cambridge Study (Farrington, 1992), a finding consistent with other studies. In other words, crime does appear to 'run in families'. This may, of course, be attributable to intergenerational styles of parenting, or criminal 'access' via the parent or older sibling, or other environmental risk factors such as living in deprived neighbourhoods. A growing number of studies however, including twin studies, now point to a key role in genetic transmission in the development of antisocial behaviour in early childhood (see Arseneault *et al.*, 2003). Heritability for *pervasive* childhood antisocial behaviour was estimated at 82 per cent in Arsenault *et al.*'s study compared with an estimate of 40 per cent heritability for adolescent and adult antisocial behaviour (see Rhee and Waldman, 2002).

This does not mean that there is a 'gene' for crime. Genetic effects operate through variations in gene clusters that influence us all. Some variations increase the likelihood of antisocial behaviour while others decrease the risk. These can influence behaviour indirectly; for example, people with certain personalities or temperamental dispositions may be more at risk of impulsive antisocial behaviour than others. Similarly, some people will be 'protected' from engagement in antisocial behaviour because they are more anxious than others, and therefore more inhibited.

Environment interacts with genes in a number of ways that can moderate or exacerbate their influence (see Rutter *et al.*, 2006b). For example, parents who pass on their genes also provide the physical and social environment in which their children grow up. Insofar as their own behaviour is antisocial, parents may both model inappropriate ways of behaving and fail to provide the kind of parenting necessary to optimal childhood adjustment (e.g. warm, problem-solving, consistent and authoritative (rather than authoritarian) parenting). Parents with antisocial behaviour are also at higher risk of family breakdown, itself an environmental stressor which may exacerbate any genetic 'risk' that a chid inherits (see Rutter and Quinton, 1984).

Genetic susceptibility can also exacerbate the adverse consequences of child maltreatment (see below). In one study children whose genotype conferred low levels of MAOA expression (the Monoamine Oxidase A gene) more often developed conduct disorder or antisocial personality disorders and went on to commit violent crime in adulthood than children with a high-activity MAOA genotype (see Caspi *et al.*, 2002). This is a complex and relatively new area of research (Rutter, 2007). It is something to keep an eye on, since although we cannot 'fix' genetic susceptibility, we may be able to counter such factors by providing targeted compensating experiences.

Low intelligence

This is clearly associated with early onset antisocial behaviour and later offending. In the Cambridge Study, low IQ at age 8 predicted both juvenile and adult convictions (Farrington, 1992), along with a range of other poor outcomes such as spouse abuse, aggression and bullying. Low school attainment predicted chronic offenders (see Farrington and West, 1993). One possible reason for the strong association between low intelligence, poor attainment and juvenile offending may be due to certain cognitive impairments, particularly the poor ability to manipulate abstract concepts (see Moffitt, 1993). Impairments in verbal skills and the ability to think ahead mean that young people will not anticipate the consequences of their behaviour (for themselves) nor will they be able to appreciate the feelings of their victims (low empathy). Unlike 'early starters', young people whose antisocial behaviour first occurs in adolescence do not differ significantly from their prosocial peers with regard to cognitive ability. It may also be that children with poor communication skills are harder to socialize and more frustrating to their parents (see Lahey *et al.*, 1999). The association between cognitive impairments and early onset antisocial behaviour is also closely related to hyperactivity (impulsiveness) and attentional problems (Maguin and Loeber, 1996).

Temperament and personality

Persistent offenders differ from others in a number of important ways. As infants, their mothers are likely to describe them as 'unmanageable' (Caspi *et al.*, 1995). They are more likely to be restless, to have a short attention span, to be oppositional, emotionally negative, less able to delay gratification (lack of control) and often to be more aggressive, particularly in relation to unprovoked aggression. Because of the overlap between measures of personality and temperament and measures of criminality, there is always a difficulty in determining independent personality effects. The above factors particularly distinguish those children whose antisocial behaviour appears early on, but aggression and peer rejection are closely related. Children who have poor peer relationships are at particular risk for developing antisocial behaviour and delinquency, even after controlling for initial levels of aggression. Peer rejection is a likely consequence of social incompetence. Aggressive children who mishandle relationships (e.g. by dealing with conflicts in an emotionally charged way) are likely both to 'lose' and to experience rejection by their peers (Dodge and Coie, 1987). An inability appropriately to process social information is likely to be a contributing factor.

Biased social information processing

In order to respond to events happening in their environments, children have to do a number of things. First, they have to recognize and interpret relevant cues. They then have mentally to rehearse the range of behavioural responses available to them, select one and implement it. Dodge (1991) has suggested that aggressive children are more likely to interpret cues as hostile (when they may be either neutral or ambiguous (e.g. the teenager who wants to know 'why' someone is looking at them 'like that', when the person is simply preoccupied with his or her own thoughts)). Further, Dodge suggests that they are more likely selectively to attend to aggressive social cues and to disattend to non-aggressive ones. In addition, aggressive children are less likely or less able to suppress hostile responses, and appear to see aggression as a normal and effective response (see Dodge and Schwartz, 1997). They are there-fore more likely simply to take what they want, or bully others into providing things. Whether such cognitive biases arise from experience (e.g. being themselves on the receiving end of hostility) or via some other mechanism is not clear, but there are parallels with the role of attributional biases in other areas such as depression (see Chapter 13). More generally the evidence may help us to understand how adverse experiences might influence antisocial behaviour (e.g. maltreatment). It also provides promising pointers for intervention (see below).

Drugs and alcohol

We earlier described patterns of alcohol and drug misuse among young offenders. Drugs are a risk factor for crime in a number of ways. First, theft and burglary may be undertaken to pay for them, particularly Class A drugs. Such crime is typically acquisitive and non-violent. Then there is the organized criminality that surrounds the drug industry. This may include gun crime and other forms of violence. Drugs may, of course, be one of a number of aspects of a deviant lifestyle. Alcohol is a more serious risk factor for any individual, not least of all because of its disinhibiting effects, but also because of its widespread availability and the frequency with which it is taken to excess.

Psychosocial risk factors

In this section we consider factors within a young person's environment that are thought to increase their risk of engaging in criminal behaviour. Distinguishing between these and 'individual risk factors' is, to some extent, misleading because, as indicated above, biological parents not only pass on their genes but also provide the social environment in which their children are raised. It is complicated by the fact that someone's behaviour can in fact shape their environment (e.g. some children elicit negative responses from their parents as a result of their own irritability and aggression). None the less, there is a substantial body of research indicating the significance of environment for antisocial behaviour. As Rutter *et al.* (1998) have pointed out in their review, the rapid increase in the growth of antisocial and criminal behaviour over the past half century could not have arisen as a result of a changing gene pool, but must reflect environmental influences or growth of opportunity.

As with mental illness (see Chapter 13), twin and adoptive studies provide ample evidence of the impact of environment on behaviour. Children in the same family can have very different childhood experiences as a result of their contacts and experiences outside of the family. Further, probably as a result of biological differences, children in the same families can experience family life differently (e.g. some children are more affected by parental discord than others; some children may be scapegoated or otherwise more victimized than their siblings). These 'non-shared environmental effects' are, in general, more influential than shared effects, though, with regard to antisocial behaviour, both shared and non-shared influences have a discernible impact. In the Cambridge Delinquency study, for example, antisocial behaviour was a feature of several children in a family rather than just one (see Farrington *et al.*, 1996). On the other hand, it is also the case that when parents are particularly negative towards one child, this can pose a more significant risk for that child than general family discord (see Rutter *et al.*, 1997).

Family factors

Here is a summary of the range of family-focused factors that appear to lead to increased risk of children developing antisocial behaviour.

1   *Teenage parenthood* is strongly associated with an increased risk of delinquency for the resultant children. The reasons why remain uncertain, but are likely to be at least partly due to the associated risks of poor educational qualifications, poverty (owing to welfare dependence and poor employment prospects), lack of social support and parenting difficulties. It also appears likely that teenage mothers are more likely themselves to have been involved in antisocial behaviour and to experience domestic violence and relationship breakdown (Maughan and Lindelow, 1997).

2   *Large family size* is also deemed a risk indicator for delinquency. This association may arise for a number of reasons including: (1) antisocial adults have large families whose children both inherit their genes and experience their parenting styles; (2) large family size impacts upon parenting, particularly supervision and discipline (it may also exacerbate the impacts of poverty); and/or (3) the influence of older, delinquent siblings (co-offending by brothers was common in the Cambridge Study of Delinquent Development – Rowe and Farrington, 1997).

3   *Family discord and conflict*, rather than single parenthood or family disruption due to divorce or death, increase the risk of antisocial behaviour and delinquency (see Juby and Farrington, 2001). This may also explain the increased risk associated with a period in public care, although adverse experiences in care may exacerbate the problems underpinning the reasons for admission (Utting, 1996).

Parenting

In order effectively to socialize children, parents have to communicate clear rules and expectations, and set clear boundaries. They have also to shape desirable behaviour and minimize or extinguish antisocial behaviours. For this, parental responses should be generally consistent and be able to divert children from pursuing actions that will lead to frustration and confrontation ('intervening in the antecedents'). Parents should be receptive to their children's needs and help them to develop a positive sense of their worth (self-esteem) and agency (self-efficacy). They have also to help children develop problem-solving skills and – over time – to internalize self-control. The work of Gerald Patterson and his colleagues at the Oregon Social Learning Center has highlighted the extent to which parents of antisocial children fail in respect of one or more of these quite challenging tasks (Patterson, 1982). Two things in particular stand out as significant because of their implications for intervention.

Coercive and hostile styles of parenting

These often include harsh physical punishment, and appear to exert a causal effect on the development of antisocial behaviour and delinquency (Haapasalo and Pokela, 1999). Child abuse and neglect represent extremes of poor parenting, so it is perhaps not surprising that they are strongly correlated with later offending, though not necessarily violent offending (Widom, 1997). It is likely that coercive parenting practices make their mark via several mechanisms. First, they may indicate a more generally poor parent–child relationship (Rutter *et al.*, 1997). Second, the inappropriate models of problem-solving to which these children are exposed may contribute to the development of antisocial ways of tackling problems, through modelling, imitation and reinforcement (Patterson, 1982). Third, harsh or neglectful parenting may also result in poor attachment, reducing the inhibiting effects of not wanting to displease or transgress social norms, first within the family and then – as a result of poor self-control and lack of feeling of belonging – society more widely (Hirschi, 1969).

Poor monitoring and supervision

These are repeatedly implicated as significant factors in youth offending. Parents of young offenders typically know less about the whereabouts and actions of their offspring than do other parents (Loeber and Farrington, 2001). Social context plays a role here – such supervision is easier for the affluent parent with a small family and enclosed grounds. The extent to which this finding is independent of the growing importance of peer associations during adolescence is unclear, but it is none the less significant and is used to inform interventions such as treatment foster care (see below).

Peer groups

These have been shown to be a powerful influence on antisocial behaviour, even after controlling for the 'selection effect' of people choosing to spend time with like-minded and like-behaving friends. Peer group influences impact more strongly upon behaviour during adolescence because of the time spent in that company and the diminution of contact with the family. Groups of antisocial adolescents are not only more likely to engage in offending or delinquent behaviour because they share each other's company, but they are more likely to be in places and situations that provide opportunities for crime. Given the predominance of groups in certain areas, this may indicate other environmental influences such as neighbourhood and social change (Osgood *et al.*, 1996). Belonging to a delinquent peer group also seems to be associated with *persistence* of antisocial behaviour. Most youth offending can be linked in one way or another to groups, but some groupings present particular concerns, namely gangs; indeed, Esbensen and Weerman (2005) have defined a gang as: 'any durable, street-oriented youth group whose involvement in illegal activity is part of their group identity'. There is some evidence that gang membership makes a unique contribution to criminal behaviour, over and above the effects of having delinquent peers (Battin *et al.*, 1998). In the UK, the Youth Justice Board (2007) cautions against the loose use of the term 'gang', noting that juvenile justice practitioners viewed gangs as (1) associated more with young adults than with younger adolescents, (2) differing in the seriousness and intensity of their criminal activity from other groups, and (3) likely to be connected with older, organized crime groups. We currently know little about what factors draw young people into gangs, or how gang membership (as opposed to other forms of group association) influences crime, and the focus on gangs may well distract attention from more significant social issues they may signify – such as social disorganization. None the less, the rise in gang-associated gun and knife crimes is focusing more and more attention on gangs as a locus of intervention (see Fisher *et al.*, 2007).

Resilience

Even when exposed to broadly similar experiences, not all children respond in the same way. Many of those exposed to a range of adverse circumstances do not go on to develop antisocial behaviour. There has been increasing interest in what 'protects' these apparently resilient children who do well *despite* their life circumstances. After discussing the methodological and intellectual challenges associated with assessing reliance, Rutter *et al.* (1998) emphasize the importance of looking at protective *processes* and the circumstances in which they operate to minimize risk. As well as increasing our understanding of causal mechanisms, this may enable us to devise potential means of prevention.

In relation to antisocial behaviour they summarize the main findings on what contributes to resilience are as follows:

- a lack of genetic vulnerability (bearing in mind that susceptibility to psycho-social hazards is also a function of experience);
- a higher IQ, and temperamental and other personality features that elicit positive responses from others;
- a stable, warm and largely conflict-free relationship with at least one parent (even in circumstances where there is a lot of family conflict), and parental supervision, particularly in neighbourhoods where community controls are weak;

- good experiences at school, probably via their impact on self-esteem and self-efficacy; a prosocial peer group may counter other risk processes;
- other experiences that provide diversionary opportunities such as academic achievement, sport, or changes in social circumstances that can point young people in a different direction ('turning points');
- a positive attitude of mind and good social problem-solving skills.

Clearly some of these potential influences are easier to 'engineer' than others, and have informed the development of some promising interventions. Rutter cautions that the studies on which these findings rest are few and far between (Rutter *et al.*, 1998).

Societal factors

Although we do not have space to discuss societal factors in detail in this chapter, it is important to emphasize the significance of influences that operate at a level beyond that of the individual and the family. These include the neighbourhoods in which people live and which provide varying levels of social support, community control, policing, opportunities or disincentives for antisocial behaviour, and so on (see Wikström and Sampson, 2003). Some of these factors are implicated in interventions that have been developed in recent years (see below) and – although our knowledge about the ways in which neighbourhoods impact upon offending is still relatively underdeveloped – an understanding of these influences informs community-based approaches (see Chapter 9). The availability of drugs, alcohol and guns and the normalization of violence through the media may all have influenced the changes in profiles and rates of crime in the UK in the past 50 years. Increased opportunities for crime also arise from the availability of sought-after goods (e.g. mobile phones) and by the steps not taken to deter opportunistic crime (e.g. inadequate locks on cars).

There are also variations in relation to ethnicity, and these are exacerbated by discrimination in a variety of enforcement processes (Phillips and Bowling, 2007). Again, we have a limited understanding of those differences that appear to exist after such external sources of distortion have been controlled out (Wikström and Butterworth, 2006). The effects of race may well be mediated by socio-economic conditions or family risk factors. One important source of bias that Rutter *et al.* (1998) and Wikström and Butterworth (2006) point out is the failure of researchers to include this dimension into much of their analyses, and, in the UK context, an over-reliance on research from the USA. Conclusions drawn from the literature as a whole must therefore be treated with some caution when applied to young people from minority ethnic groups within the UK.

What works in youth offending?

Youth justice is clearly a wide field, and one could examine 'what works' from a variety of perspectives, including the organization of services (e.g. policing, sentencing); the focus of interventions (individuals, families/parents, schools, communities); the timing of intervention (preventing antisocial behaviour in childhood, in adolescence and intervening after offending has been adjudicated); types of intervention (psychosocial, cognitive-behavioural, multisystemic) or by focusing on types of offence. Insofar as some offences appear very particular (e.g. arson), there may be some merit in focusing on offences, but, as noted above, the evidence currently points to versatility of criminal offences rather than specialization. It seems likely that common elements may need to be addressed irrespective of the nature of the offences, although considerable tailoring may be required for particular kinds of offences (such as sexual offences).

We begin with a review of three interventions aimed at preventing young people from offending before going on to consider a further three that have been targeted at young offenders. The evidence reviewed draws, wherever possible, on systematic reviews and controlled trials. Most of these studies are conducted outside the UK, most commonly in the USA and Canada, but the interventions included either resemble interventions used in the UK or are those which could be incorporated relatively easily since the focus was comparable. There are many more reports of the purported effectiveness of interventions other than those presented here. In large part this will be because of the different thresholds of evidence used. Two of the interventions considered are popular programmes in some countries, and their underpinning philosophies have influenced UK sentencing. This is why, although they enjoy no empirical support, we take stock of the evidence base – the sieve of history having such large holes.

Prevention

Because of the association between early onset behaviour problems (particularly oppositional and conduct disorders and hyperactivity) and criminal behaviour, there has been a growing interest in early interventions (see Chapter 3). These fall largely into two groups: (1) helping parents more effectively to manage their children's behaviour, and (2) working directly with children to improve those children's behaviour.

Early parent training

Bernazzani and Tremblay (2006) reviewed the available RCTs looking at the effectiveness of support and training programmes provided to families with a child under 3 years of age at enrolment. Studies were eligible for inclusion in the review, whether or not the intervention was available to the general population or to identified high-risk groups. Parent training or support was required to be a major component, although not necessarily the only one. The reviewers had initially intended to assess the impact of these interventions on delinquency, but decided to include a broader range of outcomes on finding that only one study reported on delinquent behaviour. Partly as a result of such broad inclusion criteria, the included studies, though only seven in number, were very diverse, so it was not possible to pool the data (an important means of overcoming the limitations of small studies, but only appropriate when studies are broadly similar in key respects). The reviewers' overall conclusions are that, as yet, we know too little to make a definitive judgement about the potential of these very early interventions. They suggest that what is needed is the development and rigorous testing of interventions aiming specifically at preventing disruptive behaviour.

Child social skills training

This is an intervention provided to children whose problems begin in the early years. It is based on evidence that these children often have deficits in social information processing and problem-solving skills, both of which are risk factors for later antisocial behaviour. Such programmes are relatively inexpensive, can be delivered on a broad basis (e.g. in schools) and are less prone to the difficulties inherent in delivering family-based programmes. They may be seen as a defensible educational activity, irrespective of their impact upon offending. They are largely cognitive-behavioural programmes based on social learning theory, with a major emphasis on problem-solving. There have been a number of reviews of high-quality studies of the effectiveness of social skills training, which – although the data are complex – generally point to their effectiveness in preventing antisocial behaviour and crime (see Lösel and Beelmann, 2003).

More recently, Lösel and Beelmann have conducted a review of social skills training, for children and young people aged 18 years and under, which was confined to studies that targeted young people not yet adjudicated delinquent or given a clinical diagnosis, and reported at least one measure of antisocial behaviour as an outcome to be modified (Lösel and Beelmann, 2006). They identified 55 research reports of RCTs which provided data on some 89 comparisons of the effectiveness of social skills training against either no treatment or an alternative treatment. The headline messages from their detailed review are as follows:

1   Social competence training appears to have a significantly positive overall effect on the antisocial behaviour of children and young people (although it is noted that the effects on aggressive and delinquent behaviour are somewhat smaller, though still encouraging).

2   Although follow-up periods are not as long as they might be in other areas of research, the evidence indicates that positive outcomes can be sustained over time and, given that these programmes are typically short in duration and delivered in groups, they may well be cost-effective (see Welsh and Farrington, 2001).

3   Programmes appeared to have the most impact with older youth (13 years and older), and with young people already evidencing behavioural problems, reinforcing the view that it may be best to focus our resources on high-risk samples.

4   The evidence suggests that some types of intervention are better than others, and cognitive-behavioural interventions (which comprised four-fifths of all studies) 'consistently show not only the largest overall effect but also a significant impact on all types of antisocial behaviour. These effects are relatively reliable insofar as they are based on the largest number of studies'. Most skills programmes now contain some aspects of behavioural or cognitive-behavioural therapy.

5   Although the overall effect of programmes was positive, irrespective of theoretical orientation, some programmes appear to bring about worse outcomes for those who participate in them. Care needs to be taken to ensure that the interventions provided are truly beneficial (see McCord, 2003).

Juvenile awareness programmes

The best known of these is 'Scared Straight' and they are not only ineffective but the evidence suggests that they can increase the risk of offending (Petrosino *et al.*, 2006). These programmes are designed to 'scare' at-risk young people or delinquents away from a life of crime. Young people at high risk for future offending are taken into prisons, where they are exposed to the brutality of prison life, hearing firsthand from inmates how they came to be where they are, and receiving vivid images of the consequences of their actions. Some programmes are more confrontational than others; some have a more educational emphasis. Either way, deterrence is the rationale. Petrosino and colleagues first conducted a systematic review of the effectiveness of juvenile awareness programmes in 2002 (Petrosino *et al.*, 2002). This review, which was last updated in 2006, synthesizes the evidence from nine American RCTs and quasi-randomized trials. While most study participants were juveniles, some programmes mixed juveniles with young adults up to age 21 years. Here is the authors' conclusion:

> These randomized trials, conducted over a quarter-century in eight different jurisdictions and involving nearly 1,000 participants, provide evidence that Scared Straight and other juvenile awareness programs are not effective as a stand-alone criminal prevention strategy. More importantly, they provide empirical evidence – under experimental conditions – that these programs are likely to increase the odds that children exposed to them will commit another delinquent offense.
>
> (Petrosino *et al.*, 2006: 98)

Programmes like 'Scared Straight' continue to be used, in spite of the evidence of their harmful effects, and Petrosino continues to receive enquiries from Americans wanting to know how they can get a child on to such a programme. This is deeply worrying because, as the reviewers also point out, when crime reduction programmes go wrong, their 'toxic effects' not only impact upon the participants, but 'result in increased misery for ordinary citizens that comes from the "extra" victimization they create when compared to just doing nothing at all'. Having a good and popular idea, being well resourced, well intentioned and well trained, does not guarantee a non-malign, let alone a positive, outcome.

Promising interventions with young offenders

In this section we consider two interventions that have been extensively deployed. The first – cognitive-behavioural therapy – enjoys considerable empirical support as an intervention of choice in dealing with young offenders. The second – restorative justice – has a different and wider focus.

Cognitive-behavioural interventions

These draw primarily on learning theories and cognitive psychology to understand and intervene in problem behaviour (see Chapter 7). Their rationale is the range of cognitive errors and distortions that influence the behaviour of offenders; these may include, for example, misperceptions of the motivations of others, an inability to think through the consequences of their actions, a tendency to blame others ('external attributions') and not to see their own contribution to situations.

Cognitive-behavioural programmes begin with a careful assessment of the particular problems for any individual (see Chapter 7). Typically, offenders are taught to identify the patterns of thinking and beliefs that contribute to their wrongdoing, so that they can find alternatives. Offenders often have poor problem-solving skills so they are taught to consider all aspects of a situation; to rehearse and reality test their beliefs about what is happening; to think through the available choices, the pros and cons of each, and then to select the one that – both in the short and long term – maximizes positive outcomes and minimizes negative ones. Some young people will be provided with anger management or social skills training, as necessary, and so on. All a little utilitarian-sounding perhaps, but these interventions appear to be effective.

Lipsey and Landenberg (2006) conducted a systematic review and meta-analysis of RCTs evaluating the effectiveness of cognitive-behavioural programmes with both adult and juvenile offenders from *general* offender populations (i.e. not committing specific types of offences). They identified 14 studies that met their eligibility criteria, six of which involved juveniles, and most of which focused on male offenders. The results indicated that, in line with earlier reviews, cognitive-behavioural programmes reduced recidivism rates by 27 per cent. Programmes in community settings were more effective than those in prison settings and with high-risk offenders.

The reviewers point out that most of these programmes were either research programmes or 'demonstration projects' with a strong research component. Getting things to work under mainstream conditions is often more challenging, and requires careful attention to ensuring that programmes are rolled out as they were designed and implemented, and that staff are well trained and appropriately supervised with manageable workloads. Implementation requires attention to so-called 'treatment integrity' (which is why many recommend 'manualized' approaches, where procedures are carefully documented). The resource implications can be significant, but this must be set against the long-term costs of offending, and the potential squandering of scarce resources if programmes are not delivered in the ways required to maximize their potential. Other evidence points to the usefulness of cognitive-behavioural programmes across a wide range of specific problems (e.g. aggression, substance misuse, fire-setting, indecent exposure), and with groups of different ages, cultural backgrounds and gender (see McGuire, 2000; Utting and Vennard, 2000).

Restorative justice programmes

These seek to transform the ways in which we view and deal with crime and antisocial behaviour, although there are different views as to how this can or should be done (Bazemore and Elis, 2007). Restorative justice (RJ) interventions differ in a number of ways from 'traditional' approaches. The latter are primarily focused on the offender; their disposals (e.g. prison, probation, boot camps) effectively label offenders as 'bad people' deserving of punishment, and generally deal with them in ways that make it difficult for offenders to feel part of the communities from which they came. This weakens further any sense of connection or obligations they may feel. In all of this, victims are sidelined. In contrast, restorative justice programmes are primarily focused on the victim. Programmes seek to label the offence – rather than the offender – as 'bad', and to facilitate reintegration by requiring reparation by the offender towards the victim ('re-integrative shaming': Braithwaite, 2001). Through this process, offenders are re-engaged with their communities and helped to establish a 'reformed' identity.

This usually entails bringing the offender (who must not be in dispute about culpability) face-to-face with those affected by his or her actions. This may take the form of a conference (e.g. family group conference) or an appearance before a panel (more usual in neighbourhood reparation schemes). Unlike mediation, not only do the victim and the offender meet, but they may be accompanied by family, friends, relevant professionals (including police, probation, drugs treatment personnel) or, where there is no 'direct victim' (for example, in fraud or vandalism), representatives of organizations or communities that have been affected. While it is not clear that such face-to-face encounters are essential to effective programmes (see Bazemore and Schiff, 2004), they epitomize the importance of starting with an acknowledgement of the damage to the victim and the community, giving all those who have been affected by the crime an opportunity to influence the decision-making, holding the offender to account for his or her actions in a very direct way, and identifying the steps he or she will take to make amends. In doing so, RJ programmes relocate the responsibility for monitoring and dealing with crime at a community level, and aim to develop community capacity to do so effectively. There is, therefore, an endeavour to instigate systemic changes at the macro level through restorative justice (Bazemore and Elis, 2007).

There is a large literature on restorative justice exploring: (1) the various approaches that have been taken to it; (2) its effectiveness, both from the standpoint of victims and communities and in relation to recidivism; (3) the tensions that may appear to exist between restorative justice and society's demands for retribution (see Hayes, 2007), and (4) the processes or 'ingredients' that shed light on why and when such procedures work.

Strang and Sherman (2006) identified seven completed RCTs of face-to-face restorative justice programmes. Five of these focused on crimes with personal victims and these formed the basis of their systematic review. Three studies focused solely on juveniles; two were carried out in Australia and three in the USA. The outcomes addressed were repeat offending, victim satisfaction and victim revenge crimes. They concluded that face-to-face restorative justice programmes are a promising approach to preventing repeat offending by offenders who have committed – and admitted committing – violent crimes, but not for property crimes by juvenile offenders, at least in the short to medium term. They note that victims of crime who participated in restorative justice evinced higher levels of satisfaction than those in the control groups, and indicated that they are less likely to commit crimes of retaliation.

'What works in sentencing?'

The past ten years have seen an emphasis on engaging offenders in programmes designed specifically to reduce recidivism by directly addressing their offending. The use of cognitive-behavioural interventions is one of the ten evidence-based principles underpinning the 'Effective Practice Initiative in England and Wales', with care being taken to ensure that programmes are delivered in culturally sensitive ways (Hudson, 2007). Cognitive-behavioural interventions are used both in custodial and community settings, and are aimed at improving cognitive skills and otherwise tackling offending behaviour, substance misuse, drink-driving, and violence and sexual offending. For example 94 per cent of young offenders whose sentences included intensive supervision and surveillance had offender behaviour training as part of their programme (Youth Justice Board 2004; see also Feilzer *et al.*, 2004). In general these interventions form part of broader programmes that also tackle other risk factors associated with crime, such as occupational skills deficits, unemployment, social support and integration.

The Youth Justice Board (YJB) commissioned a national evaluation (Feilzer *et al.*, 2004) of 23 cognitive-behavioural projects that they had funded (to the tune of £3.9 million). Fifteen of these projects worked with persistent young offenders and four with adolescent sex offenders; the four remaining projects were focused on education (n=2), reparation (n=1) and mental health (n=1). The overall completion rate for these very varied programmes was 59 per cent. The Youth Justice Board's own summary (2004) is upbeat:

> the findings show that cognitive behaviour approaches can reduce reoffending, even among those groups who are particularly hard to reach. By addressing offending behaviour, improving education and encouraging social interaction, these projects can go a long way to increasing the prospects of participants so that they can lead law-abiding lives.

However, the authors who conducted the national evaluation (and who are thanked in the YJB's publication) draw more cautious conclusions. They highlight the inadequate planning and poor research design (both attributable to the Youth Justice Board) which effectively scuppered the significant lessons that might otherwise have been learned from this major investment in both the programmes and their evaluations:

> Young people valued the 'different' relationship they had with the project worker, their support and respect, and reported that they had changed their behaviour and desisted from crime. Similarly, parents reported that they had noted positive change in the young people's behaviour. However, these positive notes are not reflected in the reconviction rates recorded for this study and should therefore be treated with caution.
>
> (Feilzer *et al.*, 2004: 8)

Half of local evaluators deemed questions about effectiveness were premature and declined to comment on this aspect of their projects. Those that did felt that projects had 'largely' or 'partly' achieved their aims. This is some way removed from the rigorous evidence base we need to develop in the UK.

The national evaluators undertook a very small reconviction study for persistent offenders. Those who completed a programme had a lower reconviction rate than non-completers, but the authors observe that this may have been because people completing programmes were less likely to reoffend, rather than a treatment effect. That said, the 'finding' about completers doing better than non-completers resonates with other studies, but it is also the case that there is often evidence of a 'wash-out' effect, indicating the need for follow-up or booster programmes for even these 'successful' participants (see Cann *et al.*, 2003; Merrington and Stanley, 2004).

Advocates of cognitive-behavioural programmes have never claimed it to be a 'one-size-fits-all' or 'complete answer' to offending. Given the range of influences on offending it is evident that focusing on offending behaviour without addressing other influences is likely to be ineffective, which may be one of the reasons why the results of cognitive-behavioural programmes alone are, outside of research programmes, rather modest (see McGuire, 2002). It may also be the case that the mechanisms which bring about behaviour change (e.g. empathy enhancement, problem-solving, modelling, reinforcement) are most effective as part of an approach that simultaneously addresses the societal risk factors associated with crime, and promotes social connectedness. Restorative justice facilitates this.

Restorative justice is an intuitively appealing idea with much to recommend it – even if it is no more effective than other approaches. There is a growing body of research, including some – somewhat rarely – within the UK, which is beginning to shed light on the effectiveness of these programmes, how they work and the conditions under which they work best (for whom, with whom). One of the core concepts, that of reparation, now features in a range of sentencing options in the UK. For example, young offenders who plead guilty at their first appearance in court may be given a Referral Order. This requires them to attend a youth offender panel, comprising two volunteers from the local community and a panel adviser from the local Youth Offending Team. The panel, together with the young person, the parents and sometimes the victim, agree a contract lasting between three and twelve months designed to repair the harm caused by the offence and to address the causes of the offending behaviour (see Crawford and Newburn, 2003).

Reparation also features in some aspects of cautioning, and intensive supervision and surveillance orders (ISSOs), whether as a condition of bail or part of a community or custodial sentence (see Youth Justice Board, 2002). This is an important developing area, but there is still a lack of carefully designed research that will enable the unpicking of the contribution made by restorative components in multimodal interventions such as intensive supervision and surveillance programmes.

A second principle of restorative justice, reintegration, is also evident in British sentencing policies. Enhanced 'community punishment orders' have been described as containment and reform, based on 'what works' principles (National Probation Service, 2004: 17):

> Community punishment is the sentencing of offenders to unpaid work for the benefit of the community. It is one of the most successful and popular sentences ever devised. It . . . achieved reconviction rates broadly comparable with other sentences, and at a fraction of the cost of imprisonment; and . . . can deliver the three sentencing elements of retribution, reparation and rehabilitation within a single court order and sentencing activity. In a single sentence it can meet the different needs of a range of stakeholders and satisfies these three key components of justice.

Despite their title, these orders are designed to teach prosocial attitudes and behaviour (modelled by those supervising their work), problem-solving skills and employment-related skills. They build on nearly 20 years of research which suggests that providing people with positive experiences that enhance their sense of self-worth and self-efficacy forges a sense of connectedness to society (strengthening social bonds), motivates people to desist from offending and helps their ability to establish alternate, prosocial identities. Gill McIvor, an early researcher and commentator on community sentences, summarized this process as follows:

> In many instances, it seems, contact with the beneficiaries gave offenders an insight into other people, and an increased insight into themselves; the acquisition of skills had instilled in them greater confidence and self-esteem; and the experience of completing their community service orders placed them in a position where they could enjoy reciprocal relationships – gaining the trust, confidence and appreciation of other people and having the opportunity to give something back to them.
>
> (McIvor, 1998: 55–56)

The introduction of Youth Rehabilitation Orders builds on these developments.

What works in substance use and misuse?

Reducing substance use among young people has been a major policy goal since 2003. The aim of the Drugs Intervention Programme for Children and Young People aims to reduce substance misuse, particularly (but not exclusively) Class A drugs; to reduce substance misuse-related crime, and to improve other life factors related to substance misuse and criminal behaviour.

Before we consider the elements of this programme and the evidence of its effectiveness, we take stock of the wider evidence base. In relation to drug use, much attention is given to disrupting street-level, national and international drugs markets. This résumé, in contrast, focuses purely on the treatment of individual young people. We draw primarily on two reports. The first is a review of the evidence on interventions to reduce substance use among disadvantaged and vulnerable people, commissioned by the National Institute for Health and Clinical Excellence (Jones *et al.*, 2006) with associated guidance (NICE, 2007a, 2007b). This was aimed at all those with responsibility for reducing substance use, including social care, young and criminal justice sectors. It forms the basis of much that follows. We then summarize the pertinent findings from the National Treatment Agency's review of effective interventions in drug misuse (Gossop, 2006). While this is primarily focused on adults, it contains material of relevance to young offenders, and is important information for those working in any setting dealing with people with substance misuse problems.

What is effective in work on substance abuse with vulnerable and disadvantaged young people?

The summary of findings of the 401-page report by Jones *et al.* (2006) contains little to comfort us:

> Despite a wide variety of approaches producing improvements in substance use knowledge and attitudes . . . few interventions resulted in a reduction of substance use behaviours beyond the immediate post-intervention assessment phase. It is therefore difficult to draw conclusions from the studies reviewed. Those approaches that demonstrated success tended to address a wide variety of risk factors and problem behaviours rather than having an exclusive substance use focus. However, even for these types of approaches there was not a broad evidence base.
>
> (Jones *et al.*, 2006: 286)

The report goes on to consider the evidence in relation to particular groups of children, both in terms of reducing substance misuse and of reducing the influence of known risk factors. Again, most of the included studies were not conducted in the UK, many – particularly the RCTs – being undertaken in the USA. The authors used an 'applicability scale' to indicate their evaluation of the relevance of study findings to the UK context, from 'Likely to be applicable across a broad range of settings and populations', or 'if appropriately adapted', down to 'Applicable only to settings or populations included in the studies'. We summarize the findings in relation to the groups of most relevance here:

1   *Young offenders.* The reviewers identified only ten studies examining drug prevention programmes for young offenders, five of which were RCTs of varying quality. They conclude that *multisystemic therapy* may be more effective than 'usual services' at reducing 'soft drug use' (as defined by the National Youth Survey in the USA) and substance-related arrests immediately following the intervention (see Henggeler *et al.*, 1991; Littell *et al.*, 2005).

   The *educational programmes* identified were deemed as being of 'low UK applicability' but in any case the findings did not indicate their effectiveness. Neither a modified life skills training intervention nor a combined anti-violence plus values clarification programme made any difference in rates of substance misuse, although there was some evidence from one RCT to suggest that a combined approach might bring about short-term reductions in substance misuse, in illegal and violent offences, or in school problems (Friedman *et al.*, 2002).

   There was no evidence that *juvenile drug courts* (a four-phase programme including intensive probation supervision, frequent random drug testing, judicial monitoring and the use of incentives) or a multi-component programme (a multi-agency strategy including counselling, skills building, prosocial bonding and mentoring) were effective (Stein *et al.*, 1992; Sloan *et al.*, 2004). Drug courts are none the less being piloted in England at the time of writing.

2   *Young substance users.* The reviewers looked at interventions targeted at substance users who were not substance dependent. Early usage of illegal

substances is a risk factor for later dependence and for offending. They identified four systematic reviews and 18 other studies, 11 of which were RCTs. These were divided into four groups: (1) those evaluating brief interventions/motivational interviewing; (2) those assessing family therapy interventions; (3) those examining counselling, and (4) those examining other interventions. Studies on counselling essentially compared different forms or intensity of counselling. They were not regarded as particularly relevant to the UK context and were inconclusive, so are not reported on here.

The studies on *motivational and brief interventions* concluded that the evidence suggests that these interventions can have useful short-term effects on the use of cigarette, alcohol and cannabis (Olianski *et al.*, 1997; Aubrey, 1998; Tait and Hulse, 2003; McCambridge and Strang, 2004). While in the medium term those receiving a motivational interviewing intervention continue to do better, the evidence does not reach statistical significance (McCambridge and Strang, 2005). Similar patterns hold for attitudes, intentions and behavioural outcomes relevant to substance misuse.

Family therapy. The evidence here suggests that family therapy is more effective at reducing substance misuse in young people than other types of group therapy interventions, at least immediately following treatment (Joanning, 1992; Liddle *et al.*, 2001, 2004; Austin *et al.*, 2005). Multidimensional family therapy appears to be more effective that other approaches in the short to medium term (Liddle *et al.*, 2001; Austin *et al.*, 2005). Brief family therapy appears to be more effective than group therapy in producing immediate reductions in cannabis use (Santisteban *et al.*, 2003) and overall substance use (Lewis *et al.*, 1990). The reviewers deemed these studies to be of moderate applicability to the UK context.

3 *School drop-outs, truants and underachievers.* The reviewers identified 12 studies, ten of which were controlled trials (eight randomized), and two were before-and-after studies. Ten were education-based interventions, the remaining two were multi-component. Although the reviewers group the studies into social influence (n = 6) and skills interventions (n = 4) these programmes shared common elements, such as social skills practice, motivational activities, decision-making and communication training. In general the evidence is inconsistent with regard to reductions in substance use (including alcohol and cannabis), although they may bring about changes in attitudes and knowledge. Evidence from the multi-component interventions was similarly inconclusive.

The evidence is similarly inconclusive for other groups of relevance, namely homeless young people, high-sensation-seeking adolescents and institutionalized youth. There is little evidence of any quality on any of these groups. It would be easy to be downcast by the dearth of good-quality research with clear and encouraging messages of 'what works', but it is good to be aware of the sparseness of the evidence base when this is the reality.

The broader picture of outcome research on substance abuse

The evidence from systematic reviews is shaped by the questions they are designed to address. Jones *et al.* (2006) were specifically concerned with young people under 25 who engaged in problematic use of both legal and illegal drugs (including alcohol when used in combination with other substances). Use was defined as problematic if it led to social, psychological, physical or legal problems. They included those with problems of dependence, but their review was not confined to dependence. The review by Gossop (2006) draws on a broader range of studies, covering both adults and young people. It also highlights the dearth of evidence that exists in many areas, but also the growing body of evidence that interventions for drug mis- use can be effective. The study cites a meta-analysis of 78 studies of drug abuse treatments, conducted between 1965 and 1996, which indicates that drug treatment programmes can have significant and clinically meaningful impacts upon both drug use and crime (Prendergast *et al.*, 2002). They concur that the more important questions now might be how to improve treatment, to tailor it to the needs of differ- ent clients and to make it more likely that people who need it will engage in treatment, stay in treatment, and be helped to *maintain* (vital) any improvements made during treatment.

Gossop's review is primarily concerned with adults who are dependent on, or misuse, substances. The study pays considerable attention to what differentiates apparently effective interventions from those that are ineffective. The review also contains information that is of relevance to young people with serious drug problems, including cannabis users, and encompasses medical interventions not covered in the review by Jones *et al.* We therefore summarize some of the more relevant findings from their review as an adjunct to the preceding section. Those working with young people with substance use problems are recommended to read both of these reviews, together with a review of psychosocial interventions by Wanigaratne *et al.* (2005) which reinforces most the key messages presented here and earlier. Here are the main findings from research:

1   Methadone maintenance is a well-researched intervention for opiate addiction that produces better outcomes in terms of illicit drug consumption and other criminal behaviour when compared to no treatment, detoxification-only, metha- done reduction treatments, programme expulsion or programme closure (Gossop, 2006: 6). Patients prefer injectable methadone maintenance to oral maintenance, but it costs five times more than the latter.

2   The evidence regarding motivational interviewing is mixed, and the 'effective ingredients' poorly understood. Some evidence points to its effectiveness as a stand-alone intervention, and to a 'value-added' effect when added to other treatments (see Hetterna *et al.*, 2005).

3   There is some evidence that contingency management (providing incentives and disincentives designed to make abstinence more desirable and continued drug use less desirable) can be a useful adjunct to interventions such as methadone maintenance.

4   Relapse-prevention programmes, that combine behavioural skills training, cognitive interventions, and lifestyle change procedures, can improve outcomes.

These programmes are designed to address the factors commonly associated with relapse, namely cognitions, negative mood states and external events (see Unnithan *et al.*, 1992).

5   'Twelve Steps' programmes (both Alcoholics Anonymous and Narcotics Anonymous) may be effective interventions in their own right and may enhance the effectiveness of other programmes (see Fiorentine and Hillhouse, 2000). As a form of aftercare they are also associated with reductions in drug use.

6   Studies of residential rehabilitation programmes generally show good outcomes after treatment that appear to persist over time. About half the participants in residential units in the NTORS study had been abstinent from heroin and other opiates in the three months prior to follow-up (Gossop *et al.*, 1999). Although there is no consensus over the optimum length of such programmes, good results have been obtained using short-term, residential 'Twelve-Step'-based programmes and, again, an AA approach to aftercare enhanced the outcomes for most groups of substance misusers (Brown *et al.*, 2002). These findings are the more encouraging given that those entering residential care are usually the most chronic and severely problematic cases (Gossop *et al.*, 1998).

7   The evidence on the effectiveness of brief interventions is uncertain, particularly where long-term users of illicit drugs are concerned. Treatment gains, when reported, do not always last. Brief interventions have been used with adolescent substance misusers; they tend to be based on motivational interviewing principles and have been most often used with cannabis misusers. Again, the evidence is mixed, but indicates the potential effectiveness of motivational enhancement therapy, cognitive-behavioural therapy and multidimensional family therapy. Gossop notes that for problematic cases brief interventions may be insufficient.

The authors emphasize the importance of strengthening the links between substance misuse services and psychiatric services (see Cameron *et al.*, 2007), given the range of psychological, behavioural, emotional and mental health problems associated with substance misuse.

Criminal justice and substance misuse interventions

As indicated earlier, despite the link between offending and substance misuse, only persistent young offenders appear to have problems related to the misuse of Class A drugs (Flood-Page *et al.*, 2000). Others may become involved in crime in order to obtain drugs that are otherwise outside their economic reach (Hammersley *et al.*, 2003). In addition to orders that can require a young person to attend a programme directed at factors associated with their offending, a number of initiatives have been designed to 'use the point of contact with the criminal justice system to *identify* those young people with, or at risk of developing, substance misuse problems, to assess their needs and to provide the appropriate support and treatment, helping to reduce substance misuse and offending behaviour' (Home Office Powerpoint Presentation, italics added).

Consequently, the Drug Interventions Programme (DIP) for children and young people was designed in accordance with the principles of *Every Child Matters* (DfES, 2005a). The YJB was concerned to emphasize that this programme must be integrated within the broader YJS and drug strategy, that it was not just about Class A drugs or treatment, and was not just about the extension of adult interventions to children. The pilot schemes were:

- Arrest referral schemes in ten areas for children aged 10 to 17. These schemes are designed to help identify new risks and needs and to provide young people with access to relevant support services.
- On-charge drug testing, in ten areas, of 14- to 17-year-olds under Section 5 of the Criminal Justice Act (CJA, 2003). Again, this is designed to identify young people who might benefit from substance misuse services.
- In five areas (from December 2004) Drug Treatment and Testing Requirements (DT(T)Rs) are to be attached to action plan orders and supervision orders under Section 279/Schedule 24 CJA. These were designed to improve access to services and assist in rehabilitation.

The aims of the DIP are to reduce substance misuse and associated crime. An extensive account of the pilot schemes and an evaluation of their effectiveness was published by the Home Office in July 2007 (Matrix Research and ICPR, 2007). Predictably, the data do not enable the authors to draw any conclusions about the effectiveness of these three components of the DIP. The reasons given are limitations in the design of the impact analysis and the early point of evaluation. None the less, they recommended a roll-out of arrest referral on the grounds of the positive reception, the benefits as identified by young people and other stakeholders, and the cost-effectiveness of the scheme. Drug testing appeared to add little to the benefits of arrest referral, and the authors conclude that there is insufficient evidence for extending such schemes. Stakeholder responses were mixed and there were very few positive tests, making it a costly intervention with no clear benefit. Evaluations of drug treatment and testing orders with adults found reconviction rates of around 80 per cent. Programme completion was a problem, with only 30 per cent of participants finishing the programme. The evaluation team highlight the need to enhance programme retention and completion (Hough *et al.*, 2003). The Home Office has since announced that following this evaluation, government ministers decided to wind down the pilots during 2007. A promising, if rare sign, that evidence is taken seriously.

Substance misuse – is a broader approach needed?

The interventions discussed above are only part of the broader strategy practised by the Youth Justice Board, which advised practitioners to have regard to *all* those factors that might impact upon the misuse of substances by young people, including homelessness, mental ill-health, basic skills, education and training, and peer group influences (Youth Justice Board, 2003). While it was not effective, the Drug Intervention Programme recognized the need for a broader approach to substance use among young people. In March 2007, the National Institute for Health and Clinical Excellence issued guidance to those working with vulnerable young people. They made five recommendations (NICE, 2007a). Two were concerned with developing local strategies to identify vulnerable and disadvantaged young people (under age 25) who were misusing (or at risk of misusing) substances. The approaches recommended included the Common Assessment Framework and others available from the National Treatment Agency. The other three recommendations are as follows:

1   For young people aged 11 to 16 at high risk of substance misuse, arrangements should be made to offer a family-based programme of structured support lasting two years or more, drawn up in partnership with the child's parents or carers, and led by competent staff. The programme should include at least three brief motivational interviews and parenting skills training (including enhancing parental monitoring and supervision). Those working in youth justice are identified as one of the groups that should act on this recommendation.

2   The provision of group-based behavioural treatment for persistently aggressive or disruptive children aged 10 to 12 who are considered at high risk of substance misuse, and for their parents.

3   The provision of motivational interviewing for all problematic substance mis-users, including those attending secondary schools or further education colleges. Motivational interviewing is a brief psychotherapeutic intervention. In this context it aims to help substance misusers reflect on their substance misuse in the context of their own values and goals, with the aim of motivating them to change (see McCambridge and Strang, 2004).

The anticipated cost of fully implementing these recommendations in England alone is £8,149,000 per annum (NICE, 2007b). This could, however, lead to a significant reduction in the costs associated with substance misuse. In England and Wales it is estimated that the costs per year per drug user incurred by the health sector and by social care is in the region of £11,800 to £44,000. For every pound spent on drug treatment it has been estimated that at least £3.00 would be saved on criminal justice costs and £9.50 would be saved in crime and health costs combined (National Drug Treatment Agency).

Findings from research on youth justice in England and Wales

So far we have, as befits a social work text, concentrated on strategic interventions to attenuate the likelihood of offending, and on those aspects of the formal youth justice system (such as the restorative justice initiatives) which focus clearly on the modification of offending behaviour. The system itself is considerably broader, and workers may be seeking to attend to a broad range of issues such as employment and training, basic skills, housing, family discord and so on. We conclude this section with a snapshot of effectiveness taken through a different lens, namely the value added of a youth justice system as a whole. The youth justice system in England and Wales was set a target of reducing reoffending by 5 per cent by 2006 in comparison to a baseline rate in 2000.

In 2005 the Home Office published a report of reoffending and reconviction rates of young people in 2003 (Home Office, 2005). The authors compared the profile of reconvictions over the preceding twelve months with predicted reconviction rates (i.e. the rate one would expect if one year's conviction rate had the same profile as a previous one). Note that reconviction rates are not the same as reoffending rates (the former depend, among other things, on police action). The authors also took into account the increased efficiency in processing youth cases and the greater use of pre-court disposals. The samples compared in the report covered all 10- to 17-year-olds receiving cautions, reprimands, final warnings or non-custodial court disposals, and all those discharged from custody during the first quarters of the calendar years 2000, 2001, 2002 and 2003. The authors point out that external factors cannot be ruled out, so changes may not be solely, if at all, attributable to the youth justice system, but the changes were as follows:

- The overall actual reconviction rate within one year in the first quarter of 2003 was 37 per cent. This is a percentage reduction of 2 per cent relative to the 2000 baseline (and statistically significant at the 0.05 level).
- While somewhat smaller than reductions in 2001 and 2002 (5 and 4 per cent respectively), the pattern is not significantly different. Three years is too short a period for a meaningful trend analysis.
- Statistically significant reductions were recorded in the reconviction rate for (1) first-time offenders, (2) repeat offenders, and (3) male offenders. The authors report a small, non-statistically significant reduction in female reconvictions but suggest this may to due to small sample size or normal random variation.
- In 2003, the most significant recorded reduction in reconviction rates was for offenders who received a fine for their original offence. This contrasts with 2001 and 2002 when the largest reductions were for those receiving other disposals.
- Statistically significant reductions were also recorded for discharges, referral orders, and first-tier penalties as a whole (discharges, fines, reparation orders).
- The largest significant *increase* in reconviction rates was recorded for offenders who received Curfew Orders (as in 2002). A statistically significant increase in recidivism was also recorded in 2003 for 'action plan orders'.

Not surprisingly, the reductions are generally reported as a success story for juvenile justice services in England and Wales, although unless we can proffer a convincing narrative as to *why* these changes might be expected, it is not clear that we can so read them. These appear to be encouraging findings, but the overall picture presented in this chapter augurs caution. It emphasizes the need for careful assessment, well-tailored, multi-component interventions, and more rigorous approaches to monitoring and evaluation.

13 Social work and mental health

What an awful condition is that of a lunatic! His words are generally disbelieved, and his most innocent peculiarities perverted; it is natural that it should be so, and that we place ourselves on guard – that is, we give to every word, look and gesture, a value and meaning which often times it cannot bear, and which it would never bear in ordinary life.

Lord Shaftesbury, 1844

History, ideology and politics

Is there any other affliction which creates such suspicion and wariness, so that the words of a philanthropist writing in the early reign of Queen Victoria still ring true today? Not even AIDS evokes such fear in the minds of an otherwise fairly intelligent and tolerant public. Thus, half a century's-worth of legislative reforms recently came under threat. These more liberal attitudes towards mental illness were first given expression in the 1959 Mental Health Act, with its emphasis on voluntary treatment whenever possible, and on seeing mental illness as a medical condition. Later, the 1983 Mental Health Act stressed the principle of care in the community and introduced a check on whether any restrictions on liberty were only as strong as they needed to be to prevent harm to the individual or to others. In contrast, the Mental Health White Paper (2002), now a bill, was, at heart, concerned with little else but compulsion. This, despite the fact that research indicates the adverse effects of hastily applied, risk-averse compulsion on service users that seriously threatens their future cooperation with would-be helpers. Yet these draconian proposals were defended on BBC Radio 4's *Today* programme (as authoritative a debating chamber as Parliament these days) by the Home Secretary who, at the discussion paper stage, assured us, with poorly disguised irritation, that the government would not be diverted by self-interested professional bodies and campaigning groups. But pause here and consider two things: (1) what exactly *is* the purpose of a discussion paper but to draw in informed opinion? Who else exactly was expected to comment? Biscuit manufacturers? Hairdressers?; (2) why was the *Home Secretary* routinely defending a draft bill that would normally be seen as a health matter? Well, possibly because these proposals were the progenitors of a public order bill grafted on to a health initiative. As we go to press, an alliance against this seems to have had the intended effect, in that the government has decided just to bring forward an amending act.

These new policies were based on scant evidence of an increased risk to the public from community care policies (see Appleby, 1997) and fly in the face of findings from empirical research conducted to establish the views of patients themselves about their future care (see Fisher *et al.*, 1984: Macdonald and Sheldon, 1997). Most of the draft recommendations are taken up with the establishment of new powers, reining back on consent to pharmacological, physical and even surgical treatments, and there is (rather unjustified) fear in the air. Nor is it paranoid to raise the possibility that financial incentives are at work here, since the previous two governments followed their predecessors in thinking that, given the increased efficacy of new treatments, hospital beds would become an unnecessary expense to the NHS except in emergency cases. Thus, against professional lobbying for a *continuum* of care and treatment facilities, beds were cut back, so much so that hospitals in inner London now typically have around 140 per cent occupancy rates and patients take it in turns to go in and out according to 'least worst' disposal decisions.

The explanation for this failure of political nerve lies, as in the child abuse field, with the undue importance placed upon dramatic, tragic, yet statistically rare single cases of violence and murder. These lead to journalistic feeding frenzies; to moral panic among the general public – to which concerned elected representatives then respond in a 'something must be done' fashion. Thus proposed legal change and guidance have been framed on the back of headlines featuring, for example, the random violence (everyone's worst nightmare since routine vigilance and precautionary behaviour count for little) of a very ill man, Christopher Clunis, who killed Jonathan Zito on a London Underground platform in 1992. A tragedy for the families involved, but cooler, more epidemiologically astute heads are required if we are to set such dreadful happenings in the context of the day-to-day episodes of family and domestic violence and crime featuring people who have never been near a psychiatrist in their lives.

This attitude of public fearfulness, leading to stigmatization and then repressive policies favouring invasive treatments, has deep historical roots (see Scull's excellent treatise (1993)). '*Diseases desperate grown by desperate appliances are relieved or not at all*' about sums up the standard medical view in the eighteenth, nineteenth and even in the first half of the twentieth century. The film *The Madness of King George* gives an idea of what even the King of England had to endure at the hands of his doctors. He has received a bad historical press, but was much admired by John Adams (American revolutionary and first US Ambassador to England) and by Dr Johnson. It later emerged that he was not insane but suffering from the physical condition Phorphoria, which affects the glands and hence the nervous system and so behaviour, emotion and thinking. Public disquiet at his treatment created pressure for reform among the less elevated – the removal of property rights on grounds of alleged insanity being the major cause for concern. But these bleeders (and purgers) and their successors also had other tricks up their sleeves, not solely reserved for the gentry. Patients were routinely immobilized, centrifuged, and douched in cold water (see Figure 13.1).

Later they had blood samples removed and shot back in (so-called 'protein shock therapy'). They were, slightly more plausibly, but still cruelly, deliberately infected with malaria to produce hyperpyrexia to combat 'General Paralysis of the Insane' – a syphilitic condition. Still later they were given overdoses of insulin to produce

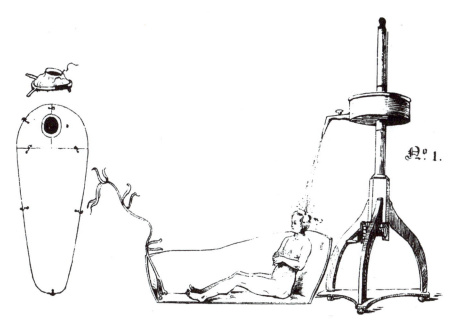

Figure 13.1 Immersion in cold water, an ancient nostrum for insanity. Aquatic shock treatment, otherwise euphemistically known as 'hydrotherapy', here takes the form of the douche.

Source: illustration from Alexander Morison, *Cases of Mental Disorder* (London: Longman & Highley, 1828)

hypoglycaemic convulsions. Then, in the 1950s and 1960s, they had parts of their brains chopped out (leucotomies and lobotomies) – to rather deleterious effect (see Valenstein, 1980). More recently, on the basis of rather equivocal evidence of comparative efficacy (see NICE, 2002), 11,000 people a year in the UK continue to be electrocuted. A systematic review of the effects of ECT (Tharyan and Adams, 2005) indicated *some* positive effects for deeply depressed patients with suicidal ideation, mainly in the form of efficiency gains over slower acting pharmacological treatments. But three things are worth noting: (1) suicidally depressed patients tend to kill themselves when on the way to recovery, when motivation returns a little; (2) there are some damaging side-effects to ECT (one-third of patients report persistent memory loss – see also Rose *et al.*, 2003); (3) the better the methodology (so that the only procedural difference is the electricity) the smaller the outcome differences (see Johnstone *et al.*, (1980) for a well-controlled study). Incontrovertibly, there is a large placebo effect at work here, and probably negative reinforcement effect too (see Chapter 7). We are no supporters of the once cultist theories of Thomas Szasz (1971) but we are reminded of his view that these procedures are a little like calling in a TV engineer or banging the television set when you dislike the quality of the programmes.

It is also interesting to note how physical treatments for mental illness tend to mirror contemporary technology: centrifugal spinning machines – as if whatever was inside could somehow be flung out – and mechanical devices for dripping cold water on to patients in the late eighteenth and early nineteenth centuries. If water was seen as a cooling palliative for 'brain fever' then why not just throw a bucketful over the poor devils, one is entitled to ask. But no, this was the 'machine age' – it had to be done 'scientifically' (see Melechi, 2003).

Why this preoccupation with shock? Perhaps it is that, despite 30 years' worth of advice from The Royal College of Psychiatrists to use with caution, ECT serves the professional identification needs of staff, connecting them, as it were, with the laser scalpel. Might it be also that the appetite of some patients for ECT is explained by the fact that they feel that something decisively medical, complicated and frightening is being done? Understandable reactions, but it is only ethical to accept them if the benefit/harm ratios are right.

Apart from the humane work of a few pioneers, notably William Tuke and his Quaker family (1732–1822) at the York Retreat, Philippe Pinel (1745–1826) in France, who pioneered psychiatry as a proper medical speciality based on individual records of aetiology, and Conolly (1794–1866) at Hanwell (see Scull, 1993) who set their faces against restraint, the mentally ill received little in the way of kindness or understanding; little that was gentle or healing was in fashion, nor, despite considerable advances in treatment and care, is it always still. Even today effective psychotherapeutic help is difficult to obtain and, where it is available, there is a persistent class and ethnic bias in who gets it. Middle-class patients are more than four times more likely to receive talking therapies than the less well-off or the elderly – though recovery rates are about equal across such groups. There are also long waiting lists to contend with, and the bulk of referrals are directed by GPs up the medical ladder to psychiatric units, and then down the social services snake to 'support'. The main message of the available effectiveness research is that those psychologists, social workers and health staff with a working knowledge of cognitive-behavioural methods should get out more (see Sheldon, 1995; NICE, 2007b).

Academic research in mental health, which influences training and policy when the results suit, remains somewhat polarized in respect of ideas about the causes of these conditions and, consequently, about what constitute effective methods of preventive and remedial interventions. Mention 'the medical model' at social work conferences and you will hear the sort of background hissing once reserved for the characters with black hats and moustaches in the old cowboy movies. The atmosphere crackles too when social scientists with bulging folders of ethnographic data from rare Polynesian cultures (who apparently prize the hallucinatory experience) and psychiatrists foregather. Thus, biologically derived models and treatments are largely seen by social workers and by most service-user representatives as an over-extended metaphor with serious implications for civil liberties – *à la* Thomas Szazs (1961), Laing and Esterson (1979) and Alain Foucault (1967). The foregoing books are still popular texts on social work courses despite the lack of empirical support for any definite propositions that they ever get close to making. Psychiatrists and nurses, on the other hand, tend to see such ideas as fanciful, and far removed from the day-to-day realities of psychiatric units and medication clinics. But then this is exactly what you get in such a broad field where passably good, but different, research ranges, for example, over studies of neurosis (anxiety-based conditions); deliberate self-harm; depression; psychosis; neurological conditions, and plausibly implicates biological, psychological, social and cultural factors all mixed up together. Different professional staff thus tend to huddle near the place on the causal and treatment continuum that training and experience make them feel most secure. What chance then of effective, genuinely integrated services?

Despite all this 'professional anthropology' there *are* signs of a *rapprochement*. Consultant psychiatrists and psychiatric nurses now receive a much broader education than hitherto, in psychology and on the social factors affecting the course of mental illnesses. The latter group are, rightly, resisting the pressures threatening to turn them into depot-injection technicians. Social workers appear less hostile to findings on genetic predispositions and the value of pharmacological treatments – when they get to hear about them that is. But of all the professional groups working in the mental health field, social workers have probably suffered the worst crisis of confidence and, on the principle that 'if you don't have plans for yourself, then you very quickly become part of someone else's' (Beck, 1976), they have often been relegated to sorting out benefit entitlements on the telephone.

Since there is undoubtedly a continuum of causes and effects, there is undoubtedly a need for a continuum of professional interventions. What, therefore, is the point of social work staff, students and their tutors complaining about the 'hegemony of the medical model' in mental health, but not equipping themselves with knowledge and skills regarding psycho-social approaches of proven worth, particularly cognitive-behavioural approaches? It reminds one of dissident politicians who seem to prefer the easy righteousness of life in opposition to the awkward compromises which power inevitably brings.

These difficulties notwithstanding, what has changed for the better? Well, diagnosis and treatment planning is now almost universally a shared activity undertaken by a team of different professionals, with constructive views from social work and nursing staff being entertained according to their merit. There is much more work to do further to merge services, but undoubtedly progress has been made, particularly in the involvement of people who use our services in planning and decision-making.

Psycho-social factors in mental disorders

The early contributions of social psychology and medical sociology to the mental health field created important insights into the following aspects of professional behaviour, namely: the influence of social context upon professional judgement; variations in diagnostic reliability, and the influence of life events, gender, ethnicity, and socio-economic status both upon illness rates, patterns of treatment, and levels of after-care. Let us consider some examples.

Rosenhan (1973) arranged for confederates (psychologists, a paediatrician, a painter and a housewife: N = 8) to pose as new patients seeking voluntary admission to 12 psychiatric hospitals. They all complained vaguely of hearing voices saying 'empty', 'hollow' and 'thud'. All but one were admitted, all acquired a diagnosis of schizophrenia, and many remained in hospital for considerable periods. The reaction of most psychiatrists to the research report that followed was that it proved only that well-meaning professionals could be fooled by well-rehearsed stooges. However, the details of the study show something more interesting going on. These pseudo-patients were instructed to behave normally on reaching the admission ward, and yet this behaviour was 'filtered out' by professional assumptions. In other words, their apparent normality tended to be regarded as deliberate symptom-masking. Their later note-taking was described as 'writing behaviour' (if you want to turn an ordinary activity into something clinically 'interesting', just attach the word 'behaviour' to the description). The well-chosen title of this study, best thought of as an empirical test of the views of Lord Shaftesbury with which we began this chapter, is 'On being sane in insane places'.

When the day-to-day normality of the behaviour of the pseudo-patients became impossible to ignore, they were given a diagnosis of 'schizophrenia in remission'. Their stay in hospital ranged from 7 to 52 days. The real patients on the ward showed greater diagnostic accuracy, however, voicing suspicions as to whether these fellow inmates were really ill at all – the nurses and doctors never did.

Follow-up studies to these experiments revealed even more pointed social influences upon diagnosis. The authors circulated copies of their paper, accompanied by an announcement that they would shortly be replicating the studies. This was not done, but pre-post measures for diagnoses of schizophrenia were taken. In all cases rates for this diagnosis fell at a level well above chance. Equally interesting was the fact that 21 per cent of real patients admitted at the targeted hospital were confidently thought to be pseudo-patients by medical staff. These findings underscore the point about the stickiness of diagnostic labels when quickly applied as a result of a single reported symptom; of lesser concern these days, thanks to DSM IVTR and ICD10 protocols, but still to be had – particularly in cases where (1) there has also been drug abuse, and (2) regarding confusional states in older people.

Negative expectations regarding remission and recovery by staff are a regular finding of research in this field, and are also a feature of studies of the discrimination and social exclusion felt by patients (see Birchwood and Tarrier, 1992; Macdonald and Sheldon, 1997; Gilbert, 2003). However, epidemiological and service-effectiveness research points to a much less pessimistic conclusion, showing that many people recover from periods of even severe mental illness, examples of which in physical medicine would be called 'cures' but in psychiatry tend to be described as 'episodes of remission' or 'dormancy'. The facts tell us that recovery is a distinct possibility.

The next important study to test the influence of psycho-social factors on diagnosis was that of Temerlin (1968). Temerlin asked psychiatrists, psychologists and graduate psychology students to diagnose someone on the basis of a sound-recording of an interview. The interviewee, played by an actor, presented as 'a normal, healthy man'. Shortly before hearng the interview, participants in the experimental condition (N = 95) heard from a high status person (acting on behalf of the experimenter) that the individual to be diagnosed 'looked neurotic but actually was quite psychotic'. Control group participants (N = 77) heard the interview either: (1) with no prior suggestion; (2) with a reversed prior suggestion; (3) as an interview assessing 'scientific productivity'; (4) part of a 'sanity hearing'. The vast majority of those in the experimental group gave a psychiatric diagnosis. Psychiatrists were most influenced towards a diagnosis of psychosis by the 'high status' suggestion (60%); graduate students least biased, and psychologists fell in between. There were considerable within group differences in diagnosis, as well as between group differences. No diagnoses of psychosis were made by participants in the control groups, and all but fifteen concluded the interviewee was in good mental health or 'sane'.

The foregoing study and others like it were designed to test the capabilities of professionals in deciding whether someone was sane or not. Ullman and Krasner (1969) collected the results of many of these projects in support of their campaign for a more rounded psycho-social approach to diagnosis. They found reliability rates for schizophrenia to be tolerably concordant (validity is a different issue, note) at 74 per cent. However, decisions regarding manic-depressive disorder, personality disorder and for neurotic conditions (much more prevalent illnesses) were 36 per cent, 66 per cent and 56 per cent respectively. Now the way in which figures are presented has a powerful effect on perception and cognition (see Chapter 4). So although 74 per cent usually represents a first-class assignment grade, it also means in this case that a quarter of patients were misdiagnosed and probably mistreated. Figures today are better, but not by as much as you might expect (see below).

Darley and Batson (1973) invited trainee priests to participate in a study on 'religious education and vocations' (p. 102). Following a group 'testing' session (in which they completed religious questionnaires) students were randomized to one of two groups. All were asked to prepare a 3–5 minute talk based on a written brief. Students in Group 1 were given a passage outlining the vocational challenges and opportunities facing seminary students. Students in Group 2 were given the parable of the Good Samaritan. After a few minutes the assistant administering the experiment told participants that, as they were short of space, they would need to go to another building to record their talks, and drew them a map of where to go. Some students were also told 'Oh you're late. They were expecting you a few minutes ago . . . The assistant is ready for you so you'd better hurry.' This was the *high hurry condition*. Other conditions, similarly constructed, were: 'less urgency', 'intermediate hurry' and 'low hurry'. En route to the recording office, students passed someone 'sitting slumped in a doorway, head down, eyes closed, not moving. As the subject went by, the victim coughed twice and groaned, keeping his head down.' Those who stopped to ask if he was all right were told by the person that he had a respiratory problem, had just taken a prescribed pill and was taking a rest, after which he would be OK. But not everyone stopped to ask. Those in a hurry were less likely to help, but the brief made no difference, although the researchers wryly observe that several of the students going to give a talk on the parable of the Good Samaritan 'literally stepped over the victim as he hurried on his way!'.

These iconoclastic studies remind us that psychiatric diagnoses, the way we view people wearing labels, and what we are prepared to do to them if pre-programmed assumptions about their behaviour take over, are, in part, socially and psychologically constructed. This research further reminds us that psychiatric diagnosis never was, nor is it yet, an exact science, even at the level of 'ill or not?' decisions, let alone regarding opinions as to the degree of 'fit' of major categories in the formulary.

The undoubted improvements in diagnostic reliability recorded in the contemporary literature are due to a few particular influences:

1   The development of diagnostic 'catalogues' based on the soundest epidemiology that we have, and upon inter-rater concordance tests. Most notable among these is the DSM programme in the USA, and the mental health section of

the ICD10 in the UK. Psychiatric diagnosis is not particularly our business but, because we have to implement programmes of care based upon them, we need to understand their implications for what we are trying to achieve. One often hears staff on training courses discussing the plight of people with 'mental health problems' or, vaguer still, as having 'mental health issues' (who of us would ever consult a garage mechanic regarding 'issues around the front brakes'?). Intendedly non-discriminatory – but technically useless. Diagnoses matter; they should inform care and treatment approaches, and if discrepant information regarding symptoms comes to light, social workers should be bold enough to encourage a rethink by medical colleagues.

2   Reliability checks between different checklists to aid accurate diagnoses are now in place. Accuracy rates are improving, since some of the more fanciful background factors have been dropped in favour of Schnieder's first-rank symptoms (see Gelder *et al.*, 2001).

3   Time limits and frequency rates have been introduced over the years so that single episodes, short-term aberrations or low-level symptoms are noted, but contribute less to the final classification.

Where the, admittedly less than perfect, protocols discussed above have not been fully introduced (e.g. in France, Italy and other parts of continental Europe), diagnostic reliability rates have remained (1) dismal, and (2) very influenced by theory (particularly psychoanalytic theory) as opposed to empirical research. Thus the early opposition to diagnostic formularies as likely to cramp the natural style of staff (perish the thought) has not been supported by the evidence.

4   The other noteworthy development in psychiatric practice has been an increased willingness to see these categories as provisional only, and to recognize a degree of overlap between them – as something more akin to a spectrum, with, say, blue for schizophrenia and red for mood disorders occasionally merging into purple rather than belonging neatly in box one or box two.

Socio-cultural factors

People of African-Caribbean origin or their children, particularly young men, are much more likely to be diagnosed as suffering from a serious mental illness – schizophrenia predominating; are more likely to be admitted to hospital under the compulsory sections of the Mental Health Act; are less likely to have the involvement of a family doctor in the process (the preferred option under the Act); are more likely to have a 'dual diagnosis' (serious mental illness made worse by substance misuse), and are much more likely to experience admissions to hospital involving police officers (Section 136). Further, black patients are more likely to have cautionary notes about potential violence entered on their case records; are more likely to have been physically restrained; are more likely to be confined in secure psychiatric units, and are more likely to receive pharmacology-only treatments or ECT. They are *less* likely to receive counselling, psychotherapy or cognitive-behavioural therapy; are less likely to receive 'half-way-house' discharges; have lower levels of follow-up contact, and, above all, receive far lower levels of services intended to prevent future relapses (see Davies *et al.*, 1996; Bhugra *et al.*, 1997; Boydell *et al.*, 2001; Chakrabarty and McKenzie, 2002). A bleak picture based on considerable forensic evidence. The question is, why? Social work authors quickly made up their minds about this problem years ago. It is, they asserted (largely on the basis of unrepresentatively small samples), the psychological fall-out from the effects of endemic racism. Well, possibly; why shouldn't it be? Imagine being subjected to routine disrespect; then add in the more pointedly rejecting experiences of active discrimination; mix well with institutional antibody reactions, which, whether consciously in place or not seem designed to exclude, stereotype and marginalize, and how would anyone feel? But then, empirical findings suggest that there are more complex combinations of hypotheses to be considered. Here are the main contenders:

1   *That people of Afro-Caribbean origin have in their population a stronger genetic predisposition for schizophrenia and that people of South Asian origin, who are over-represented in suicide statistics, have a stronger inherited predisposition to severe depression and subsequent self-harm.* The problem with this hypothesis is that surveys of the prevalence of severe mental disorder in the countries of origin show that, for example, rates of schizophrenia there are either lower or about the same (see Bhugra *et al.*, 1997). One has to be cautious about such observations however, in that they are influenced by the availability of psychiatrists to diagnose these conditions, but then psychosis is hard to ignore, and more reliable community samples produce comparable figures.

2   *That there is something different about migrant populations and that this select group of first-wave immigrants who came to Britain were (1) either especially genetically vulnerable, or (2) found themselves under such stress here that those who were biologically predisposed had higher rates of precipitation, or (3) that sensing their vulnerability, they thought they might be better off in the fledgling NHS.* This cluster of hypotheses are readily refuted by the 'healthy migrant' results of studies of these populations. That is, research studies show that those with the courage and capacity to venture abroad tend to be healthier both physically and psychologically than the home population (see Ferrardo, 2002). Further, it was not the first-generation immigrants who are over-represented, but their sons, daughters and grandchildren. They were born here, but it is *they* who account for the epidemiological 'spikes'. Hypothesis (3) above can be disregarded since the facilities available for psychiatric care in the 1950s were not sought but avoided by almost anyone who had the option.

3   *That those in this sub-population who do present with severe mental disorder are misunderstood and miscommunicated with, and therefore over-diagnosed and thus over-represented.* This is a possibility, particularly regarding the use of compulsory treatment orders, restraint and confinement. But the proposition is largely defended via case studies in otherwise theoretical books. However, to offer up a counter-case study, one of the present authors was chair of an inquiry into the death of a patient of African-Caribbean origin who blundered into an armed robbery being committed by people he knew. He had a criminal record himself, and, when questioned by police as to his identity, described himself as 'the son of an Ethiopian Prince'. He was thinking of Haile Selassie in his role as founder of Rastafari. A psychiatrist and social worker were called to the police

station and the patient was sectioned. But then all sociological fancifulness evaporates, for he was frankly deluded; had a history of violent attacks on his (very supportive) family; was high on crack cocaine, and had stopped taking his psychotropic medication (see Richard Phillips Inquiry).

Similarly, investigations of compulsory admissions regularly show good evidence and clinical cause for detention, and thus do not support the cultural miscommunication hypothesis – though such factors probably make some difference regarding disposal.

4   *Greater involvement in drug use (known to exacerbate psychotic breakdown in those vulnerable to it) may account for the excess figures.* Census changes and the lack of secure comparative research mean that we cannot readily test this hypothesis via relatively small clinical populations (prevalence comparisons are 1 per cent for the UK generally, 2 to 3.4 per cent from studies of African-Caribbean populations) against a general population 'noise level' of 58 million in the former case, and 17 million in the latter. Nevertheless, we do know from studies of drug misuse, including (we are afraid) cannabis, that there *are* substantial concentrations of drug misuse in our inner cities where minority ethnic communities often live. We know too that drug dealing is concentrated in these urban areas; and we have good evidence on the negative effects of prolonged drug use on later relapse. We do know also that drug dependency tends to lead to florid exacerbations which are likely to lead to urgent, police-assisted admissions; we also know that 'dual diagnoses' are increasingly prevalent in our inner city psychiatric units and we also know that friends and relatives supply narcotics to inpatients, necessitating screening precautions. This hypothesis is thus plausible as a contributory factor in these illnesses and disposals (see Arsenault *et al.*, 2002).

5   *That the experience of racism in its direct and institutional forms constitutes a series of provocative life events and that such factors are all the more pernicious because they are continuing rather than episodic stressful events.* The argument here is that such oppressive experiences may precipitate serious mental illness among biologically vulnerable sub-populations, some of whom would otherwise escape the worst effects. Well, given what we now know from many studies of the social and psychological effects of racist attitudes on stress levels and on any sense of inclusion, we must conclude that such factors are very likely to tip the balance in cases where there is a background genetic vulnerability (see Fernando, 2002).

6   *That immigrant families tend to be larger, thus increasing the chances of the phenotypic expression of underlying psychotic conditions.* There is little evidence to support this statistical hypothesis, since there are other populations (e.g. on the Indian subcontinent) where large families are still the norm but where rates for some serious conditions are lower. In any case, given the comparative rarity of severe illnesses in large populations, it would be almost impossible to prove (see Bayes, 1763/1958).

7   The hypothesis that readily stands up, particularly if we add in the stress effects of racism, is that *minority ethnic clients are far less likely to have had access to culturally sympathetic preventive services.* Thus, screening, early intervention,

suitable medication and relapse-prevention follow-up are much less likely to be present in such cases.

8   Finally, we must consider whether the additional stresses of living in pressured, inner city environments, with poverty, urban decay and poor housing in the background, account for the excess. These social factors accord closely with known risk factors. This too then is a likely hypothesis – particularly when international comparisons of precipitation and relapse rates are added in – in that studies show that clients in stable social circumstances, who live in arguably less stressful rural environments, produce significantly lower incidences of precipitation and relapse.

These are complex and entangled matters, but the arguments presented above amount to our best empirical research-derived picture of what is going wrong and why.

Psycho-social factors in diagnosis and treatment will continue with us for the remainder of this chapter. However, findings will necessarily be mainly condition or illness-based from here on. We shall concentrate on research findings and their implications for practice in the main diagnostic groupings most likely to be found on the case lists of mental health social workers and child and adolescent mental health services staff (CAMHS). We begin this exploration with the commonest mental disorder and include an account of what it feels like to have it.

Depression

Louis Wolpert (a distinguished embryologist who suffers from depression himself) had this to say in his book *Malignant Sadness*:

> It was the worst experience of my life. More terrible even than watching my wife die of cancer. I am ashamed to admit that of my depression but it is true. I was in a state that bears no resemblance to anything I had experienced before.
>
> (Wolpert, 1999: viii)

Clinical depression is the generic term used to distinguish this from episodic, depressed mood plausibly related to a particular personal event (e.g. loss of a close relationship, redundancy, bereavement), though these are known to play a part as triggering and/or maintenance factors. It is quantitatively different in extent, and qualitatively different from routine unhappiness owing to the sheer depth of feelings of hopelessness, inadequacy, unworthiness and all-pervasive pessimism that they bring.

The DSM IV TR (2000) criteria for major depressive episodes are:

1   A period of at least two weeks in which there is either depressed mood or loss of interest or pleasure in nearly all activities (anhedonia).
2   At least four symptoms from the following list: changes in appetite, sleep pattern (including early morning waking); lack of interest in social interaction (which

adds up to sitting slumped for large parts of the day, finding nothing pleasurable to look forward to, and preferring to be alone); decreased energy; feelings of guilt and/or worthlessness; having difficulty in concentrating and making decisions; thoughts of death or suicide; irritability and/or inability to sit still in some cases – particularly in younger people (see Hawton and Van Heeringen, 2002). These symptoms must persist for most of each day in nearly every day of each week for at least 14 days. Contributory factors towards diagnosis are: avoidance of recreational contact with friends and relations; having no time for children; avoidance of, or a fear of, or lack of interest in, occupational tasks, and loss of interest in previously not-too-demanding domestic tasks. Differential diagnoses include substance misuse-induced conditions; reactions to bereavement, and serious physical self-neglect.

The lifetime risk for a major depressive disorder, from large community samples, varied from 10 to 25 per cent for women and 10 to 12 per cent for men, with an average age of onset in the mid-twenties. Worryingly, increasing numbers of depressed children are being seen who meet these criteria. The disorder is episodically persistent, with 60 per cent further relapse rates, and 15 per cent to 18 per cent figures for suicide. So mental illness can kill, and should be taken more seriously alongside potentially life-threatening physical disorders.

Studies such as that conducted by Brown and Harris (1979) on social factors affecting health reveal that certain life events and circumstances are strongly associated with depression, namely:

1 Class position, and all that goes with it, emerges as major epidemiological and aetiological factors, not sufficient in themselves to produce clinical depression, but constituting a powerful mixture of 'provocative' agents in the absence of protective social factors, and associated with a doubling of the rates of continuing depressive illness.

2 Poverty is a major predisposing factor in both mental and physical ill-health (see Black *et al.*, 1980; Acheson, 1998), as the room for counteractive measures and the retention of a sense of self-control is so restricted.

3 Bereavement, and loss, particularly when still a child, and particularly involving the loss of a mother prior to, or during, adolescence, also produced a noteworthy, statistical association in these data (see also Rutter and Hersov, 1987).

   Here are some typical comparison figures for those suffering from depression who did or did not have major life events (e.g. bereavement, divorce, abuse, loss of employment) in their lives, and who did or did not have compensatory sources of support. There has been much wrangling over these statistics (see Brown and Harris, 1979) but the differences are so large as to be unlikely to be accounted for by collateral factors. We are quoting this 30-year-old material since it is (1) the most comprehensive, and (2) the most scientifically robust we have.

4 Single parenthood or semi-single parenthood, particularly if there are two or more young children, constitute the next set of factors in this research. Halsey and Webb (2000) documented the effects of being a poor, lone parent in an admirably non-judgemental way, via a series of well-conducted studies and

Table 13.1 The relationship between life events, social support and depression in women

	Social support (% depressed)	*No support (% depressed)*
No life event	1	3
Life event	10	23

Source: Cleary and Kessler (1972) quoted in Brown and Harris (1979)

reviews (see also the work of Jordan, 1996). They were pilloried for pointing out the obvious fact that bringing up children alone is in most cases doubly demanding, and that there are measurable effects on social mobility, education, social exclusion, future employment and later entanglements with the law. Halsey never said it *couldn't* be done: many pull it off; he just argued that it was much more difficult.

5   Unemployment emerges as a provocative factor in a number of studies and has also been associated with suicide in young males. It is a major factor in the lives of aound 80+ per cent of those surveyed with a history of serious mental illness. Apart from its raw economic consequences, it affects any sense of personal control, self-esteem, choice, family relationships, and both mood and behaviour. We currently have around one million people unemployed in Britain (most of them, thankfully, in the short term). However, a much larger group of individuals is not counted since they are the recipients of incapacity benefits.

It is estimated that 110 million working days are currently lost per year in Britain due to depression alone (see Thomas and Morris, 2003), at an estimated cost of £9 billion per annum if we combine treatment and care costs with lost economic output.

6   Happily, alongside provocative factors, there also exist protective ones, most notably in the form of a confiding partner – or even a reliable friend. These counter-effects seem to derive from emotional intimacy, practical support, and a willingness to listen and stay involved through troubled times.

7   Practical provision, housing and basic income support. These have all improved over the past 20 years, but at the expense of emotional support and advice from social workers.

8   We know from epidemiological research that women are more likely to seek help with emotional problems and depression than men; and from psychological research that they are more likely to blame themselves for the negative circumstances in which they find themselves. The problem is that if a woman presents repeatedly with symptoms that, even though their effects may be blunted by medication, are beyond the immediate reach of routine pharmacology, then they will tend to be referred to a psychiatrist, and thus some of the labelling factors discussed earlier come into play. From other studies we know that for men, who often delay seeking professional help, chronic stress at work is a strong contributory factor, leading to significantly higher suicide rates (see

Lester, 2000). So, stiff upper lips, though occasionally useful in life, may sometimes be fatal.

Although vulnerability to depression – particularly in its severer forms – appears
from twin studies to be genetically endowed to the tune of about 30 per cent,
environmental circumstances, life events and personal crises therefore play much
stronger precipitating and maintenance roles. Furthermore, depression has social
and psychological effects of its own upon those nearby, particularly upon young
children.

All forms of mental illness have a severe impact upon families, but depression,
particularly in mothers, and if chronic, has the most insidious effects upon children. They need reflections of personal worth as much as they need vitamins, and yet
such emotional engagement and encouragement is exactly what depressed people
find most difficult to give. Children of pre- and early school age are likely to attribute
the blame for its absence to themselves (see Piaget, 1958). Depression, unlike
schizophrenia, is thus quite 'catch-able'. Social workers need to reflect this in their
practice, however much current policies encourage them to work with one designated
client for very short periods.

Thus, in the absence of, or in support of, the protective factors reviewed above,
social workers have two main functions in cases of depression: (1) Advocacy, i.e. to
act as negotiators with the various services, including medical and nursing services,
which can play a crucial role in recovery. This function is highly valued by clients (see
Macdonald and Sheldon, 1997). It is also worth remembering that not everyone has
a GP, and that those who do may sometimes be *persona non grata* with them; not
all GPs will undertake reviews of medication unprompted; and not all workplaces
live up to their published aims regarding employees' welfare and employment conditions. Therefore, having someone on side to mediate regarding these crucial factors
is perceived time and again in client opinion studies to be vital. (2) As practitioners
we can work directly with children and with families to explain the mechanics of
this illness, and help to dispel common myths. We can also attempt to remove some
of the inappropriate self-blame which goes with this condition. We can also help in
harnessing the available resources of family and friends to meet the needs for the
support of clients.

Epidemiological and treatment research shows that depression peaks in early
adult to mid life, but that, in a smaller number of cases, can occur in childhood and
adolescence, where the simple use of antidepressant medication has come under
critical scrutiny as a result of systematic reviews (see Garland, 2004). The evidence
on the general effectiveness of SSRIs (selective serotonin re-uptake inhibitors) (e.g.
Seroxat) in children and younger adults has allegedly been distorted by disattention
to a 'grey literature' of negative results. Such medications may thus help some, but
may induce suicidal behaviour in a minority. At the other end of the age spectrum,
depression in elderly people is under-diagnosed in primary care almost 50 to 80 per
cent of the time, possibly due to the masking effects of other physical conditions and
to ageism (see Chapter 15).

Effective treatments for depression

The main trends from interventions research suggest the following to be the more effective treatments for depression:

1   Pharmacological treatments are, again, not strictly our business, except that when social work and nursing staff actually encourage compliance with the medication prescribed, noting and passing on information about side-effects (the main reason for relapse) and encourage regular medication reviews, something better than 'prescribe and forget' approaches can result.

   The first generation of effective antidepressive medications were the Tricyclics. The dosage safety margins and the side-effect complications were, however, rather challenging for prescribers. These medications have now been largely replaced by a new generation of treatments (pills) (the SSRIs), though both Tricyclics and the earlier Monoamine Oxidase Inhibitor drugs still have a role with patients who simply do not respond to the (usually safer), less side-effect burdensome medications. SSRIs act upon mood centres in the brain by reducing the rate of neurotransmitter 'recycling'. They are an effective treatment, though some dependency effects are now beginning to emerge. However, they are better tolerated than earlier medications, have fewer side-effects such as lethargy or agitation – but are slower acting, which can be a problem in urgent cases. Combinations of psychotherapy, counselling and support, plus appropriate medication, appear to be particularly effective in complex cases (see Craighead and Llardi, 1998; Nemerhoff and Shatzberg, 1998; NICE, 2006).

   Research tells us that it makes no sense for GPs and psychiatric nurses to concern themselves exclusively with medication (though work pressures encourage just this) or for social workers to concern themselves only with psycho-social influences. Integrated services work best.

2   *Other psycho-social approaches.* Group therapy achieves mixed results – depending on what goes on in the groups; client or patient-led support groups show scattered gains against very forgiving evaluation protocols.

Case example

Mrs M (44) was referred for CBT and 'social support' by her psychiatrist. Her life experience closely encapsulates the research findings discussed above, in that she had (1) a series of sad and threatening life events: she was an adopted child (probably her intended role was to thaw out a frozen marriage). She was raised in a distant, arm's-length way; she later had two violent marriages herself; was raped; suffered the loss of her 18-year-old daughter in a car accident and had to make the decision to switch off the life-support machinery; (2) she later, understandably, had occupational difficulties, made worse by the current, 'if officially ill, stay away; if officially well, come in and perform to standard' policies which pass for 'human resources management'.

Scores on the Hamilton and Beck Depression Inventory Scales showed her to be in the most serious 1 per cent of cases, with suicidal ideation a daily pre-occupation. Medication made her sleepy and unable to function. She was therefore likely to alternate between feeling that nothing mattered much, and occasional bursts of agitation: 'Like being on your way somewhere important but "dozing off at the wheel" ', she said.

The cognitive component of work with Mrs M concentrated on the following factors:

1   That her brittle sense of gratitude towards her adoptive parents – 'they told me I was special because they *chose* me, but then they sent me to a boarding-school three miles down the road and didn't often have me home'. As an adolescent she kicked over of the traces, this behaviour leading to expulsion from school. In her parents' view, and note, in *hers*, this amounted to ingratitude. Similarly, that her interest in her natural mother's fate amounted to a 'betrayal of trust'.

2   That her early sexual experimentation ('I knew how to get boys to give me what I wanted': *Social worker*: 'What was that?' *Answer*: 'Attention, affection') was the result of: 'bad blood'.

3   That her desire to find a 'strong man or two' who would protect her – which led to two violent relationships (the attractive macho behaviour was not supposed to be brought home) – was a result of her 'stupidity'.

4   That she should have performed some routine checks on the state of her daughter's car (e.g. tyre pressures, brakes) before she set off on her fatal journey, even though she had absolutely no mechanical expertise.

5   That the person who followed her and raped her had 'had his fuse lit' by her, and that she should have known better what flirting would lead to.

6   That getting better meant abandoning her daughter's cherished memory and 'moving on' without her, and so would constitute another betrayal. The approach used was to persuade her to take her daughter's love and the memories of her with her throughout life. She seized upon the idea.

7   That her present, loving partner, whom she thought 'too kind for his own good', was only displaying sympathy or at best short-term love, and would leave her when he found out more about her (they are now happily married).

The behavioural components in this case were based on the idea of 'scheduling pleasant events' against a desensitization hierarchy (see Chapter 7). The principle here is to encourage reality testing (i.e. will the meal with friends *really* be a disaster; will the movie *really* not be enjoyable; will trips to the keep-fit club *really* not result in weight loss; will confiding in your partner *really* distance him more than will the 'partner-management scheme' currently in place; does bad, manipulative sex with previous partners mean that nothing more meaningful is possible with someone quite different?).

This work led to substantial reductions in depression scale scores in 11 one-hour sessions, noteworthy experimentation (at work) and trying out a different, less pessimistic and fearful lifestyle, and to a substantial fall in preoccupations with suicide. A fluke? Not so. That this client is able to laugh again; able to work full-time; able to reconcile herself with her other, somewhat estranged, child, and is willing to contemplate further developments in her recovery, is not unusual in this literature. Gaining access to such help is the ongoing challenge and we surely cannot leave this work to psychologists with one-year waiting lists, or to psychotherapists with a charge of £80 per session and so excludes most Social Services clients. So get trained in CBT, but ask yourself why you weren't/aren't being, in the first place.

Bipolar disorder

Another mood disorder, also known as manic-depressive illness. This is a devil's bargain of a condition; the uplifted mood, the energy, and the false or real sense of creativity that it brings make it addictive. Before, that is, the collapse into despair and self-loathing occurs. Byron, Van Gogh, Virginia Woolf, Picasso, Sylvia Plath and Winston Churchill are among a long list of historical figures who suffered from this condition and ascribed many of their achievements to its (transient) blessings. The downside was described by Churchill as 'the black dog'.

Kay Redfield Jamison's compelling book *An Unquiet Mind* (1997) gives frank and deep insights into what it is like to live with extreme mood swings. She is herself a sufferer/beneficiary, but she is also a professor of psychiatry, and a co-author of the standard textbook on the illness (see Goodwin and Redfield Jamison, 2004):

> The war that I waged against myself is not an uncommon one. The major clinical problem in treating manic-depressive illness is not that there are not effective medications – there are – but that patients so often refuse to take them. Worse yet, because of a lack of information, poor medical advice, stigma or fear of personal and professional reprisals, they do not seek treatment at all. Manic-depression distorts moods and thoughts and incites dreadful behaviours, destroys the basis of rational thought, and too often destroys the desire and the will to live. It is an illness that is biological in its origins, yet one that feels psychological in the experience of it; an illness that is unique in conferring advantage and pleasure, yet one that brings in its wake almost unendurable suffering and, not infrequently, suicide.
>
> (Redfield Jamison, 1996: 6)

The prevalence rate is around 1 per cent. About 15 per cent of people who suffer from it kill themselves, but this is, statistically, the iceberg tip of the misery it brings; it can also lead to aggression towards loved ones, financial ruin and occupational disasters. Twin studies show a strong familial inheritance pattern, with risk figures of around 70 per cent; higher, note, than for schizophrenia.

The symptoms (especially for full-blown bipolar disorder – there are other less extreme 'mixed' manifestations) are straightforward, though there are also studies showing confusion with florid schizophrenic episodes, particularly where young people and ethnic minority patients are concerned. The essentials for accurate diagnosis are:

1   One or more manic episodes – characterized by highly elevated mood, alongside a major depressive episode.
2   Erratic and untypical behaviour.
3   Risk-taking well outside the norms of previous behaviour.
4   Racing thoughts and irritation at the 'slowness' of other people.

During such near-manic episodes, sufferers feel highly creative and full of energy (read the actor Stephen Fry's accounts of it) until mental exhaustion sets in (see Müller-Oerlinghansen *et al.*, 2002). The depressive episodes that follow (one or more is necessary for the DSM IV TR criteria to be met) are a cruel anticlimax to this and are often anticipated by patients. Therefore, in this illness, there is, on the way down, or on the way up, a window of insight, and it is at these transition points that suicide risks increase.

As to causes, anyone who has personally encountered this condition will, if rational, abandon notions that these problems are anything other than brain disorders; the effects are so severe and so independent of social circumstances.

Neuroscientists are making steady inroads into an understanding of mood disorders (see http://www.brainexplorer.org/bipolardisorder-aetiology.shtml). A range of neurotransmitter chemicals such as noradrenalin, serotonin and dopamine have been the subject of research studies. The basal ganglion and the limbic system (the mood control 'thermostat' sites at the back of the brain) have been implicated. But then the cortical areas seem to be the location for the negative thoughts that compound depressed or elevated mood.

Pharmacological treatments

The reason for the inclusion (above) of a little information on what is known on the effects of brain chemistry on disturbed mood (much isn't) is because pharmacological treatments (an attempt to control imbalances in this very biologically driven illness) and cooperation with such medical regimes is probably the best hope for recovery – providing, that is, that there is sufficient psycho-social support to make compliance tolerable. Kick and McElroy (1998), in their authoritative review of intervention research, pick out Lithium salts as 'the pharmacologic cornerstone of treatment for patients with bipolar disorder'. It is a chemical element, not a high-tech pharmacological formulation, and has been in use since the 1970s to good effect. However, this optimistic statement, based on (to date) ten controlled trials and one systematic review, requires two riders:

1   Lithium does not suit all patients, the effective dose being uncomfortably close to the toxic dose, and there is a new generation of atypical anti-psychotics with fewer side-effects – except for high weight gain, which is itself not without physical and psychological consequences.
2   The problem with these treatments is that many patients fail to take them. In other words, in the manic phase they dislike the idea of being less 'alive' (even

though such feelings are usually regarded by friends and relatives as illusory, self-damaging and unsustainable). Therefore the regular matching of dosage to psychological and social circumstances is time-consuming, but crucial. Our proposal is that all staff, from consultants to GPs to psychiatric nurses to social workers, need to involve themselves in such treatment programmes with the aim of securing the best trade-off between mood stability and toleration of side-effects.

Here is an account of what this process of accurate dosage – with an eye to coping with current environmental stresses – feels like from the inside:

> The too rigid structuring of my moods and temperaments, which had resulted from a higher dose of Lithium made me less resilient to stress than a lower dose, which, like the building codes in California that are designed to prevent damage from earthquakes, allowed my mind and emotions to sway a bit.
>
> (Redfield Jamison 1996: 67)

Psycho-social interventions

From follow-up research, between 30 per cent and 40 per cent of precipitation and relapse in bipolar disorder occurs as a result of environmental factors. Therefore, since we can do little at present other than to counter biological factors through medication, what useful alterations can we make to these psycho-social pressures?

The research literature currently contains nine randomized controlled trials (RCTs) testifying to the additional usefulness of psycho-social interventions in mood disorders, enough evidence to be going on with, particularly if considered alongside promising but less robust trials and alongside insights from qualitative, client opinion research (see Milkowitz *et al.*, 1996; Craighead *et al.*, 1998). Our best bets regarding such approaches may therefore be summed up as follows:

1   There is good evidence regarding the efficacy of psycho-education; that is, simply holding sympathetic dialogues with clients and their families to explore the nature of the disorder and alerting them to early signs of relapse.
2   Most studies on relapse prevention in this field feature variants of cognitive-behavioural theory and family therapy.
3   Social workers have a role to play in limiting the harm, both to clients and to their families. In the manic phase sufferers are very likely to, for example, give away their money and to ruin their employment prospects or their businesses. Families, though they usually understand that something is wrong, nevertheless often attribute such behaviour to malign intent. Therefore, in the early stages, probably the most beneficial interventions that social workers can make is via a family conference where early signs of mood disturbance, damage limitation and family support are near the top of the agenda.
4   Social workers also have a role in preventing and containing the financial ruin referred to above. There is a Court of Protection, purpose-built for such

problems – though research suggests that social workers and families often apply to it too late, when most of the damage has been done.

5   Bipolar disorder can do terrible damage to marriages and partnerships. Not only is this condition very hard to live with, but understandably, high levels of criticism and emotionally charged interchanges are also linked to relapse (see Milkowitz *et al.*, 1996). Therefore, counselling and psycho-education approaches for partners may have an immunizing effect against relapse and help to retain the support of the family.

6   Because we in social work have been artificially divided between 'adult care' and 'child care' functions there is a danger that cases which overlap these categories are dealt with by one division or the other, but not by both. In short, people with mental illnesses often have children, and their safety, their development and their life chances are much affected by the fact.

Case example

Mr R was a 'self-made man', as he often liked to remind his family. He had in his terms 'clawed his way up' from casual taxi driving to owning his own small fleet. He had two failed marriages behind him, both of which had collapsed owing to his 'tyrannical' behaviour. He had one (estranged) daughter of his own, and had acquired a new wife and two late-teenage stepsons.

   Everything came to a head late one Saturday evening, after a week of rows with his family and with his bank manager. He was discovered in his yard by police at 11.30 p.m., naked except for a pair of boots, painting his seven black cabs matt white – including the windscreens – and railing about the injustices he had suffered. He was sectioned (136) and removed with considerable difficulty to a psychiatric unit. A diagnosis of manic episode resulted. Later histories revealed that his mother had also suffered from manic depression and had killed herself when he was 16. In addition, he too had experienced milder forms of mood swings, but had not revealed the fact to his new family. Pharmacological treatment was by Lithium, to which, after adjustments, he responded well. The social work input to this case was successful, if slower, and took the following forms:

1   Seven family meetings, one with Mrs R and her two sons, and thereafter with Mr R included, took place. The aim here was (1) to explain in some detail the nature of this illness; (2) to disconnect recent florid episodes from any supposed misgivings about his new family and his role in it; (3) to give Mr R a chance to speak about his own earlier experiences to his wife and family, and (4) to negotiate a way forward.

2   Mr R's elder stepson now runs his (steadily reviving) taxi company; his younger stepson received some financial help in order to go to college.

3 The approach used here was family therapy (see Chapter 8), but not the kind that looks for *causes* in family conflicts for this strongly biological disorder, but to salve old grievances, to harness what support is left, and to make more rational plans for the future.

Schizophrenia

An awkward term, but we have been stuck with it since Bleuler first coined it in 1908. It means, literally, 'split mind', and refers to a disconnection between thinking, emotion and environmental experience. Epidemiological studies show a worldwide prevalence of just below 1 per cent. However, such cases amount typically to 40 per cent of the case loads of mental health social workers. Social anthropological research shows that all cultures have a name for it, whether with benefit of psychiatry or not, and these cultural definitions place emphasis on delusions, social disconnection, and on unwanted feelings of external control, which are seen not to be the fault of the sufferer. An eighteenth-century physician referred to it as 'the most solitary of afflictions' (Scull, 1993). The condition has been known throughout history, and a number of famous and talented people have been afflicted. The nature poet John Clare (1793–1864) – though there is more to him than that – was probably a sufferer, though schizo-affective disorder (a mixture of manic depression and schizophrenia) is more likely. He spent much of his life in the Northampton asylum, and now psychiatric wards across the country are named after him.

John Clare's life bears testimony to the fact that there is something innate at work in the condition (before we had a name for it) but that also environmental/ experiential influences are at work. He had a lost love, 'Mary', who was, in his imagination, half mythical, half real, and to whom to his dying day he was sure he had married. That he felt himself too sensitive to live in the rough world is evident in his poems. This feeling of social disconnection and differentness is at the centre of this condition, and the first generation of psychiatrists were aptly called *alienists*. Here is a verse from John Clare's poem 'I am':

> Into the nothingness of scorn and noise,
> Into the living sea of waking dreams,
> Where there is neither sense of life nor joys,
> But the vast shipwreck of my life's esteems.
> > (Clare, 1864)

So much for the inside-out experience, but if we want to help, we have to turn next to outside-in factors.

Diagnostic criteria

The first thing to note is that we are not dealing here with a single illness, but with overlapping syndromes. However, there *are* core characteristics.

Schizophrenia is a major, debilitating mental illness. It is a set of psychotic conditions, in that the client's insight into it, the false perceptions which accompany it, and the irrational attribution of symptoms and their original causes, are, to an extent, impermeable to rational discussion. We say 'to an extent' because one regularly meets patients who, if one accepted the first premise – 'my body is being interfered with by outside forces'; 'people whom I have never met mean to destroy me' – then their odd-seeming, precautionary measures can look like rational defensiveness.

This condition comes with *positive* and *negative* symptoms. The former reflect overt distortion of normal functions (e.g. bizarre and grossly inappropriate behaviour; disturbed speech which is tangential and illogical; false beliefs, and in the most serious cases, a tendency to act upon these beliefs). The term 'negative symptoms' refers to an absence of, or a severe diminution of, normal behaviour (e.g. social withdrawal, a flattening of affect and a lack of volition), so that there is little to sustain ordinary social interaction.

The more specific DSM IV TR criteria regarding positive symptoms for this illness should guide our understanding:

1   Hallucinations, i.e. seeing things that are not objectively there; smelling odours that no one else can smell; feeling bodily intrusions that no one can find any cause for; or most commonly, hearing voices which seem to the patient external, but no one is there.

2   Delusions, i.e. thoughts which sometimes carry imperatives for behaviour. These are often bizarre, erroneous beliefs, which are often strongly held and resistant to reason. They may be persecutory ('people follow me wherever I go'), or they may take the form of 'ideas of reference' wherein commonplace objects and events acquire special significance. In a case known to us, the sight of a salt cellar on the breakfast table meant 'I have been "assaulted" in the night', 'a salt . . .' and so on. The differences between our own everyday tendencies in misinter-preting stimuli and those in schizophrenia are (1) the degree of bizarreness; (2) its imperviousness to later reflection; (3) its persistence in the face of contrary evidence, and (4) a sense of loss of control over the processes of mind due to external, manipulative forces.

3   Thought insertion, i.e. ideas that are felt to be *put* inside the head from outside; or thought withdrawal, the idea that private thoughts are being *removed* and possibly broadcast to others.

4   Incoherent speech is often a manifestation of thought disorders and false perceptions. Typically, patients lose control of the structure of any particular narrative, going off track, failing to complete points, or exhibiting loose associations which have considerable meaning for them but not for listeners: 'word-salad'.

5   Schizophrenia can also manifest itself in grossly disturbed behaviour, from childlike silliness to extreme agitation without apparent external provocation.

As to negative symptoms (i.e. the absence of usual and appropriate behaviours), the following patterns are regularly seen:

1   Affective (emotional) flattening, i.e. the blunting of the usual forms of emotional expression. Often there is a lack of facial expression (but note that this may also occur in cases of clinical depression); reduced body language, and general social disconnection.
2   Apathy, and an avoidance of stimulating circumstances, particularly an avoidance of emotionally demanding social circumstances.
3   Withdrawal from close contact with family and friends, however helpful and supportive they have been.

Within this general picture several aetiologically and epidemiologically distinct subtypes of the condition may be perceived (Table 13.2).

Table 13.2 Symptoms of subtypes

Subtypes classification	Main symptoms
Paranoid type	Persecutory ideas and feelings and/or profound jealousy without cause; religiosity or grandiose behaviour.
Disorganized type	Disorganized speech and/or behaviour, inability to engage in everyday tasks; strange speech patterns, inappropriate laughter.
Catatonic type	Marked psycho-motor disturbance, immobility, echolalia-repeating whatever is said by another person.
Undetected type	All of the above symptoms may play a part but are mild or episodic in their presentation.
Residual type	This diagnosis requires at least one episode of schizophrenic behaviour, but is without prevalent psychotic symptoms, though with some negative symptoms such as poverty of speech, flattened affect or avolition.

Source: from DSM IV TR (2000).

4   A further problem with diagnoses based partially upon negative symptoms relates to the effects of pharmacological treatment itself. First-generation, neuroleptic medications were notorious for producing side-effects which many patients regarded as worse than the disease, namely weight gain, heart problems, salivary dribbling, tardive dyskenesia (strange, high-stepping gait) and neck rigidity. Second-generation medications have fewer side-effects but are more expensive, and are still not always prescribed early enough. Relapse rates with such treatments are 20 per cent per year; but 80 per cent per year off them. Dosages and tolerance levels need to be regularly reviewed. Social workers have a role in alerting health colleagues to such problems.

Causes

The first point to acknowledge is that there is much that we do not know. Of all the mental illnesses this one has been the most controversial. There are (not very convincing to us) social-anthropological and sociological studies which have sought to depict schizophrenia as a form of socio-cultural rebellion and a better manifestation of true sanity than most of the bourgeoisie (anyone else) can rise to. The Marxist philosophers (Foucault, Sartre) depicted the condition as a psychological *cri de coeur* against the alienating pressures of what they called 'late capitalism'. The psychoanalysts vaguely saw the condition as rooted in childhood psycho-sexual conflicts (what isn't, for them) but now steer well clear of these patients since the symptoms are, clinically, too extreme to justify even their less fanciful notions as to aetiology.

The problem facing attempts to disentangle the strands of biological inheritance and environmental inheritance is that usually the parents who confer the genes also provide the upbringing. Thus, even though studies have concluded for decades that mental illness runs in families, and that the greater the consanguinity (blood-relatedness) the greater the risk, we could never be sure what the transmission routes were. More secure data come from three different sources: (1) mono-zygotic versus di-zygotic twin studies: comparisons between identical twins with 100 per cent of genes in common, versus fraternal twins with 50 per cent in common, but the psychological experience of 'twin-ness' still present; (2) adoption studies, wherein identical twins have been placed in different family environments from birth; (3) cross-fostering studies, wherein (approaching the question of genetic versus environmental influences from the other direction) children with no known genetic vulnerability have been adopted into families where a surrogate parent acquires a diagnosis of schizophrenia (see Gottesman, 1991; Sheldon, 1994). The other possibility is that this is an *in utero* disorder; in other words, something happens to the embryo – which could be an environmental cause – that delays and disrupts certain patterns of brain development. We don't know. However, it appears from these later data that you cannot 'catch it' – though one could well have one's life chances severely influenced by the social, psychological and economic consequences of it – as is the case of any serious disability. However, symptoms of schizophrenia in parents seem to be recognized by children as something completely different, troubling but non-rational, and so not always a cause for self-blame.

To get some idea of the physical versus environmental patterns we are dealing with, look at the pair shown in Plate 13.1. These identical twins, separated at birth, met by accident at a volunteer fire officers' convention when someone who knew one of them asked the other how he had managed to get into the bar since he had just passed him walking in the opposite direction. Both are firemen, both are married to primary school teachers; both wives are called Doris, both of whom are teachers; their hobbies are identical, the books they own are amazingly similar, and they are both halfway through building the same kit canoe for the hunting trips that they both enjoy.

The question is: Supposing that one of these twins (and others in a large sample) had a secure diagnosis of schizophrenia, what would be the chances of the other acquiring one? Table 13.3, typical of many others, shows levels of actuarial risk for schizophrenia.

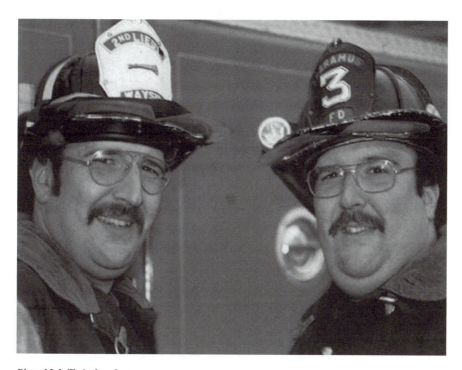

Plate 13.1 Twin brothers

Source: Reprinted courtesy of The Image Works/Encarta

Table 13.3 shows three things: (1) that the greater the level of consanguinity, the greater the risk of a diagnosis of the same disorder in a relative; (2) that there is a substantial leap in risk for M^z twins versus D^z twins which is well beyond chance or environmental influence (see line six of the table), but that (3) this still leaves around 40 per cent's worth of environmental factors to be accounted for. Social workers are educated to look preferentially at environmental influences for their clues as to what to do about problems, though it is worth noting that society has made less progress with completely environmental problems such as racism, ageism and gender-discrimination than with some largely biologically inherited ones (e.g. diabetes or psoriasis, both of which conditions have social consequences).

But let us look next at how physiological and social factors *interact* – for this is the key word – to produce precipitation and relapse. The best model of such interaction we have was thought up by mathematicians familiar with psychiatric data – a good example of the benefits of disciplinary conscillience.

Figure 13.2 is best thought of as a 3D graph in the shape of a piece of paper with a fold in it. The three axes are (1) genetic burden, from low to high; (2) environmental stress levels, from low to high, and (3) the actuarial likelihood of being counted among those diagnosed as schizophrenic. Better still, think of the surface plane in terms of the coordinates that could be drawn across it. Thus if a line is extended from the genetic axis, and intersects a line drawn from a point on the environmental stress axis, where they cross, and how close to the 'snowbank'

Table 13.3 Level of risk to relatives of schizophrenics

Relation	Risk (%)
First-degree relatives	
Parents	4.4
Brothers and sisters	8.5
Brothers and sisters, neither parent schizophrenic	8.2
Brothers and sisters, one parent schizophrenic	13.8
Fraternal twin, opposite sex	5.6
Fraternal twin, same sex	12.0
Identical twin	57.7
Children	12.3
Children – both parents schizophrenic	36.6
Second-degree relatives	
Uncles and aunts	2.0
Nephews and nieces	2.0
Grandchildren	2.8
Half-brothers/sisters	3.2
Third-degree relatives	
First cousins	2.9
General population	0.86

Sources: Based on figures from Slater and Cowie (1971); Zerbin-Rüdin (1967); Shields and Slater (1967): Tsuang and Vandermey (1980).

precipice they are, determines the likelihood of precipitation or relapse. We can do little as yet about the genetic axis beyond the suppression of effects by psychotropic medication, but we can do something about the other dimension.

The stress axis in Figure 13.2 is made up of secure results from medical sociology (see Brown and Birley, 1968), psychology and social psychiatry (see Falloon *et al.*, 1984; Birchwood and Tarrier, 1992). For although it would be very easy to gather the impression from station bookstalls that 'stress' is a condition that afflicts mainly the employed middle class, in fact, stress – that is, being required to come up with demanding behavioural responses against a short time-scale, against which circumstances conspire, and therefore feeling disablingly emotionally aroused, worried and fearful about failure – falls disproportionately upon the poor, the psychologically troubled, and the physically or mentally disabled. Socio-economic findings also show that if one was not poor before becoming mentally ill, one is very likely to become so afterwards. Indeed, the social conditions in which most seriously mentally ill people live add up to: being on one's own; probably without a partner; with few if any friends; with no occupation; with few relatives or carers to lend support; subsisting in a voluntary housing scheme; being welfare benefit-dependent, and on the receiving end of a meagre 'care in the community' service (see Leff, 1997; Macdonald and Sheldon, 1998). Where the experience is that one has few options, and that little that one does will have an impact, becomes internalized, it also becomes a self-fulfilling prophecy.

However, there is another type of stress, more psychological than the socio-economic factors co-represented along the top axis of Figure 13.3, which is called *expressed emotion* (EE). A concordant finding emerged in early psychiatric

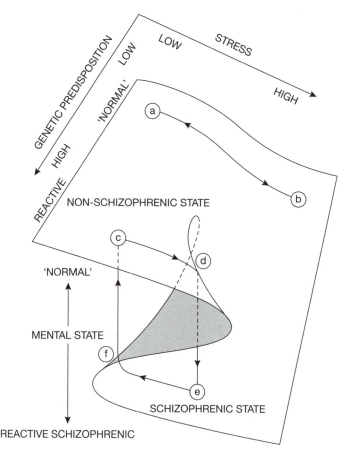

Figure 13.2 Relative impact of genetic and environmental variables in reactive schizophrenia

Note: This model encompasses the suggestion that a high level of genetic predisposition requires only a middling level of environmental precipitation to produce a strong risk of disorder (c-d-e). Similarly, a middling level of genetic burden requires a high level of precipitating stress to manifest the disease (a-b). When the stress is relieved the patient returns to a period of relative normality (e-f-c).

Source: Woodcock and Davis (1978). Reproduced by kind permission of the Penguin Group.

rehabilitation studies (see Olsen, 1984) when relapse rates were found to be higher among those patients returning home to their families as opposed to sheltered accommodation or boarding-houses. On the whole, families care for as long as they can, and they naturally want to encourage away a condition which strikes at the heart of family life. The result is emotional pressure, which is exactly what people with schizophrenia find most difficult.

Expressed emotion can even be measured. Where up-against-it families and carers score highly on EE scales, the stress, as measured by galvanic skin response (GSR) reactions (a measure of electrical conductivity changes in the skin due to arousal) goes up, and stays up even when such encounters are over (see Birchwood and Tarrier, 1992). Relapse rates in high EE environments were found to run at 50 per cent, but only at 9 per cent for low EE subjects in one study (see Falloon *et al.*, 1990). Therefore this is no vague sociological concept like *anomie*; it affects physiology, psychology, measurable social well-being and relapse rates.

Let us turn now to experiments which have tried to lower stress in living conditions resulting from too much emotional demand. We have a dozen or so of these, all with positive results (see Falloon *et al.*, 1990; Pharoah *et al.*, 2006). Figure 13.3 is one such example; it contains a comparison between a family-based education and EE-lowering programme, and routine, individual, after-care. The difference in relapse rates is obvious. Such interventions, though known about for some years, are not routinely available in the UK outside specialist centres.

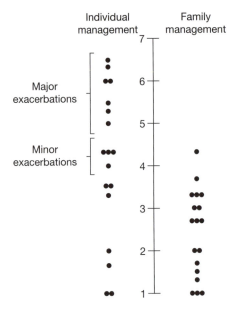

Maximum target rating (blind) during the 9 months of treatment

Figure 13.3 An experiment with expressed emotion

Source: Tsuang and Vandermens (1980). Reproduced by kind permission of the *International Journal of Social Psychiatry*/Oxford University Press.

Case example

Mr A (23) was referred to Social Services for after-care following discharge from a 16-day stay in a psychiatric unit. He was admitted via section 136 of the 1983 Mental Health Act after shouting at passers-by and standing dangerously (at night, and in the rain) in the middle of a dual carriageway, trying to stop traffic and tell his story to the occupants of cars. It emerged that he was struggling to cope with his job where his colleagues were allegedly signalling details of his latest incompetence to each other via notes and special glances. He was, in fact, regarded as a quiet but basically efficient employee, until he began to laugh and look meaningfully at people in a very out-of-context way. He was convinced that his flat was bugged and that people were following him home from work, and he took elaborate precautions to throw off his 'pursuers'.

The diagnosis was paranoid schizophrenia, in that he felt himself persecuted but could give no reason as to why. He responded well to medication, returned to work, but relapsed within two weeks. His father's attitude was 'pull yourself together', in contrast to the perhaps over-doting behaviour of his mother. They both came to be seen as part of the conspiracy. After a fierce and tearful row, he attacked them and was sectioned again, this time for a longer period.

The role of Social Services was:

1   To secure half-way house accommodation away from the over-demanding circumstances of home life.
2   Then, as he improved, to secure a housing association flat.
3   Then, via an employment rehabilitation scheme to get work experience on an environmental project – at which work he excelled.
4   Then, to get a part-time job – at which he also did well. So well, in fact, that he was given a position of responsibility over other staff. He relapsed within three weeks, but after a brief stay in hospital was reinstated to his old job, which he was still doing seven years later.

This case demonstrates well the 'thermostatic' character of schizophrenia, wherein a biological predisposition is clicked into life by an increase in expectations and associated stress.

Psychosocial interventions

We have close on 100 randomized controlled trials, plus systematic reviews of these investigating the effects of psycho-social interventions, most reporting worthwhile results. Below this level, non-randomized trials, pre-post tests and client-opinion studies are available showing similar, if less secure results (see Kopelowicz and Liberman, 1995, 1998). Therefore, these interventions are not simply residual or palliative – though there is nothing wrong with stopping things getting worse, providing that this emphasis is not based on myth and institutional pessimism. For schizophrenia is, analogously, closer to diabetes than appendicitis. It requires treatment, but then, as importantly, management and support. Here is a commentary on the most promising interventions drawn from the literature:

1   Social work support, such as befriending, advocacy on behalf of clients regarding social security and housing matters and regarding access to medical and other social services, is highly valued by clients. There is no bottomless well of need here; client opinion studies regularly reveal a simple wish for continuity

of support by a known and trusted person (see Macdonald and Sheldon, 1992).

2   However, serious mental illness also has its acute phases and its florid relapses, and in the past approved social workers have, for good reason, seen their main role as the protection of the clients' civil liberties (see Hewitt, 2004). Nevertheless, there is also a compelling case for early, decisive treatment. 'Assertive outreach' programmes have done well in recent research studies. We are uneasy about the term, and prefer the use of 'preventive' instead, but the principles of these projects are valid (i.e. not to wait around before ensuring that suitable medical treatment takes place, and to think about rehabilitation from the start).

3   Rehabilitation from psychiatric units is no small issue. Stays in hospital are now relatively short, but insufficient attention is paid still to the circumstances to which patients return, and which may well have played a part in what sent them into hospital in the first place. It is important to meet clients prior to discharge and discuss their worries and concerns; ensure that they are psychologically prepared for leaving, and that everything necessary to meet their immediate social and material needs is prearranged. Where coordinated schemes are in place, future relapse is less likely, but as things stand this is a lottery.

4   Community care for mentally ill people looks to those of us who worked in the old mental institutions like a policy success. Thousands of patients who pose limited risk to the wider community (but note that it might pose one to *them*) have been successfully resettled. What they tell us they would like amounts to a modest shopping list of adaptations: day centres to be open, not 9 to 5, but at the weekends too, and during the main holidays when lonely people feel vulnerable; for such centres to be judged not by programmes and activities but for their welcoming, non-stigmating approach (see Macdonald and Sheldon, 1997).

5   Serious mental illness threatens the humanity of sufferers, and anything that can be done to empower clients and those who help care for them (1) to understand these conditions and (2) to counteract the negative symptoms of loss of social skills, anhedonia, and loss of interest in either meaningful occupation or employment (where it is available) is not only clinically worthwhile, but is also an ethical obligation. Where social skills training groups are in place the results are good, and have been for some time. Social workers acting as advocates on behalf of clients regarding employment possibilities also produce positive results; in fact, sheltered, sometimes part-time, but *real* work, following preparatory placements perhaps, and with support services in place, greatly influence lives for the better – not only materialistically, but through increased self-esteem (see ODPM, 2004).

6   Staff in relapse-prevention schemes, and practitioners generally, should also consider the psychological needs of clients alongside their material ones. We have already reviewed the results of interventions to lower expressed emotion. These are moderately effective but costly (in terms of success rates) – but then the wider economic costs of schizophrenia are wildly expensive in comparison. Would anyone grudge funding a scheme that produced a one in four or five recovery rate in cases of life-threatening *physical* disease? In any case, with practice we

might get better at predicting the outcome (see Rollinson *et al.* (2008) for work in progress).

7   Delusional thinking, more threateningly, *acting* upon delusional beliefs, is a major diagnostic feature of schizophrenia. Until recently, thanks to a hangover from psychoanalytic theory, they were seen as 'functional' (i.e. as safety-valve expressions), and staff in the mental health field were sternly cautioned not to meddle with them for fear of making things worse. Many pioneering cognitive-behavioural therapists have challenged this view over the past decade, and have achieved compelling results which are now being replicated with auditory hallucinations (see Chadwick *et al.*, 1996: 69). We have both, against the established rules, noted positive effects from a gentle, evidential challenge to delusional beliefs. The approach, now finding favour in the literature, has four components: (1) counselling clients to regard strong beliefs as nevertheless hypotheses which can be tested; (2) the introduction of the idea of taking a few risks to test them; (3) to encourage clients to ponder plausible connections with their own life histories and current levels of self-esteem; and (4) to encourage them to note when and where delusional thinking is either higher or lower and to make connections between circumstances and thoughts.

Obsessive-compulsive disorder

We all have small obsessions in our lives (think back to childhood), but the lives of some individuals are completely taken over by them. This is the fourth commonest mental disorder, with a lifetime prevalence rate of 2.5 per cent, and it can have serious effects on the quality of life of both sufferers and their families. The condition occurs in both males and females with typically an early *first* onset in males (6 to 13 years) and a later onset in females (20 to 29 years).

Diagnostic criteria

To meet DSM IV TR criteria, clients must have experienced the following:

1   Repetitive behaviours (e.g. hand washing, constant, driven checking, or a rigid observance of strange rules and rituals). Minimally, these must occur for at least an hour a day.
2   These behaviours and their obsessive cognitive components – which can be just as distressing – are aimed at preventing some dreaded event (such as contamination, infecting loved ones, or not preventing disasters). Thus there is a strong negative reinforcement element, in that behaviour is precautionary well beyond cultural norms or half-way rational approaches to risks, but if nothing bad happens they 'work' (see Chapter 7).
3   At some stage, most sufferers recognize that these compulsions in both their cognitive, behavioural and emotional forms are unreasonable and excessive – but nevertheless feel imprisoned by them.

Causes

These are not fully known, though there are candidate areas in parts of the brain thought to control impulsivity and alertness. There is also a strong familial pattern, with large increases in vulnerability according to kinship. Monozygotic twins have a much higher incidence than do dyzyotic twins and so it is reasonable to conclude that this is partially an inherited disorder (see Franklin and Foa, 1998; DSM IV TR, 2000) but also one in which stress factors play a part.

Pharmacological interventions

There are effective medical treatments, and there are many randomized controlled trials testifying to this fact. The prime indications are for SSRIs and trycyclic medications. Up to 60 per cent of patients respond well to these, but numerous studies also show that cognitive-behavioural approaches and social support schemes enhance their effectiveness considerably.

Psycho-social interventions

Cognitive-behavioural therapies are the methods of choice (see NICE, 2007b), and, as with panic disorders and phobias, virtually amount to an ethical, let alone a technical imperative for professionals to carry out.

Case example

Mrs R, a single parent with two children aged 6 and 9, came to the notice of a Social Services CAMHS team because of concern expressed by teachers that they seemed preoccupied with cleanliness and would not touch everyday objects. After a brief assessment it became clear that their mother was imposing these rules by reason of her own obsessive-compulsive disorder. The history revealed that she had, since her late teenage years, engaged in ritualistic behaviour regarding contamination – not sitting on toilets, washing her hands 30 to 50 times a day, employing disinfectants even to polished furniture, and using TCP to wipe down her children's hands and faces before she was able to express any physical affection towards them. She also felt compelled to line up chairs and curtains to some imaginary perfect position; to check that lights were *really* switched off at night. All this was exhausting, and it drove her to seek treatment. However, Mrs R was also obsessional about her obsessions and, although prescribed appropriate medication, often refused to take it.

Social work and health staff came up with a detailed approach to this problem which, given a long and chequered history of treatment, concentrated on her family as a somewhat untapped resource. The features were:

1 A behavioural family therapy approach which allowed the children (aged 6 and 9) and their (somewhat alienated) father to express their views in a

---

controlled environment. This produced the conclusion that the children really did not fear contamination and were complying (1) because it was 'the routine', and (2) because not to do so would upset their mother.

2 A social worker and CPN working together persuaded Mrs R into a programme, based on desensitization and response prevention. This interim approach worked quickly, the problem with obsessions, anxieties and phobic reactions being that very little reality testing ever takes place, so strong and reflexive are the avoidance procedures.

3 A medication review with a psychiatrist at which was recommended a lower dose of anti-anxiety medication, producing fewer side-effects.

4 The husband was persuaded to think in less 'all-or-nothing' ways about contacts with the children, to which change of heart the children responded well.

The children no longer carry out cleanliness rituals; the mother has abandoned many of hers (though as she puts it, she still 'itches').

Eating disorders

These involve deliberately restricting the consumption of food, or binge-eating and then vomiting (bulimia). The commonest condition is anorexia nervosa.

Diagnostic criteria for anorexia nervosa

1 Refusal to maintain body weight at or above a minimally normal weight for age and height (e.g. weight loss leading to maintenance of body weight less than 85 per cent of normal; or failure to make expected weight gain during periods of growth).

2 Intense fear of gaining weight or becoming 'fat', even though patently underweight.

3 Disturbances of the way in which one's body weight or shape is experienced; undue influence of body weight or shape on self-evaluation, or denial of the seriousness of the current diagnosis.

4 In post-menarcheal females, amenorrhoea (i.e. the absence of at least three consecutive menstrual cycles – possibly a motivational (negative reinforcement) factor).

Types

• *Restricting type:* During the current episode of anorexia nervosa, the person has not regularly engaged in binge-eating or purging behaviour (i.e. self-induced vomiting or the misuse of laxatives, diuretics or enemas) but continues to restrict the intake of food.

- *Binge-eating/purging type:* During the current episode of anorexia nervosa, the person has regularly engaged in binge-eating or purging behaviour (i.e. self-induced vomiting or the misuse of laxatives, diuretics or enemas). This eating disorder, which predominantly affects young women (at a figure ten times greater than in males) and has a death rate through self-starvation approaching 20 per cent, has been heavily politicized in the past, with feminist psychologists seeing it as a form of 'hunger strike' against patriarchy. Questions have also been raised regarding the influence of advertisements featuring sylph-like models who are obsessive about their body shape.

It is interesting to note that in countries where the food supply is precarious, anorexia is much less common, even though it does have a strong familial pattern worldwide. Twin studies show predisposition levels of around 70 per cent (see Tierney, 2004). In much of the literature, there exists a false dichotomy between biological/developmental influences and socio-cultural ones. Genes produce a wide range of phenotypical expressions. Heretofore, the 'ideal shapes' in the old 'Bollywood' films favoured 'rounded bodies', since this was a sign of wealth. Then as economic prosperity improved, Western-style thinness became more fashionable. Biology, culture, societal factors and psychology thus all interact here, as they do throughout the spectrum of mental health problems.

Psychological studies of starvation effects (interestingly, conducted on conscientious objector volunteers in the US during World War II) revealed that the first few days of food deprivation are characterized by intense feelings of hunger; by dreams about food; by conversations about little else, and even by visual hallucinations about it. Then, steadily, appetite recedes and a state described by some as 'ascetism' or as 'transcendental' takes over – as recorded by practices of fasting for religious reasons throughout the ages. Alexander Solzhenitsyn (1974) recalls the experience in the Gulag of being put into solitary confinement on 'punishment rations' (a small bowl of gruel once a day) and hearing urgent, whispered advice from the next cell not to eat it lest the pangs of hunger become intolerable. Complete abstinence for a few days would make the desire for food less preoccupying. Something similar to this extinction of appetite effect may occur in anorexia.

Effective interventions

We now have good systematic reviews of interventions for anorexia nervosa and its close cousin, bulimia nervosa – which is typified not by not letting food in in the first place, but by binge eating followed by self-induced vomiting and purging (see Wilson and Fairburn, 1998; Tierney, 2004).

Pharmacological interventions for bulimia nervosa are much more methodologically secure than for anorexia nervosa. This is probably because the latter condition was long seen as primarily a psychological condition.

Antidepressant/anti-anxiety medications are widely used for the treatment of anorexia nervosa, often in combination with family therapy and increasingly cognitive-behavioural therapy. But whether single interventions in either direction are superior to combinations is as yet unclear. Qualitative studies of the experiences of clients undergoing treatment reveal the following common features:

1   Diagnosis is often faltering, as clients regularly attribute their weight loss to external factors (e.g. to problems at school, failed relationships, disagreements with parents). These are as likely to be symptomatic as causal.

2   Family therapy and cognitive-behavioural approaches (see Chapters 7 and 8) are most effective when the diagnosis is firm and the focus is on harm reduction.

3   Family therapy approaches which carefully expose the various 'games' and avoidance strategies usually at work in this disorder are often (though sometimes retrospectively) valued. That is, if a loved one is apparently starving herself to death in front of her parents, then the temptation to become increasingly coercive, or to feed by stealth, is understandable but is likely to be viewed by the young person as the *cause* of her aversions.

4   Therapeutic regimes must, of course, allow the experiences of all parties a certain priority, but weight gain and improved body mass index measures *must* be the final measure of improvement, not self-reported well-being, lest this too becomes part of a manipulative trade-off.

5   The factors associated with effective psycho-social outcomes reviewed in Chapter 3 also apply in the face of this complex disorder; that is, time-limited, focused, quite intensive interventions do better than less structured interventions (see Crisp *et al.*, 1991; Tierney, 2004).

Case example

As a keen amateur ballet dancer, Sarah, aged 15 years, decided further to restrict her diet for art's sake. Over a few months people started to comment on her dramatic weight loss. It eventually came to the point that she was made to see her GP by her parents. He diagnosed her as anorectic, an opinion that was hard for Sarah to accept:

> I didn't think there was anything wrong. I couldn't understand what all the fuss was about.

Despite Sarah's unwillingness to acknowledge that she had a problem, her GP suggested she saw the practice nurse. However, Sarah did not find this particularly helpful:

> She wasn't really experienced in treating people with anorexia. She just talked to me about what I should be eating but I ignored what she was saying because I thought she just wanted to make me fat.

When Sarah's weight loss continued, her GP realized that she needed more expert assistance. Therefore, she referred Sarah to a specialist eating disorders service, where she received cognitive-behavioural therapy. Sarah found this helpful because it challenged her negative thoughts and encouraged her to think about things differently. It also made her feel that she was regaining some control of her life. Sarah also noted that it helped to talk to someone who understood her condition:

> She [the therapist] didn't just think I was attention-seeking or dieting. She knew that this was a real problem for me and that made me realize I had to do something about it.

The specialist service also arranged for family therapy sessions which she found helpful, though there were times when she felt the experience artificial, with everyone being 'on their best behaviour'. But then:

> In family therapy I was able to say things to my parents that I hadn't said before. They listened to me instead of shouting and they started to understand what I was going through.

Six months on, Sarah is still receiving individual therapy, but is gaining weight. She also still attends regular group sessions at which she meets other young people with anorexia to talk about her problems.

Let us now move on to another condition that usually manifests itself in childhood and adolescence.

Asperger's Syndrome

> I see everything. But most people are lazy.
> They never look at everything. They do what
> Is called glancing.

> Mark Holden, *Sunday Telegraph*, 2002: 2

This disorder is named after Dr Hans Asperger (1906–1980) who first identified it in his clinical practice and research. It is a milder form of childhood autism, without the severe communication difficulty and delay in language acquisition which accompanies that even more disabling condition. It often crops up in the case loads of CAMHS social workers and so is included in this digest. Another reason is that this syndrome has in the past been under-diagnosed and misattributed to simpler behavioural problems, problems in education, and to the effects of family breakdown.

Diagnostic criteria

1   A qualitative impairment in social interaction, as manifested by at least two of the following:

- marked impairment in the use of multiple non-verbal behaviours such as eye-to-eye gaze, appropriate facial expression, body postures, and gestures to regulate social interaction;
- failure to develop peer relationships appropriate to the age/developmental level;

- a lack of spontaneous seeking to share enjoyment, interests or achievements with other people;
- lack of social or emotional reciprocity.

2 Restricted, repetitive and stereotyped patterns of behaviour, motor clumsiness, and at least one of the following expressions:

- An all-encompassing preoccupation with one or more stereotyped and restricted patterns of interest that is abnormal either in intensity or focus;
- apparently inflexible adherence to very specific, non-functional routines or rituals;
- stereotyped and repetitive motor mannerisms (e.g. hand or finger flapping or twisting, or complex whole-body movements);
- persistent preoccupation with parts of objects, not wholes;
- significant impairment in social, occupational or other important areas of functioning.

There is no clinically significant general delay in language (e.g. single words used by age 2, communicative phrases typically used by age 3. There is no clinically significant delay in cognitive development in childhood, or in the development of age-appropriate self-help skills, adaptive behaviour (other than in social interaction) and curiosity about the environment. A recent experiment, one of many, gives an insight into the cognitive distortions of autism spectrum disorders. Many people suffering from autism see themselves as blessed with greater acuity of perception. The experiment involved showing a picture of a rural scene to young people with a diagnosis of Asperger's Syndrome and to matched controls. The controls typically said: 'It's a country scene with some cows in a field'; the experimental group typically said things like; 'there are twelve black and white cows in the field, four of these facing to the left, eight to the right; there are hawthorn hedges, and there is a plastic bag discarded in one of them; the church is flat-topped and has no spire . . .'. Acuity of judgement is, in some circumstances, helpful, but in this condition often leads to social paralysis.

There is a strong genetic element to this disorder, but the best available solutions come from changes in the local environment.

The research trends in this field are increasingly methodologically robust, and show strong signs of convergence regarding findings concerning the best available medical and psycho-social interventions. Here they are:

1 Early diagnosis in childhood prevents misunderstandings and misattributions by family members – on whom the best outcomes depend.
2 There has been an upsurge in the literature of authors who themselves have this syndrome writing about their experiences and what they feel like, and about what forms of help are most appropriate and effective.
3 The available pharmaceutical treatments for Asperger's Syndrome are symptomatic only. In other words, if the condition leads to depression then antidepressants might help; if it leads to obsessive-compulsive behaviour, then there are other medications which might help (see Nathan and Gorman, 1998).

4   The most effective psycho-social interventions are based on old-fashioned behaviour therapy – simple, reward-based, desensitization programmes implemented by parents under professional guidance (see Chapter 7).

Case example

John was always regarded as a difficult child by his (dedicated) parents. His failures at school led to interviews with educational psychologists and family therapists who automatically assumed that his obsessive, often antisocial behaviour must have its roots in his home life. Only at age 14 was he properly diagnosed with Asperger's Syndrome. By that time, he was unable to eat when other people were present; couldn't sleep in his bed, which he thought contaminated by germs; was unable to use a public telephone; and couldn't turn on a tap for fear of contamination. When he became a student, reading physical sciences, he required two assistants to carry out experimental work. When referred for CBT, he usually turned up two hours late, and was more interested in why the wallpaper was striped or why a computer was unplugged. The cognitive part of this CBT programme was not helpful; the only thing that worked at all was desensitization therapy designed to get him to test out what would actually happen if he failed to disinfect the taps before and after using them, or slept in his bed (see Chapter 7). The answer, he eventually agreed, was 'nothing'. Having taken graded, small steps towards overcoming his obsessions he obtained his physics degree, thanks mainly to his parents and to the understanding approach of the university.

Personality disorders

These conditions have long been recognized as syndromes but the debate as to whether they are 'genuine' mental illnesses has never gone away. The Royal College of Psychiatrists played the 'treatability' card a few years ago, i.e. since no effective treatments exist, and since these conditions are largely exacerbations of normal personality characteristics, these patients should be passed on to Social Services. In the new mental health legislation this position has rightly been reversed – since there are many medical conditions for which no effective treatments exist, but which are still attended to.

Personality disorders may be defined as:

A severe disturbance in the characterological constitution and behavioural tendencies of the individual, usually involving several areas of the personality, and nearly always associated with considerable personal and social disruption. Personality disorder tends to appear in late childhood or adolescence and continues to be manifest into adulthood. These types of conditions comprise deeply ingrained and enduring behaviour patterns, manifestations themselves are inflexible responses to a broad range of personal and social situations.

(ICD-10)

'Personality' is a construct, a recognizable pattern in behaviour, inferred cognition and inferred emotional patterns which are semi-independent of environmental circumstances. H. J. Eysenck (1965) has produced the most enduring and empirically tested set of dimensions. You have to imagine, not a 2D bell-shaped curve, but actually a 3D bell shape; from side to side lies the introversion (stimulus-shy), extra-version (stimulus-hungry) continuum – the nearer the middle, the more statistically typical. From back to front lies the neuroticism/psychoticism continuum. It is on the statistical shoulders of the bell's curves that the serious cases of personality disorder exist, so that on one side there is a pervasive withdrawal from recognized social responsibilities, and on the other an aggressive, manipulative urge towards self-gratification at almost any cost. In the middle section is something called 'normality'.

The underlying feature of these conditions is the failure to develop an adequately functioning conscience; that is, a lack of moral conditionability. This evidence also indicates a strong environmental component. Soldiers can, after all, be trained into something close to psychopathic behaviour in the circumstances of conflict. Young people, whose status in gangs boosts their fragile identities, can behave in un-characteristically depersonalized and aggressive ways, the point at issue being that, even in extreme environments, not *everyone* does.

Personality disorders have been shown from large community samples to have a lifetime prevalence range of 0.5 per cent to 3.5 per cent with more men than women affected – a wide variation made worse by low inter-reliability rates. Today they produce around only a 58 per cent diagnostic agreement (see Dowson and Grounds, 1995). This situation persuaded the authors of earlier versions of the DSM to conclude that this was 'almost a diagnosis not worth making' but that we are still stuck with the problem and have to live with this 'almost'.

Effective interventions

There are few. Behaviour-modification regimes (see Sheldon, 1995) such as token economies worked moderately well in closed institutions in the 1960s and 1970s, but then – unsurprisingly – since lack of generalized conditionability is at the heart of these problems – on discharge most patients/clients reverted to doing what came naturally. Cognitive-behavioural approaches are making limited but clinically noteworthy inroads today (see Dowson and Grounds, 1995) and are cautiously challenging the 'untreatability' orthodoxy.

There is a further set of considerations regarding the support of people with personality disorders that is worthy of discussion. These clients, whether intentionally or not, and whether they know it or not, can sometimes exploit and misuse health and social services support. This consumes considerable energy and resource, and in effect can result in entire organizations – if not careful – being subject to intermittent punishment, negative reinforcement, plus small rewards, and responding accordingly, and not always helpfully or effectively (see Chapter 7).

Case example

In a recent case, primary care services were bombarded by urgent requests for further tests and treatments for 'low blood sugar' from a young woman and her parents. A number of persistent attention-seeking problems, and episodes of antisocial behaviour, were attributed to this condition, except that multiple tests revealed that blood sugar levels were normal. Just at the point where it was being suggested that the patient might be happier at some other surgery, the complaints stopped. But then they started again (this time backed by large internet searches on this condition) with the local hospital. When they tired of it, the patient was referred to – guess where? – Social Services, who, because there was the welfare of a small baby to consider, started the whole investigative process all over again.

Case reviews and family meetings also ended in acrimony. In effect, the various sources of potential help were being targeted in rotation to the point where each *nearly* gave up, and then the focus shifted elsewhere. Only a meeting of *all* the professionals involved, so that findings and experiences could be shared, produced a cast-iron service regime – not based on organizational respite. In the face of this, the patient moderated her demands and started to receive help when she was not stridently demanding it. There are indeed cases of medical misdiagnosis; there are indeed some cases in which clients rightly fight to claim their due rights to effective services, but there are also some cases where *nothing*, however well problems are assessed, however well provided services are, will *ever* satisfy a few personality-disordered people. Oppositional behaviour becomes, in effect, a 'career' and a complicated form of avoidance behaviour.

Conclusions

These can be briefly summarized: first, since mental disorders are more or less (depending on the condition) bio-psycho-social problems, they require bio-psycho-social solutions. The clearest evidence is that where health and social services personnel collaborate, the results are better.

Second, we have seen that risk dominates the way in which people with a psychiatric history are perceived. There is a new review (DoH, 2007) headed up by Louis Appleby (see also Appleby, 1997) which suggests that ex-mental patients have committed 400 murders in the past eight years (one a week). These are high figures, but the way in which some of the detail is presented in the report gives cause for concern, e.g. '5 per cent of all killings were committed by people with a diagnosis of schizophrenia' (so 95 per cent were not – though there is an over-representation here); 25 per cent (of the 5 per cent) had stopped taking medication' (so three-quarters had not). 'In many cases, 29 per cent in the confidential enquiry, patients had probably been seen in the previous week before the murder, and so therefore risks had been negligently underestimated'. Now you just cannot have it both ways. If they *hadn't* been seen this would amount to a scandal, and if they *had* been seen it amounts to a different sort of scandal.

A few dreadful attacks on complete strangers are conflated in the latest and the previous figures, but then most violence takes place against family and people well known to those who commit it – and often under the influence of that fatal combination: hard drugs and mental illness. However, official statistics now confirm that you are close to three times *less* likely to be attacked by a person who has been or is mentally ill today than you were in the 1970s, before the community care policy was implemented.

14 Social work with people with disabilities

In all societies of the world there are still obstacles preventing persons with disabilities from exercising their rights and freedoms and making it difficult for them to participate fully in the activities of their societies. It is the responsibility of states to take appropriate action to remove such obstacles.

Bengt Lindqvist, Special Rapporteur on Disabilities,
United Nations Commission for Social Development, 2000

Care needed?

It is beyond dispute that people with disabilities continue to be economically and socially disadvantaged (see Burchardt, 2003; Jenkins and Rigg, 2003; Russell, 2003; Preston, 2006). Social work can be *one* of the means whereby states deliver their commitment to removing such inequalities, but it can also be one of the barriers that disabled people encounter when seeking to exercise their rights and freedoms. Understanding and thinking about social work's role in this regard requires a vigilant approach both from individual professionals and from organizations.

Social work with disabled people has largely reflected the ways that they have been viewed by society as a whole. Historically, they have been viewed as people marked by personal tragedy and who find it difficult fully to participate in society. Disabled people are thought of as dependent on others; in need of 'care'; intrinsically of less socio-economic value than non-disabled people, and as a group of people for whom separate provision – of a kind that we would not accept for non-disabled people – is deemed a reasonable response:

> The very language of welfare provision continues to deny disabled people the right to be treated as fully competent, autonomous individuals. Care in the community, caring for people, providing services through care managers, case managers or even care attendants all structure the welfare discourse in particular ways and imply a particular view of disabled people.
>
> (Swain *et al.*, 1993: 268)

Locating problems *within* disabled people themselves ignores the ways in which the social, physical and economic environments impact upon them and create barriers to their participation. None the less, it has been the dominant way of conceptualizing disability, and continues to exert considerable influence in practice in both health and social care. It is often referred to as the 'medical model' of disability.

The social model of disability

Although its origins stretch back to the 1960s (see Hunt, 1966; UPIAS, 1976), it was Michael Oliver who first articulated what was to become known as the social model of disability (Oliver, 1983). Put most concisely, it sees disability as the social consequences of having an impairment. Within the social model, the main causes of disability lie, not with someone's impairment, but in the pervasive economic and social barriers which prevent disabled people from securing a reasonable quality of life (see Oliver and Barnes, 1998). These barriers are the consequence of a world organized by non-disabled people around the needs of non-disabled people. They reflect values and attitudes that disabled people encounter on a daily basis, both from other individuals and from institutions, and which run counter to the project of citizenship and social justice for disabled people.

There is a growing body of empirical evidence to support this analysis. Using the social model as an analytic lens, disabled activists have reshaped the discourse within which disablement is discussed and disabled people have brought about significant changes through political activity. They have, for example, been responsible for initiating significant changes in legislation, in policy and in practice. Disability discrimination is now illegal. Independent living is recognized as an important organizing principle of welfare (e.g. DoH, 2005). Choice and dignity are terms that are now appearing routinely in policy documents (e.g. DoH, 2004). This is in contrast to the decades in which their interests were represented largely by non-representative organizations run by non-disabled people (see Hasler, 1993). One vehicle for this has been the Disabled People's Movement, a network of organizations run by disabled people for disabled people.

These changes, while long overdue, have taken place in a relatively short period of time. They mark, however, only the beginning of a process. For the majority of disabled people there continues to be a gap between the rhetoric of politicians, and professionals, and the reality of their daily lives.

Social work and disabled people

Writing in 1983, Michael Oliver identified social work as the occupational group most likely to be able to work alongside disabled people to challenge the barriers they faced in achieving citizenship and social inclusion. In the second edition in 1999, Oliver and Sapey note that this anticipated role contribution had not materialized. In the 2006 edition the authors conclude that:

> the individual model of disability is so embedded in social work practice that in its current form the profession is unlikely to retain its role of working with disabled people as citizens. The citizenship approach to welfare seeks to change fundamentally the relationship that disabled people have with the welfare state, and this requires the administrators of welfare also to change fundamentally.
>
> (Oliver and Sapey, 2006: 189)

They remain hopeful that social work will rise to the challenge, but note that time is running out and the organization of social work and the discourses that shape it run somewhat counter to the changes needed. Their strategy for fostering a citizenship approach, based on human rights, is to develop an approach to professional social work that facilitates the challenging 'of oppressive social policies, but which does so *with* disabled people rather than *for* them' (Oliver and Sapey, 2006: 183, italics added).

An inclusive approach

The social model of disability was first articulated by people with physical impairments, but its relevance to those who find themselves disabled as a result of other forms of impairment, whether intellectual or mental, visible or invisible, has long been recognized. The social model of disability is not compatible with an approach that groups people according to type of impairment, as this is inherently the core of the clinical approach to disability. This is not the same as saying that it is not important for professionals to have a good understanding of the nature of impairments that people experience. For example, those working with the deaf need to understand hearing impairment, what this means for hearing-impaired people and what is important to them.

Social work with people with profound and complex needs raises particular issues and we note these as they arise. For the most part, however, the focus of this chapter is primarily on the role that social workers can play in maximizing the quality of life of all disabled people and their families. This entails working within an ethical framework that seeks to promote the human rights of disabled people, their entitlement to equal opportunities, and to self-determination. The evidence base of most relevance to social workers in this regard is that which casts light on what disabled people say about their lives and their aspirations; what they want or need from professionals, and how they experience services. Much of this work has been undertaken by disabled people themselves, and this chapter draws heavily on their work and on research which reflects their views. We look first at the social work with disabled children and their families.

Disabled children

The UK is a signatory to the UN Convention on the Rights of the Child. Article 23 states that signatories:

1   Recognize that a mentally or physically disabled child should enjoy a full and decent life, in conditions which ensure dignity, promote self-reliance and facilitate the child's active participation in the community.
2   Recognize the right of the disabled child to special care appropriate to the child's condition and to the circumstances of the parents or others caring for the child.
3   Recognize the special needs of a disabled child; assistance should be extended in accordance with paragraph 2 of the present article and shall be provided free of charge, whenever possible, taking into account the financial resources of the

parents or others caring for the child, and shall be designed to ensure that the disabled child has effective access to and receives education, training, health care services, rehabilitation services, preparation for employment and recreation opportunities in a manner conducive to the child's achieving the fullest possible social integration and individual development, including his or her cultural and spiritual development.

In other words, a disabled child has the same entitlement to a reasonable quality of life as a non-disabled child. He or she may need additional support to access those opportunities routinely available to non-disabled children. Although not generally enforceable in law within the UK, the Convention provides an internationally agreed benchmark on children's basic rights, and as such provides a template for thinking about public services to children, and the goals to which social workers should aspire when working in partnership with children and families.

Parents and families of disabled children

Poverty, poor housing and social isolation all make parenting more difficult. Families with disabled children have been shown to have lower incomes than other families (see Gordon *et al.*, 2000) and face additional expenditure as a result of their child's disability (see Dobson and Middleton, 1998). Mothers of disabled children are less likely to be in work than their peers, and therefore less likely to have the social and financial benefits associated with employment (see Baldwin and Carlisle, 1994). They also have a higher risk of becoming lone parents with all the consequences that brings.

The additional challenges that being the parent of a disabled child can bring means that parenting can be more than usually stressful. Precisely what people find stressful and how well they cope varies enormously. Our experience of stress is, in part, a function of the appraisals we make about our circumstances and what is happening, but it is also a function of the choices available to us (see Lazarus and Folkman, 1984). Even the appraisals we make and the coping strategies we deploy, while in large measure a consequence of our learning histories, are also a function of material, physical and social factors. Having friends, being able to buy help, and having access to good housing and transport can make a huge difference to one's experience of stress. The reality is that the choices available to disabled children and their families are far fewer than those available to others, and the hurdles are considerably greater.

Feeling in control can make an enormous difference to people's ability to cope (Bandura, 1969). Parents value professionals who can go beyond the rhetoric of working in partnership and work in ways that help parents make informed choices and achieve what they want for their children, drawing on their expertise and knowledge of their child and their family (Russell, 1991; Appleton *et al.*, 1997). Unfortunately, study after study has shown that the picture of provision for disabled children and their families continues to be one of fragmented services, poorly organized and difficult to find out about, even more difficult to access, and generally providing too little and too late (Audit Commission, 1994, 2003; Beresford, 1995; SCOPE, 2003). Parents have often to fight tooth and nail for basic help and have often to exaggerate the extent of their problems and inability to cope in order to meet eligibility criteria. They frequently experience professionals as being negative and unhelpful (see Scope, 1996; Baxter *et al.*, 1990). Often they bring to their inter-actions with parents attitudes based on a view of disability as an individual tragedy. Professionals who hold such negative views about disability are unlikely to convey to parents a sense of their child's worth or of being there to help. It is little wonder that parents' experience of services is that, rather than enhancing their sense of control over what is happening, they find it is eroded (Beresford, 1995).

Like other children, disabled children's quality of life reflects, to a large extent, the quality of care they receive (both from their parents and in other key settings) and the opportunities they have to participate, to make friends and to achieve. The social model of disability focuses attention on the ways in which social, material and environmental factors can impact upon the well-being of children and their families. It highlights the important role that social workers could play in helping them increase their options and gain more control over their lives.

In the UK, these aspects are increasingly reflected in legislation, policy and guid-ance that emphasize the rights of disabled children to live as ordinary a life as possible (e.g. DfeS ECM; CA, 2004; DH Quality Protects and Assessment Framework). This is coupled with an emphasis on what is called an outcomes-based approach, namely approaching the business of assessment, planning, monitoring and evaluation, and the process of working, in terms of the outcomes desired by people who use our services, rather than a focus on the service inputs. There is increasing emphasis on 'bespoke' arrangements, often achieved by providing families and older children or adults with money to organize services in the ways that best suit them. These have the added benefit of placing parents or children in the 'driving seat' with professionals in a supporting role (DoH 2000 Guidance, and see below).

Listening to disabled children

Since the ratification of the UN Convention on the Rights of the Child (Article 12, UNCRC, 1989), little progress has been made (talk is cheap) in developing an approach to services for disabled children that realizes their right to express their views about things that affect them (see Cavet and Sloper, 2004). This is particularly true in relation to children with intellectual impairments or communication difficulties (see Morris, 2003). Too often, these factors are cited as reasons for not engaging directly with children. Sometimes the possibility is not even considered:

> In some instances, disabled children may not be heard because it is assumed they have nothing to say.
>
> (Russell, 1998: 23)

Social workers working with disabled children may need to be tenacious in ensur-ing that children are involved in decisions and plans about their lives. As Read *et al.* (2006) observe, this is important because as well as providing information for people to act on, the 'process of being heard in your own right accords value to the things that you think and feel' and 'can make a vital contribution to growing maturity' (p. 139).

Social workers working with children who do not use speech for communication will need to develop other communication skills. This might be in the form of British Sign Language (the main form of sign language for deaf, deafened or hard-of-hearing people people: www.british-sign.co.uk), Makaton (speech combined with signs (gestures) and/or a symbol picture: www.makaton.org), or Bliss (meaning-based symbols: www.blissymbols.co.uk). In some circumstances, it might involve working closely with those who have specialist skills or those who know a child sufficiently well to be able to interpret their body language or facial expressions, or other means of communicating such as the use of pointing (with the head or eyes). The challenge is to *find a way* of communicating (see Rabiee *et al.*, 2005)

What families want

Families are clear about what they want and what they value. In this section we review some of the things that families have repeatedly said are important to them. It is a major indictment of services that these 'ingredients' of effective service provision have been known for so long, but are still not routinely in place (Audit Commission, 2003; CSCI, 2005).

Information about impairment

The difficulty of accessing good-quality information in a form that is accessible is a persistent problem throughout social care, but nowhere is it more acute than for parents with disabled children. Parents want as much information as possible about their child's condition and what it means for their son or daughter and for themselves. They also need time to absorb it and review second and third thoughts. This means that social workers and other professionals need to think carefully about how they provide information. Face-to-face meetings are essential but few people can retain a mass of detail, particularly in times of stress. People therefore need further opportunities to talk about what has happened and think about the implications. Writing things down can take the pressure off parents having to try to remember everything that is said. Published information in the form of leaflets or web addresses can be shared with others in a similar situation and often leads to other sources of support. Then there is the need to provide information in minority languages and the careful use of interpreting services for families whose first language is not English.

Information about services and other resources

A common complaint from parents is that it is hard to find out what services are available and harder still to gain access to them. Public bodies are not adept at making available information about their duties and responsibilities for supporting children in need (CSCI, 2005). Agencies that directly provide services often have limited means to advertise them, and may well be reluctant to stimulate demands they cannot meet. Local and national voluntary organizations are important sources of information, but many families may not be aware of them. The internet is becoming an important means of broadcasting advice on what is available and what people are entitled to, but it is not a panacea. A survey of carers' use of the internet suggests that socio-economic inequalities may impact upon the extent to which the internet can be the key source of information, and indeed as more reliance is placed on the internet as a repository and source of important information then those who do not, or cannot, access it will become further disadvantaged (see Blackburn *et al.*, 2005). Individual social workers therefore have a responsibility to ensure that the families with whom they work are aware of all possible sources of support.

Access to relevant services

Like all parents, those caring for disabled children need some form of support, but unlike other parents they may need additional kinds of support that are not routinely available or not needed by most parents. They may also need support for longer periods of time. There is a clear expectation in UK law that disabled children are, by definition, children in need. They and their families are therefore entitled to a careful assessment of their needs. The practice guidance on the scope of that assessment (DoH, 2000a, 2000b) seems ideally placed to address the social and environmental barriers identified within the social model of disability, covering as it does:

1   *A child's developmental needs.* In this domain, the assessment is geared towards reviewing the child's health, education, emotional and behavioural development; the development of their identity; family and social relationships, and their social and self-care skills. Research with disabled children and their families highlights particular issues of importance. First, parents are concerned that children receive the kinds of services that can help them to reach their developmental potential (see Read, 1996; Hall *et al.*, 1997). This should not be confused with 'curing' impairment. Enabling children to communicate, however profound their disability, is a priority in this regard (see Russell, 1998). There is a growing literature on how this can be achieved, but the basic moral starting point is that it is essential that children should be enabled to express their views and wishes about their lives, their preferences and their experiences of services (see Beecher, 1998; Morris, 1988). Second, in families where there are other children, the assessment should address their needs too, as well as those of the parents. Particularly as they grow older, the needs of disabled children may be at odds with those of their non-disabled siblings; parents may need additional support to cater for the needs of all their children. Siblings *may* need support in their own right, to do things they might otherwise not be able to do. The assessment should therefore explore the impediments to parents' ability to balance such competing needs. These may be financial or reflect limited social resources, an inadequate level of support services or ill-health. They may reflect an absence of a safe physical environment in which to play.

2   *Parenting capacity.* This covers basic care, safety, stimulation, guidance and boundaries and stability. 'Capacity' generally refers to individual abilities to provide these things for children, but in assessing families with disabled children social workers need to focus on the additional demands this places on parents and what could be done to address these demands. The parents of disabled children have often to provide considerable help with personal care, well after the time that most children acquire self-care skills. Care may need to be provided

24 hours a day, and may become more physically demanding as children get older – and bigger. Many children present complex communication, social and behavioural challenges that parents have also to manage. Sleep problems are commonplace. Enabling children to participate in leisure and play activities, and even doing ordinary things such as shopping or keeping clinic appointments, can require substantial logistical planning. Finally, researchers have also high-lighted the risks of ill-health and stress to parents and other carers that come in the wake of coping for long periods, sadly with minimal support (see Beresford, 1995; Russell, 1998).

3   *Family and environmental factors.* Family functioning, housing, employment, income, social integration and available community resources are all areas in which disabled children and their families may be seriously disadvantaged. Social workers can and should ensure that families are getting all the financial support to which they are entitled, that they have access to any equipment they need and can take advantage of community resources such as play groups and other activities which non-disabled children might access. Above all, assessments need to be family driven, reflecting their priorities and desired outcomes. They should focus on reinforcing and enhancing the strengths within a family and helping them to live the lives they want, in the ways they want and that work for them. Not all people react to the same experiences or circumstances in the same way.

The assessment framework emphasizes the importance of involving children in the assessment, and indeed regards this as essential (DoH, 2000: par. 3.41). Research also suggests that while social workers may be getting better at involving children in their assessments, disabled children are less likely to have their views heard. This is particularly the case with children who have profound and complex disabilities, or who have communication needs that social workers are unable routinely to address.

In short, a detailed assessment conducted through the lens of exactly what is needed to remove barriers to participation and inclusion, and undertaken in collab-oration with parents and children, is best placed to ensure that disabled children and their families receive the support they need and that will make a real difference to their quality of life.

Children and education

For parents of school-aged children, making decisions about where and how their children should be educated can prove particularly taxing. The responsibility for assessing children's educational needs and making appropriate provision lies with the local education authority (LEA). LEAs vary in the extent to which they make helpful information available, and they also vary in the range of educational options they provide, from separate schooling provision to support in mainstream schools. The choices available to parents will therefore also vary and the legal processes underpinning the decision-making processes can be complex and intimidating (see Wright and Ruebain, 2002; Read *et al.*, 2006). LEAs are however required to provide a designated officer to assist parents and also make provision for independent advice and support, but this quality of provision also varies considerably. It is therefore important for social workers to be familiar with the local policies and procedures, as well as the relevant legislation, in order to help families who may not otherwise be adequately supported, to advocate on their behalf and be aware of independent sources to which parents can turn (e.g. the Advisory Centre for Education (ACE) and the Independent Panel for Special Education Advice (IPSEA)).

Key workers

Disabled children and their families may need services from a range of health care, housing and benefits agencies, education and Social Services, to name but a few. Many of the support services available to them are provided by voluntary or private sector agencies. Effective multi-agency working remains elusive and the exception rather than the rule (Audit Commission, 2003; CSCI, 2005). At an organizational and planning level, effective commissioning requires collaborative working across agencies, organized in ways that can overcome some of the perennial barriers to joint working, such as: separate funding streams; differences in professional cultures; differences in the way organizational performance is assessed and budgets allocated; and competing priorities within and across agencies. In the absence of 'joined-up' approaches at the organizational level, multi-agency working at the individual service level is challenging and relies on the quality of individual working relationships which, though laudable, are precarious (Cameron *et al.*, 2007). In England the creation of Children's Services Departments (covering education and Social Services) and Children's Trusts (incorporating health functions), together with inspection arrangements that look across a range of agencies, may go some way towards improving this but these changes are not UK-wide, and it remains to be seen whether reorganizing organizational boundaries will make much difference.

In such a complex organizational world parents often find it difficult to understand the system, navigate around it, and get the information and support they need, when they need it and in a form they can use. In 1976 the Court Report recommended that services be coordinated through a single point of contact for parents – a 'key worker'.

> **Key working** . . . encompasses individual tailoring of services based on assessment of need, inter-agency collaboration at strategic and practice levels, and a named key worker for the child and the family. Families with disabled children should only have a key worker if they want one.
>
> **A key worker** is both a source of support for disabled children and young people and their families and a link by which other services are accessed and used effectively. Key workers have responsibility for working together with the family and with professional services and for ensuring delivery of an inter-agency care plan for the child and the family.
>
> (Care Coordination Network UK)

There is considerable potential value of such a role for those families who wish to use them (see Beresford, 1995; Tait and Dejnega, 2001) and, some 30 years on, key working is beginning to become more widespread. The precise scope of the key worker role varies across services (see Townsley *et al.*, 2004) but, minimally, key workers are expected to: know what is available, both within their own service and elsewhere; be knowledgeable about the range of needs that families have; be able to access and to coordinate services for them; provide emotional support and advice when necessary, and act as an advocate. It is important that key workers frame their role as an enabling one, working in partnership with disabled children and their families to achieve the outcomes *they* wish. In adult services, some have argued that it is disabled people themselves who are best placed to hold the key worker role, with professional staff acting in a supportive capacity (Oliver and Sapey, 2006).

A handful of research studies suggest that, as well as enhancing rates of satisfaction among parents, key workers can make a substantive difference to the extent to which families' needs are met (see Glendinning, 1986; Sloper and Turner, 1992; Liabo *et al.*, 2001). Sloper *et al.* (2006) examined the characteristics of key worker services to which these better outcomes may be attributable. Their results (which are in keeping with the standards proposed by the Care Coordination Network UK) suggest that good outcomes are associated with the extent to which key workers were seen to have carried out the following aspects of key working, namely:

- providing support
- providing information about services and the child's condition
- giving advice
- identifying and addressing needs of all family members
- speaking on behalf of the family when dealing with services (advocacy)
- coordinating care services
- improving access to services
- providing support in a crisis.

(Sloper *et al.*, 2006)

Levels of unmet parental need appeared to be lower for those families who judged their key workers to have 'appropriate amounts of contact' with them. Sloper *et al.* interpret this as meaning that they had enough time to carry out the role properly. This in turn was associated with regular key worker training, supervision (focused specifically on the key worker role) and peer support. There was very little association between these or other factors and the extent to which children's needs were met. Sloper *et al.* suggest that this is because these lay outside the key worker's control (e.g. limited resources for children, including access to play and leisure facilities and social networks). They conclude that it underlines the need for key worker services to focus explicitly on children as well as on parents, and observe that key workers themselves have indicated that they need more training in communicating and working with disabled children (Greco *et al.*, 2005).

The transition to adulthood

Most young people and their parents associate adulthood with increasing independence, moving on to further education, or to paid employment, and with new living arrangements with friends or with partnership and marriage. These things are linked to financial independence and a greater reliance upon others for emotional support. Making these 'taken-for-granted' markers of adulthood a reality for disabled young people requires careful planning that needs to start early in order for appropriate arrangements to be made and in place. The reality for many young disabled people is that:

- statutory procedures are followed but real planning does not take place (see Felce *et al.*, 1998; Audit Commission, 2003);
- planning takes place without the involvement of the young person and his or her carers (see Morris, 1998; Beattie, 1999);
- arrangements and advice are geared towards existing services rather than what the young person wants for him or herself (O'Brien and Lovett, 1992);
- plans are written up but are not followed through (Radcliffe and Hegarty, 2001; Mansell and Beadle-Brown, 2004).

This particular transition is a critical one for young disabled people, and for those young people who are in placements outside the family home (e.g. foster care, residential special schools, boarding-schools, health settings). Decisions taken at this time can have long-term consequences for their economic, health and social well-being. They can impact upon the extent of their achieved independence and their perceived level of social inclusion.

Children's services cease to have responsibility for young disabled people when they reach 18 years of age. Those in special education provision will be handed over to adult Social Services for their continuing care. Those with a children and families' social worker will probably be passed on to someone in a disability or adult social care team. This is more than just a change of staffing and departments. The shift in legal status and responsibility can result in a loss of services that young people and their families have been accustomed to and on which they depend (e.g. respite care, speech and language therapy, access to leisure facilities).

For those children who have been 'statemented' (whose special educational needs were assessed and identified during childhood) there are statutory provisions designed to ensure that the handover of responsibility from the education authority to Social Services is well managed. Those whose legal status is uncertain may miss out on such arrangements. Either way, this is a risky time:

> All the indications are that unless very positive and proactive steps are taken, certain things may happen by default or design which do not augur well for both the young people concerned and their families.
>
> (Read *et al.*, 2006: 166)

Read and Clements summarize a study of around 1,000 young people in adolescence and young adulthood, half of whom were disabled (see Hirst and Baldwin, 1994). While a number of disabled young people in the study moved into employment and achieved a measure of independence and social integration, between 30 per cent and 40 per cent were more likely to experience difficulties in becoming independent adults when compared with their non-disabled peers. These difficulties included:

- securing employment
- long-term dependence on benefits which left them economically less well-off than young people in general

- more restricted social lives
- inadequate health care provision/coordination
- lack of continuity of therapy or paramedical services after leaving school
- increased risk of low self-worth, particularly among those who had attended special school.

Mainly owing to the impact of (un)employment, the differences that Hirst and Baldwin identified increased as young people grew older. An important finding from their study is that while those with severe and multiple impairments were particularly disadvantaged, this was not a 'group' effect. Rather, it reflected differences in the levels of support offered to these young people and their families, suggesting that the expectations professionals bring to transition planning can have serious consequences in relation to the options presented to these young people. A key role for the social worker is to ensure that transition planning for young disabled people embraces the broadest possible horizons and that no option is automatically excluded simply due to the nature and extent of a young person's impairment. Social workers also have an important role in ensuring that the planning is geared towards the young person's personal aspirations. This means making sure that plans address what is important to disabled people and will maximize their full inclusion in society.

Effective transition planning

The local education authority has a responsibility to arrange for a transitional plan to be produced for every child aged 14 who has been assessed as having special educational needs. This is scheduled to coincide with the first annual review that takes place after the child reaches 14. The LEA is expected to invite the child's parents, relevant members of staff, Social Services, the careers service/Connexions, and anyone else deemed appropriate by them or by the headteacher. Other professionals should be consulted as appropriate. Provision *must* be made to ensure that the young person's views are taken fully into account, either through attendance at the meeting or via representation by someone she or he trusts to represent them (Code of Practice, 1994).

This meeting represents the beginning of a process designed to facilitate a smooth ('less than tough' would be a more honest term) transition to adulthood over the subsequent two to four or five years. It should pay particular attention to ensuring that the young disabled person has the same opportunities as non-disabled young people to pursue further or higher education, find meaningful work, enjoy leisure opportunities and generally make choices for themselves and exercise control over their lives. Many disabled young people need housing support and personal assistance in order to live independently from their parents or within the community. Such options are often few or far between and may need to be developed if they are not available in a given area (CSCI, 2005). It is important not to rule out any options simply on the grounds of a young person's impairment. Those with profound and complex needs, particularly those in residential special schools, are particularly at risk of being placed in residential care 'by default', not least of all because a significant minority have little contact with friends or family, or may be in care (Morris, 1999). Those who choose to continue to live with their families, who require or who opt for some form of residential or group care, may still be supported to exercise choice and independence in respect of social activities, short breaks and so on.

There have been a number of initiatives designed to ensure the appropriateness and effectiveness of transition planning (see Jenkins *et al.*, 1988), individual service plans (Emerson *et al.*, 1987), and case management (see Challis and Davies, 1986). All these approaches aim to ensure that plans reflect the unique circumstances in which individuals find themselves and that services are provided that best meet individual needs. Person-centred planning – designed initially to improve the planning process for people with intellectual disabilities – differs from its predecessors in that it is intended to be more flexible, and is desirable to:

1   Pay attention to aspirations, in contrast to focusing on 'needs' which can all too easily deteriorate into plans based on the limited services readily available – or not.
2   Involve and mobilize a person's information support networks, as well as looking at what support is available or required from agencies. This recognizes the importance of friendships and the role of families and friends in social support.
3   Focus attention on the 'supply side' of the planning process; that is to say the supports that are needed to enable individuals to do what it is they wish to do.

Proponents of the person-centred approach – a key plank of government policy for learning-disabled people (DoH, 2001c) – argue that it is more than just a different method of planning. It is underpinned by a different philosophy – one that seeks to address power imbalances between professionals, disabled people and communities (see Sanderson, 2000). It is also an approach that is now being advocated more broadly than its use with learning-disabled people, and early research suggests that it is a promising one (see Robertson *et al.*, 2005).

Mansell and Beadle-Brown (2004) sound some important notes of caution however, not about person-centred planning per se, but about any policy initiative that is sold as a solution to problems that are more complex, and which may indeed themselves carry risks. Analysing the reasons for the failure of previous initiatives in relation to people with learning disabilities (e.g. individual service plans) they identify the following:

1   Resource constraints that mean care managers do not have the freedom to design individually tailored programmes of support, even though this is a key feature of effective case management (Challis and Davies, 1986).
2   The lack of a legal mandate for individualized service plans in the UK, unlike some other countries. This means that individuals are unable to seek redress when plans are not acted upon. Mansell and Beadle-Brown point out that even where there is a statutory responsibility to establish a plan, as with transition planning for young people with special educational needs, the dearth of resources are used as a rationing mechanism.

They argue that unless the impact of resource constraints within services is addressed, person-centred planning – as it becomes more widely adopted – will be similarly constrained. They also point out that the emphasis on informal care within person-centred planning may make it likely that support that would previously have been funded might come to be seen as the responsibility of a person's circle of support. The strategies they propose that might ensure that services – rather than planning processes – became more person-centred include:

1 Affording person-centred planning legal weight.
2 Separating funding decisions from individual planning and giving individuals a social security entitlement based on assessed status. They suggest this would help professionals focus on the content of the plan, rather than rationing a finite resource.
3 Increasing the use of direct payments and user-controlled trusts/independent living trusts (see below) for people with both severe and moderate learning disabilities.
4 Framing national policies such that the resourcing and achievement of personal goals and plans was expected. They point out that at present person-centred planning is a policy priority but Social Services are not held to account for delivering it.
5 Refocusing government attention from the number of plans produced to their quality.

Again, these options are generally not within the gift of the individual practitioner, but we take the view that it is important that social workers understand the organizational, legal and policy contexts in which they operate. In some circumstances it may provide some leverage (e.g. advocating for someone to receive a direct payment and organizing things so that they can do so effectively). Minimally it should inform an honest and transparent way of dealing with people without the need to collude with organizational excuses.

Disabled adults

> If independence is defined as self-sufficiency then it fits well with the doctrine of individualism. If, however, independence is defined as having control over one's life then the involvement of other people may be vital to achieve that end.
>
> (Swain *et al.*, 2003: 78)

Most people, including professionals, think of independence as the ability to do things for oneself. Those of us who, through impairment, are unable to do certain things for ourselves are seen as 'dependent' – dependent on the state, on 'carers', on professionals. This is the discourse that has shaped service provision for disabled people and the way professionals have thought about their roles. In social work, this is exacerbated by the fact that Social Services are means tested, rather than universal, services. Disabled people's social care requirements have therefore been framed as the need for services constrained by entitlement. As gatekeepers to limited resources, social workers have viewed the world through 'dependency lenses', in relationships that are by definition unequal. As a result, disabled people have often to accept services they would not choose and that do not address their needs as they perceive them. Indeed, such paternalism has resulted in a profile of services that no able-bodied person would accept for themselves or for their able-bodied friends or relatives: segregated schools, 'sheltered' work settings paying pocket-money rather than a real wage, home care and personal care services provided at times to suit the providers and often delivered in ways that undermine people's dignity and self-esteem (CSCI, 2006).

People without impairments, but with purchasing power, often choose to buy help with a variety of life's tasks such as childcare, domestic help and, at least historically, the very rich have also commanded high levels of personal care, but they have rarely been seen as 'dependent' because they have used their resources to buy services tailored to their needs, defined in terms of lifestyle and options rather than personal care and safety. The reality is that we are *all* dependent on others, economically, physically, socially and emotionally. It is the balance and interplay that change over time and in different circumstances. For many, the transition to increased economic and social independence begins during adolescence as we establish our own social networks, obtain employment, and move increasingly away from dependence on our families of origins, sometimes to other, mutually dependent relationships. Such changes bring with them an increasing ability to exercise choice and control over how we live our lives, and it is choice and control that are at the heart of independence, rather than 'doing things for ourselves and by ourselves'.

Some of the peculiar challenges facing disabled people have been discussed above (*Transition to adulthood*), but there are others. The organization of the physical and social world is such that employment is not readily available to many disabled people, and opportunities to establish and maintain social networks and therefore to establish long-term relationships are often limited. Children leaving residential schools often leave behind their friends and their social lives; many are faced either with institutional care or a rather isolated life in their communities of origin. Physical needs may be addressed, but social, economic and emotional aspirations are rarely seen as central. In institutions, disabled people may find themselves at risk of physical abuse. In the community they are at risk of social neglect. In reframing the nature of disability as one of disabling barriers within the physical and social environment, the social model of disability challenges social workers and organizations to think about services and support in terms of their ability to enable disabled people to participate in society as citizens rather than as dependants.

Social work and disabled people – the reality gap

Disability activists and researchers have laid down a gauntlet for social work. Put simply it is 'be relevant or be gone'. It challenges social workers to reflect on their role in relation to both disabled people and the state and calls the bluff in much of the rhetoric behind 'empowerment' and 'working in partnership' – in other words, asking professionals to 'walk the walk', rather than just 'talking the talk'. Bridging the gap requires changes in social work education and social policy as well as in social work practices.

Promoting the human rights of disabled people as citizens and facilitating their social inclusion should be at the heart of social work. That this has not been so is evident from the many critiques that have been made of key policy developments impacting upon the role of social workers. Oliver and Sapey point out that the policies of the New Right emphasized individualism and a residual role for the Welfare State.

New Labour, while talking the talk of social inclusion, has generally crafted its policies in ways that target individuals rather than the social systems that exclude them (Oliver and Sapey, 2006).

Education tends to reflect the predominant social and policy contexts. Social work education has still to take on board the implications of the social model of disability for the way it organizes its curricula and to take as its starting point the need for social workers to challenge existing social relationships. In contrast to some (e.g. Froggett and Sapey, 1997), we would argue that competence, knowledge, skill and expertise are important and that to lay the blame for the lack of change within social work education at the 'competency door' is inappropriate (cf. Froggett and Sapey, 1997). It is none the less the case that what an emphasis on competency translates into will depend on its philosophical underpinnings:

> The problems of disabled people, or social workers, are not resolved by the incorporation of empowerment as an instrumental competence within the curriculum.
>
> (Oliver and Sapey, 2006: 175)

Quite so. Adding 'advocacy', 'empowerment' or 'working in partnership' to the competency list will not bring about change unless students understand how people are disabled by their physical, social and economic environments. To achieve this, social work courses need to provide a sound grounding in what the social model of disability means, alongside disability equality training.

Auditing the curriculum in the light of the core tenets of the social model would do much to shed a spotlight on the wider role of social work as an agency of social change. Oliver and Sapey note that to date, few degree courses teach disability studies, and there is relatively little take-up of postgraduate courses on disability studies:

> As a consequence, social workers continue to make applications for their clients to enter residential and nursing homes, and managers continue to spend very large proportions of their budgets on such unwanted services, while local authorities continue to argue that they lack the funding for the services people in fact want. If social workers and their managers are to act differently in their professional lives, they need to be educated differently.
>
> (Oliver and Sapey, 2006: 185)

Direct payments – potential for change

Direct payments are available to disabled people, carers, parents of disabled children, and young people aged 16 and 17 years old. In April 2004, partly because councils made it so difficult for people to choose cash in lieu of services, local authorities in England and Wales were required to make direct payments available to anyone eligible for, or already receiving, community care services. People can now choose to have directly provided services or to organize their own personal assistance. At the time of writing, local authorities retain the responsibility for assessing need and eligibility for services, but this is set to change.

The provision of direct payments provides a mechanism for restructuring the relationships between professionals, disabled people and the state. Minimally, they enable disabled people to organize the support they require in ways that are most effective and desirable for them. In itself, this can transform people's lives, offering choice, control and increased flexibility, as illustrated by the following quotes from recipients of direct payments:

> 'Direct payments give me control. I now have a say in what I eat and drink, when I have a bath, what I do and when I do it. I can choose carers that can help me to live my life. I can have continuity instead of a different carer every day.'

> 'I live alone and I wouldn't be able to do this without the direct payments scheme.'

> 'Direct payments have been brilliant. The children have been able to live a normal life and my husband has not had to give up his job.'

> 'Direct payments are great, they're fantastic. It's everything that goes with them that is the drawback.'
>
> (CSCI, 2005)

The last quotation highlights one of the reasons why the take-up of direct payments has been slower than anticipated. The 2005 Report by the Commission for Social Care Inspection identified a range of impediments to the take-up of direct payments:

- lack of clear information;
- low staff awareness of direct payments and what they are designed to achieve;
- restrictive or patronizing attitudes about the capabilities of people who might use a direct payment and a reluctance to devolve power away from professionals to the people who use the service;
- inadequate or patchy advocacy and support services for people applying for and using direct payments;
- inconsistencies between the intention of the legislation and local practice;
- unnecessary, over-bureaucratic paperwork;
- problems in recruiting, employing, retaining and developing personal assistants and ensuring quality.

In addition, Glasby and Littlechild (2002) also point to other issues such as council concerns with containing expenditure and social workers' concerns about the risks they perceive as inherent in independent living (not all of which are imaginary). An Audit Commission report in 2006 found that direct payments were a net cost for each of the ten councils studied, largely due to the costs of supporting users and providing training to staff (Audit Commission, 2006). The concern, voiced by Mansell and Beadle-Brown (2004), is that in order to contain costs the value of direct payments may be reduced as take-up increases. However, some costs may come down and if councils were able to extricate themselves from their large financial commitment to the residential sector then their expenditure might be more easily managed than by deterring people from taking up direct payments. Worry about risk is a reflection of paternalistic attitudes that are themselves often shaped and reinforced by the organizations for which social workers work. The challenge for social workers is to work with disabled people to ensure that risks are appropriately identified, mitigated where possible, and that disabled people are as able as social workers to take whatever risks they deem appropriate.

The future

Social workers stand at the interface between the individual and the state. Those employed by local authorities or health and social care trusts are typically cast as gatekeepers to services. Further, the cumulative effect of changes in policy and education over the past 20 years has been to define social workers as administrators of the Welfare State, rather than advocates for social justice, and we have not always been brave enough to challenge this. Insofar as social work is a product of a broader policy context, there is clearly a limit to what it can achieve without root-and-branch changes to the welfare infrastructure. However, if they are to remain relevant, then social workers need to consider what they can do within these structures to promote change, and what they can do outside of them to lobby for change as citizens themselves. Oliver and Sapey provide a useful prescription:

1   Social workers need to develop an approach to their professional identity that rests not on 'expert knowledge' alone but on their ability to support disabled people to realize their own aspirations by (1) minimizing or removing barriers, and (2) advocating on their behalf for the supports disabled people regard as important. This has implications for training.
2   Social workers need to be staunch advocates for schemes that promote independent living, such as direct payments or individualized budgets (see DoH, 2005). They need to be active in removing the barriers that prevent or deter people from gaining access to such schemes.
3   Where conflicts arise over assessments of need, social workers need to 'adopt a position of "determined advocacy" in relation to supporting the rights of individual disabled people to participate and to define their own needs' (Oliver and Sapey, 2006: 186). Oliver and Sapey note that this does not mean relinquishing professional judgement, but instead helping people to reach informed decisions about how best to proceed.
4   Within a social model of disability, social workers should use their counselling skills to enable individuals to regain control of their lives, and 'to empower themselves through practical, emotional and social means'. This is an important function and skill given the disempowering experiences that many disabled people have at the hands of social workers and other professions.
5   The social model of disability highlights the central role played by the social barriers that create disability. In this context, social work needs to rediscover its community work origins. Social workers need to work alongside disabled people to effect change. Oliver and Sapey point out that in order to be effective, social

work needs to use its influence within the Welfare State and, in order to do this in an informed way it needs to be aligned with collective organizations of disabled people. It may, in Finkelstein's (1994) terms, need to become a profession 'allied to the community', rather than one 'allied to medicine' or (better) to choose both.

15 Social work with older people

They are waiting for me somewhere beyond Eden Rock:
My father, twenty-five, in the same suit
Of Genuine Irish Tweed, his terrier Jack
Still two years old trembling at his feet.

My mother, twenty-three, in a sprigged dress
Drawn at the waist, ribbon in her straw hat,
Has spread the stiff white cloth over the grass.
Her hair, the colour of wheat, takes on the light . . .

They beckon to me from the other bank.
I hear them call, 'see where the stream path is!'
Crossing is not as hard as you might think.

I had not thought that it would be like this.
                              Charles Causley, 1992, vs. 1, 2, 5 and 6,
                                      by kind permission of the author

Before turning to the substantive issues of social work with older people, including what is known about the effectiveness of services designed for them, we examine some of the facts that determine the experience of old age and the demographic trends that drive some aspects of service development.

Perceptions of old age

Cultures vary in their attitudes towards old age. Broadly, in the developing world and in the East, ageing is associated with wisdom and authority; the bargain is that, in adverse circumstances, where children have been nurtured and close family ties have been established, there are moral obligations to reciprocate later. The Chinese proverb 'Sow some young saplings, feed, water and care for them while you are able; then shelter under their boughs when they have grown into strong trees' sums up this older set of family relationships. In the West the sociology is different. The second thing that any stranger wants to know about you after a name is your occupation, and, by implication, your current socio-economic status.

The family unit in Britain (1) is predominantly 'nuclear'; that is, it often has limited 'liability contact' with relatives; (2) revolves around one or two adults working relentlessly to pay increasingly high housing, fuel, living and childcare costs; (3) may include biologically unrelated adults – which sometimes works well and is sometimes more complicated, and (4) tends to value 'independence' above family and community ties. In such a cultural climate older people are often viewed as a spent force, 'dependent', a 'burden' on family and society who 'should quietly stand aside'. Respect is therefore by no means automatic, though condescension often is. We have a fast culture which rates speed over experience; ageist stereotyping in the mass media, and all too often, disrespect in the streets.

Older people needing support are increasingly referred to in political discourse and by journalists in demeaning, and ageist language (see Thompson 2001; Means and Smith, 1998). We speak of 'the burden' of an ageing population and of services being 'swamped' – though many of the current generation of people over 80 fought to secure our democracy; campaigned for the welfare state and the NHS, and had the political will to tolerate high taxes at a time of austerity to achieve all this. We describe chronically ill older people who need time to convalesce as 'bed blockers' and, under the Community Care (Delayed Discharges etc.) Act 2003 (DoH, 2003), effectively fine Social Services departments if they do not conjure up safe(ish) landings elsewhere at short notice – though this often results in them ending up on a different target list later.

An experiment by the psychologist Pat Moore (1990) provides an insight into what it is like to be an older person going about their daily business. She (a young woman) wore a grey wig, old-fashioned clothes; ageing make-up; cloudy contact lenses; bound her joints and fingers to simulate arthritis; impaired her hearing using ear plugs, and then walked around 100 American cities just doing everyday things and trying to be as much like her real self as possible (see Plate 15.1). Here is a summary of her experience:

> This 'old lady' struggled to survive in a world designed for the young, strong and agile. She couldn't open jars, hold pens, read labels, or climb up bus steps. The world of speed, noise and shadows frightened her. When she needed

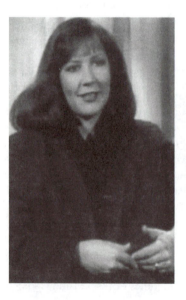 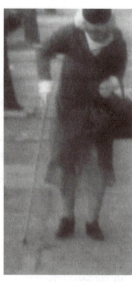

Plate 15.1
Pat Moore (left); on the right she is disguised as an elderly woman

Source: *Discovering Psychology* (1990), Program 18.

Courtesy of HarperCollins

assistance, few ever offered it. She was often ridiculed for being old, slow and vulnerable and was even violently attacked by a gang of adolescents.

(Moore, 1990: 18)

Perceptions shape people's realities. This study shows how older people can come to feel surplus to requirements; are invisible to the busy employed, and a source of frustration to people who think they need something *right now*. There was also evidence of the stereotypical association between apparent physical infirmity and mental infirmity (ask any deaf or physically disabled person).

The question of quickness versus intellectual slowness has been investigated by psychologists using the Weschler Adult Intelligence Test, a measure of abstract problem-solving abilities. Age comparisons show that intellectual ability appears to decline between 20 and 80 years if the usual time-limited version of the test is used. However, if older respondents are given as much time as they need to finish the test (which is typically not *that* much more time) then the decline in performance in older age groups is minimal. Many of us have this experience as we get older; watching the *University Challenge* quiz and feeling that we *just know* many of the answers and much else besides but fail to beat the *speed* of the undergraduates (see Rabbitt, 2005).

Ageism is not the only form of injustice that impacts on older people. In old age people continue to experience those forms of oppression they have experienced in earlier years, *plus* ageism. It is only relatively recently that Social Services have sought routinely to establish culturally relevant services for minority ethnic groups. These have often been underrepresented in preventive services, and in the 1970s and 1980s the fact that only very few members of minority ethnic groups signed up for day care centres or requested assistance at home was attributed to the 'fact' that they (admirably) 'looked after their own'. The idea that these services were not sought because they were not appropriate to the needs of these fellow citizens dawned upon managers only later, when these communities responded to the absence of relevant services by setting up their own. Similarly, the largely automatic assumption that older people are asexual or, if not asexual, then heterosexual, can lead to adverse consequences for those gay and lesbian older people who need social care services (see Bayliss, 2000; Langley, 2001). Ageism and other forms of prejudice impact not only on older people, but also on professionals and care workers; it impacts on the development and delivery of services.

Before moving on it is worth pausing to think about a concept that underpins services to older people, namely 'caring'. A commonplace term, it is easy to assume that we know what it means (we probably do, though we may all think of it in slightly different ways) and that it is straightforward. Feminists would not agree – caring is itself a highly contested concept, and one that influences the way we think about social care and about carers themselves. Some have argued that it is at odds with notions of human rights, advocating its replacement by the term 'help' which has connotations of friendship rather than dependency (Shakespeare, 2000). Others have proposed reconceptualizing care as something that is fundamental to all our experience, rather than something only relevant to the frail (Williams, 2001). Lloyd (2006) points out that while some acknowledge our inherent, mutual dependency, the latter is not viewed at all positively in the West where it is associated with loss and worries about becoming a burden. She points out that the meaning of concepts like dependency and choice depend on one's social position. For the wealthy, a decision to enter residential care may be a genuine choice: they may be used to 'buying help'. Those who are dependent on the state may have no choice, and fewer safeguards. How we think about care inevitably shapes how we approach older people; how we think about assessment and how we think about services (see also Minichiello *et al.*, 2000). How we perceive older people, frailty, and need will influence the nature of our practice: how well we communicate and what we communicate, and the extent to which we ensure that social work is person-centred.

As we shall see, while in recent years there have emerged some very positive trends in the approach of government to older people, the drivers for change often have as much to do with the imperative of containing and reducing the costs of health care services to this group (particularly those of acute health care) as they do with social inclusion, much though the latter is to be applauded (see e.g. Petch, 1993). Before turning to services for older people we first take stock of some key demographic trends.

Ageing and older people

We are all getting older. Britain now has a population of around 60 million, with 16 per cent of people over the age of 65; the United States has a population of around 296 million, with 12 per cent over 65. In the Western world the numbers in this age group are steadily growing because of three sets of factors: (1) the demographic 'bulge' following World War II; (2) better nutrition, improved public health and clinical services, and (3) increased economic prosperity. The downside is that many people are now living to ages where brain disorders which earlier death would have pre-empted are taking their toll. This is why the dementias (see below) are increasingly prevalent, bringing with them high dependency states and increased demand for social care.

Figure 15.1 gives the population trends which some have referred to as 'a demographic time bomb'. By 2026, one in five people in England will be age 65 or over. Of these, some will still be in work; the vast majority will be in quite good health; most will still be active, and many will be making a contribution to their families by caring for children, acting as volunteers, sitting on the boards of community bodies and so on. There *is* a strong relationship between age, dependency and social need at the top end of the age scale, but below this level the picture is more complex. By the same time, the percentage of people aged over 85 will have increased by two-thirds, compared with a 10 per cent growth in the population as a whole.

How many older people will require social care due to frailty or disability is uncertain (Wanless, 2006). Trends between 1981 and 2001 indicate that increases in *total* life expectancy are not mirrored by increases in *healthy* life expectancy (see Mathers, 1999; ONS, 2006). In a review prepared by Jagger *et al.* for the Wanless Review (2006 – see below) the researchers estimated that the number of disability-causing diseases will rise by 57 per cent on the most optimistic of three scenarios used in their predictive model, the 'improving population health' scenario. This assumes (1) a decline in risk factors, particularly smoking and obesity, and (2) a responsive health service with high rates of technology uptake for disease prevention

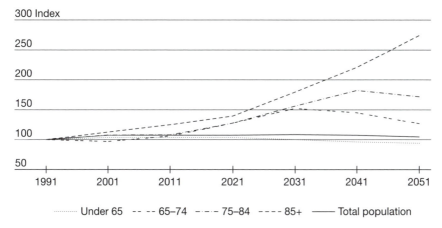

Figure 15.1 Demographic trends and age distributions

Source: Office of Census and Population Studies [OCPS] Royal Commission on Ageing)

(e.g. treatments for hypertension). 'No change' and 'poorer population health' scenarios yielded estimated increases of 67 per cent and 79 per cent respectively.

Wanless and colleagues used the 'improving population health' scenario as its 'base case scenario' when modelling the likely future need for social care in England. Using five dependency classifications based on activities of daily living (being able to wash, dress, feed, toilet, walk and so on) combined with various degrees of cognitive impairment as measures of disability, the Wanless review forecast changes in levels of need between 2002 and 2026. Based on this definition of need, around 900,000 older people were considered to have high levels of need in 2002. By 2026 they forecast:

- a 44 per cent increase in those who do not require care;
- a 53 per cent increase in the number of older people with some need;
- a 54 per cent increase in the numbers of people with high levels of need.

Given a dearth of relevant data and the uncertainty around the assumptions being made, prediction will always be an imprecise science. However, it is clear that rates of impairment and dependence are set to grow significantly, increasing the demand for services (Wanless, 2006).

Social care for older people

Despite uncertainties, data from general population trends should, long ago, have allowed us time to anticipate and plan for a predictable expansion in the need for social care services. We did not. Impediments to planning include: (1) the fact that, unlike health care, social care is not a universal service; (2) governments are elected for four to five years, with few incentives to invest in solutions for which political and electoral credit will be long delayed, and (3) at a local level, the fact that social services have many competing demands on their budgets and are currently under immense pressure to 'deliver' against some (rather dubious) targets across a swathe of governmental initiatives.

In England alone, more than one million older people aged 65 and over use publicly funded social care services, and a further large group pay privately for domiciliary and residential care. Most people prefer to stay in their own homes and would like community-based services that enable them to do so (CSCI, 2004). Despite clear preferences to the contrary, residential and nursing home placements currently account for half of the total net expenditure on social care for older people (2004/2005). Of course this reflects the cost of residential care, but it also reflects the slow development of community care (Department of Health Act, 1999). The percentage of over 65s receiving formal home care in England remains considerably lower than many other countries, although allowances need to be made for differing definitions of home care (see Gibson *et al.*, 2003). Further, there is evidence that, as a consequence of targeting those in most need, there has been a significant reduction in the number of people receiving home-based support: only 354,500 households received home care in 2005, compared with 528,500 in 1992 (CSCI, 2006). There is evidence that this means missed opportunities to prevent crises and more generally to promote the well-being of older people.

The 'baby boomers' – about to hit old age around 2015 – are likely to be more demanding than their predecessors (see Huber and Skidmore, 2003). Such a change of attitudes is symptomatic of a wider shift in expectations of services that is indicative of increased emphasis on human rights. It is also reflected in the government's intention to reform public services. In the Green Paper on adult social care, published in March 2005, the government set out its vision for the future of adult social care in England. This includes making services more personalized and offering 'true choice, excellence and quality'. Perhaps because many in the Labour government are themselves 'baby boomers', the document – unusually – talks about social care as being something to do with everyone:

> Social services and social care for adults touch all our lives at some point or another and, because of that, they are not about 'other' people. They are about families and friends, neighbours and communities, in the towns and in the countryside in every corner of England.
>
> (Department of Health, 2005: 5)

The government has set a target to increase the proportion of those supported intensively to live at home to 34 per cent of all those being supported at home or in residential care (Department of Health, 2005). This is not simply designed to shift the balance of care between residential and home care services, but to improve outcomes in seven domains of well-being for older people:

- improved health;
- improved quality of life;
- making a positive contribution;
- exercise of choice and control;
- freedom from discrimination or harassment;
- economic well-being;
- personal dignity.

Central to the ensuing White Paper was a focus on 'fitting services around people not people around services' (Department of Health, 2006). This will require not only a change in the balance and mix of social care services, but also their content and quality.

Care management

> Social workers can be care managers, but care managers can't be social workers.

This was the mantra of one director of Social Services who introduced care management ahead of the implementation of the Act that provided a statutory basis for this role (the NHS Community Care Act, 1990). It aptly summarizes the dilemmas that face social workers currently working in the field of community care for older people, to which we return later.

The Act followed on from the White Paper *Caring for People* (Department of Health, 1999b), which itself built on the review of community care policy undertaken by Sir Roy Griffiths (Griffiths, 1998). Griffiths was charged to review 'the way in which public funds are used to support community care policy' and to recommend how resources could be used more effectively. The Thatcher government was keen that perverse and costly incentives towards residential care should be removed. The rapid growth in (and expenditure on) private and independent sector residential care since 1983 resulted from the fact that those entering these care homes could do so with their care fees paid through the social security system. This provided little incentive to local authorities to assume the costs associated with community care, which came from their limited budgets, albeit residential care might not be most people's preferred option.

Following Griffith's recommendations, the NHS and Community Care Act 1990 gave local authorities the lead responsibility for assessing and planning for community care needs, in cooperation with health service partners. The role of local authorities was to be the commissioner rather than the provider of services. Care managers (who might or might not be social workers) would assess needs and arrange packages of care. The emphasis was on the mustering of practical services to enable people to live independently in the community. As the earlier quote indicates, there was little room for addressing ('managing') people's emotional and psychological needs. Since 1990, there has been considerable growth in private and independent agency provision of community care services, as well as residential care, with a concomitant shrinkage in services provided by the local authority (CSCI, 2006).

Community care, as defined in the White Paper *Caring for People*, was designed to provide services that:

- respond flexibly and sensitively to the needs of individuals and their carers;
- provide a range of options;
- concentrate most help on those with greatest need;
- intervene no more than necessary to foster independence (Department of Health, 1989).

As indicated earlier, the resourcing of community care was not addressed and remains so. Although social care funding has increased, it has arguably not kept pace with need (however tightly defined) or with demand. As a result, eligibility thresholds for services have risen, and – for any one individual – the quantity and range of services available are often severely limited.

Social work with older people

Pressures on budgets and strict eligibility criteria now leave social workers (where they are employed as care managers) with limited scope for manoeuvre, and with potential conflicts between organizational policies and procedures and their professional values. They are likely to result in a focus on formulaic assessments of risk rather than empowerment, important but contentious (Macdonald and Macdonald, 1999b; Jordan, 2004). Deadlines for assessments exert pressure to 'speed up' contacts with older people, rather than slowing them down and providing the space and permission to say what they want. As Lloyd observes, social work encounters with older people often take place at times when older people's capacity to engage in decision-making is seriously compromised by significant life events, such as bereavement, illness, impairment or moving house (Lloyd, 2006). In such circumstances people need time to reach considered decisions. It is difficult to talk through very personal issues with someone with whom a prior relationship has not existed. In costing 'time', the process of care management is not facilitative of the establishment of relationships, traditionally seen as a hallmark of social work practice, and shown by research to make a difference to the effectiveness of community care arrangements (Challis *et al.*, 1990; Marshall and Tibbs, 2006). In all, such circumstances do not make the exercise of choice or empowerment easy, and the 'Restrictions on resources and eligibility, together with charging policies, have a counter productive effect on aims to promote sensitive and individually tailored services' (Lloyd, 2006: 1178).

Surveys continue to highlight the fact that, while appreciative of home care, for example, older people do not like the 'pressure' associated with a service that is too often poorly timed (carers coming when it suits their timetable rather than when it suits the older person), unreliable and 'peremptory' (CSCI, 2006). Older people feel 'rushed' as a consequence, often because domiciliary care agencies are short-staffed, and commissioning arrangements are such that only the bare minimum is commissioned, with impossible times attached to tasks:

> 'The carers are very good but the managers change the times that the carers are due to call without telling us.'

> 'the main problem was always that they didn't have time to get from one person to the next, so 30 minutes became 20.'
>
> (CSCI, 2006: 42)

Research confirms that the needs of human beings are complex, encompassing emotional and psychological and not just *practical* needs as so often defined within the terms of community care provision (see Nocon and Baldwin, 1998; Johnson, 2005). Even in relation to practical help, older people do not always want what the local authority has commissioned:

'They [volunteers] do all the things that paid carers can't or won't do . . . The big difference is that the carers come and do what someone else has decided I need, and the volunteers come and ask me what I want.'

(CSCI, 2006: 37)

Mass, automated, basic provision to sustain life-and-limb – though better than nothing – can deny older people a sense of valued identity. In arranging care packages, social workers (and councils with Social Services responsibilities) need to ensure that community care services are person-centred, that cultural factors are at the core of the process, and that people who use them have a sense of control over their circumstances and what is done on their behalf. The importance of this is not just an ethical one, but is associated with good outcomes (see Seligman, 1975; Tanner, 1998; Lee *et al.*, 2002). Achieving this is no mean feat, but it can be done. The CSCI report on home care cites a range of examples of innovative practice, including person-centred commissioning, effective interprofessional working, and culturally sensitive practice and initiatives to improve the competence of social care staff (see also Patmore, 2002). Finally, one of the areas that social workers need to know something about in order to make good-quality assessments and provide sensitive services is the psychology of ageing (see Biggs, 1993; Coleman, 1993).

Health and social care

Health and social care needs are inextricably intertwined. Politicians and managers – who once chose to separate them – are now trying to find reverse gear (see below). In the case study below, as in others, there is a clear degree of untreated depression – from anhedonia to more serious clinical conditions. Research testifies to the ability of simple health procedures to produce large benefits (e.g. sorting out spectacles, ear and hearing aid problems; ensuring dentures fit – because if they don't it makes eating difficult; chiropody services which help maintain mobility; advocating reviews of the 'cocktails' of medication which may be adversely interacting since they have been prescribed over the years by different GPs). Confusional states in older people, for example, are often as much to do with malnutrition, self-neglect and misprescribing as early dementia. Our needs do not come packaged as 'social care' needs or 'health' needs, and the way we have organized services makes little sense (and is of even less interest) to those people who need them.

A key obstacle to coordination has been 'professional anthropology', that is, 'tribal' identity and a sense of different expertise under threat from interlopers (see Dalley, 1989). There is ample evidence of the positive effects of a less defensive pooling of skills (see Challis *et al.*, 1998; Henwood, 2000; CSCI, 2006). By way of conveying some flavour of the real personal issues and experiences which underlie and motivate this discussion of coordination, consider the following case study.

Case example

Mrs W and her husband had escaped from Poland just before the German invasion. The rest of her extended family decided to stay in Krakow and ride out the storm. They all perished in a death camp, something about which she felt guilty on grounds of a failure to persuade them to leave and (actually) a lack of any means to get them out. Mr W was an aeronautical technician and was employed at an RAF base in Surrey; he then trained as a sergeant pilot and flew a Hurricane.

Mrs W was a piano teacher and found it hard to get work at first but gradually built up a group of students. After the war she and her husband bought a small house and lived quietly there until her husband died of a stroke and she, for financial reasons, had to move to a small flat. Mrs W then developed a late-onset diabetic condition and also increasingly disabling arthritis, which meant she could no longer play the piano – a cause of great distress to her. This incongruously large instrument dominated her small room, but one quickly gathered that its continued presence was psychologically essential.

The purpose of the research project was to test consumer reactions to a new joint health and social care assessment process. On the whole, Mrs W thought well of these services and, in particular, valued the kindliness of the care assistants and community nurses. However, when asked about what services she received, Mrs W explained that they amounted to one vacuum clean per week, plus dusting; meals on wheels (which she described as 'almost uneatable'); help with washing two days per week, and the occasional health check. When asked to rank the importance of these services, she put help with personal hygiene at the top, cleaning in the middle, and help with shopping and meals at the bottom. When asked (carefully and with explanations) which service she could do without at a pinch, she said, 'help with washing'. The reason for this surprising nomination was that she felt sorry for the young girls who had to do it against an unforgiving time-scale. 'They come in; I don't always know them. They tick the sheet on the wall and then I have to strip in the bathroom. They don't even have time to let me do my own private parts – it's not their fault, but if you understand, I feel very undignified.'

(From Sheldon and Macdonald, 1996)

In the case of Mrs W, three groups of professionals had assessed her needs. Indeed, more work went into the assessment than into subsequent service provision. However, despite considerable investment by the authority in producing an 'integrated' system, most staff concentrated on their own area of expertise and ignored the rest. For example, back-up from her GP helped to stabilize Mrs W's diabetic condition, and she was also prescribed for her arthritis. However, her repeat prescriptions were difficult to obtain due to a very creaky home delivery scheme run by local chemists. Mrs W also received meals on wheels, but found them unpalatable and disguised the fact that she was not eating them. Thus the insulin was going in, but the blood sugar level it was supposed to control was dependent upon her willingness to eat the food supplied. Recent audits (BADEN, 2008) show that one-third of new admissions of older people to hospitals and care homes are suffering from malnutrition: 'starvation in the community'? The professionals involved tended to see this problem as belonging to someone else.

It was the researchers who referred Mrs W to a voluntary association for people of Polish origin who agreed to collect her by car and take her to their centre where she could eat the kind of food she liked and talk to people with whom she had something in common.

Promoting partnership working

As well as stating its intention to put people who use services at the 'centre of service provision', the 'New Labour' government committed itself to removing 'the Berlin wall' that existed between health and Social Services (Department of Health, 1998). This is part of a long line of initiatives and commitments undertaken since 1948 to encourage inter-agency working and improve inter-professional collaboration. To date, these have comprised exhortations to improve working relationships, to undertake joint planning and joint commissioning, and (voluntarily) to pool budgets. In the face of a complex organizational world in which departments undertake a range of different functions, have different management structures, different funding arrangements, and employ different professional groups, stirring exhortation has proved of limited usefulness:

> The fundamental conflicts between agencies that are financed separately, administered separately, staffed by different professions and run within different statutory frameworks are so great that no joint commissioning or joint planning has much hope of succeeding.
>
> (Lewis and Glennerster, 1996: 185)

New Labour did not see the solution to these problems in the reorganization of services either. It saw reorganization as a distraction and potentially a destabilizing influence. Instead, what was advocated was a 'new spirit of flexible partnership working'. There is evidence to support the effectiveness of integrated approaches in reducing acute hospitalization rates and long-term institutional care, and improving satisfaction and outcomes (see Johri *et al.*, 2003). Making it happen is the challenge.

The Health Act 1999 made provision for joint working by removing legal obstacles that had previously existed. Health and Social Services departments can now (1) pool budgets; (2) make arrangements whereby one agency can take the lead in commissioning services on behalf of both, and (3) merge services (Health Act, 1999: S 31). These so-called 'Health Act Flexibilities', some of which have enabled the innovative practices cited by CSIC (above), remain 'permissive powers' rather than duties. In reviewing the history of partnership working, Wanless observed that the enduring presence of this objective (along with the goals of promoting independence and developing intermediate care):

> is testimony to the difficulties in achieving the significant changes required to deliver the objectives. It also points to the fact that increasingly the difficulties of managing two parallel but separate systems of health and care are being managed by strategies that attempt to integrate their respective agendas as far as possible.
>
> (Wanless, 2006: 17)

Indeed, partnerships have become more extensive and more complex. Other government departments now hold key responsibilities for the welfare of older people (e.g. the Department for Work and Pensions is now the lead department for older people; responsibilities for communities reside with the Department of Communities and Local Government, and responsibility for social care lies with the Department of Health where leadership resides in the new, 2006, post of Director General of Social Care).

The joint health and social care White Paper (DoH, 2006) continued the emphasis on improving partnership working, but introduced some changes in the means to deliver on these aspirations. These include:

1 Outcome measures by which both health and social care will be assessed through inspection and performance assessment.
2 The alignment of budgetary and planning cycles of the NHS and local authorities.
3 Local Area Agreements – which replace multiple national performance frameworks – in which local authorities and partners will identify priorities and establish three-year agreements between all main public sector agencies in the area and with central government.
4 'Local Strategic Partnerships' – which provide the forum for collectively reviewing and allocating public resources in local areas. LSPs are non-statutory bodies (sometimes simply referred to as partnerships) which bring councils together with other local services, including the police, health services, local businesses and the community and voluntary sectors.
5 A single assessment framework.
6 Encouragement of multidisciplinary teams and networks between PCTs and local authorities, and gathering services altogether in one building.

All of these initiatives (and similar developments in other UK countries) are to be welcomed, but good, integrated service provision on a tight budget, within a means-tested system that many see as unfair, will continue to prove elusive. In 2005 Derek Wanless was commissioned by the King's Fund to determine how much should be spent on social care for older people (in England) over the next 20 years and what funding needed to be in place to secure its availability and the provision of high-quality care, focused on securing good outcomes for older people (Wanless, 2006). The review also considered how social care should be funded. In May 2008 the government launched a six-month consultation on the future funding of social care, recognizing that in England the system was heading for a £6 billion funding gap in the absence of radical reform. This follows a Royal Commission on the funding of long-term care which reported in 1999, and which recommended that personal social care should be free (a proposal that was rejected by the government in England, but implemented in Scotland, though the cost of this appears to have led to rationing of the service – see Audit Scotland, 2008). Wanless concluded:

> the potential to achieve economically justifiable outcomes is not currently being realised. Unless society is less inclined to support the same improvement in outcomes from social care as it would from, say, health care, then more should be spent on social care for older people.

However, additional funding should not be forthcoming without a commitment to reconfigure services, demonstrating value-for-money and fairness. This would include an increase in the size of community-based care packages for all those needing care, particularly the middle-dependency group; an improvement in carer support services; and the tailoring of care-with-housing services for those with significant cognitive impairment.

(Wanless, 2006: xxviii)

We return to issues of the scope and targeting of care services below.

Direct payments and individualized budgets

Direct payments (Community Care (Direct Payments) Act, 1996) were made available to older people in 2000. The underpinning philosophy is that direct payments enhance choice and control, and maximize independence – a principal aim of community care policy (see CSCI, 2004). Direct payments cannot be used to purchase services from a local authority, but can be used – by those deemed able to use them – to pay for personal assistance, and care from close relatives and friends who do not live in the same household. Internationally, cash payments are generally used to pay for informal care, including from cohabiting relatives, rather than for the purchase of formal services (see Poole, 2006a).

Older people value the sense of retaining control, to the extent that they may be willing to trade this off against amount of services when the latter are worth more than the cash benefit on offer (see Geraedts *et al.* 2000). Research by Clark *et al.* (2004) indicated that older people receiving direct payments reported themselves as happier, more motivated and enjoying a better quality of life than before.

In 2003 local authorities were mandated to offer direct payments to all people in receipt of community care services, and councils now have their performance monitored in relation to this, but even this move has resulted in only a marginal increase in the numbers of older people opting for direct payments rather than a menu of services organized by the council. Only 7,000 older people in England were using direct payments to purchase their own care by the end of 2004, compared with over 300,000 receiving state-funded home care, 0.03 per cent of expenditure on adult social care (CSCI, 2006). Barriers to the take-up of direct payments by older people include:

- Lack of clear information for people who might take advantage of direct payments.
- Low staff awareness of direct payments and what they are intended to achieve.
- Restrictive or patronizing attitudes about the capabilities of people who might use a direct payment and a reluctance to devolve power away from professionals to the people who use the service (see Hasler *et al.*, 1999; Poole, 2006a).
- Inadequate or patchy advocacy and support services for people applying for and using direct payments.
- Inconsistencies between the intention of the legislation and local practice.
- Unnecessary, over-bureaucratic paperwork.

- Problems in recruiting, employing, retaining and developing the careers of personal assistants. (CSCI, 2004).

The introduction of individual budgets, whereby service users complete a self-assessment and are then allocated a budget which local authorities hold on their behalf, thereby removing many of the hassles associated with direct payments, may encourage more older people to exercise more direct 'purchasing power'. They may also provide a 'correction' to any apparent bias in the take-up of direct payments that favour the more able and middle class (see Leece and Leece, 2006). Unlike direct payments, individual budgets may be used to purchase services from the council. These schemes are being piloted at the time of writing.

It is doubtful, though, whether significant change will occur in the absence of a radical rethink and reorganization of funding for social care. An inquiry into care services in London, conducted by the Kings Fund in 2005, concluded that neither direct payments nor individual budgets would succeed unless there were sufficient services of the right kind which people wanted to buy. The authors noted that older people and their carers were faced with (1) limited access to services, (2) limited choice, and (3) financial hardships attributable to inadequate funding and lack of clarity about which service was financially responsible for what (and disputes between them). These problems are not confined to London, and without serious development of the 'care market' (itself a demeaning phrase) older people will not be able easily to secure the right kinds of services of the right quality (Robinson and Banks, 2005).

What works for older people?

Much of our discussion so far has been about the organizational context of services for older people and a range of factors that can influence them, including funding, inter-professional working, and professional attitudes and perceptions. These are important as they impact directly on older people, their carers and families and on those paid to provide services, including social workers. In this next section we look specifically at what is known about the effectiveness of services designed to help older people remain in their own homes, to return to their own homes following admission to hospital and – if necessary – to make a satisfactory transition to residential care. Rarely are social workers directly involved in working with older people, except at the stages of assessment, monitoring and review – and all too often monitoring and review fall off the agenda of social workers, despite the fact that this is a statutory responsibility (see CSCI, 2005). None the less, as case managers, social workers need to know what the evidence base is about the various services they might seek to provide, including what older people say about their value and what works in relation to the *delivery* of services.

Supporting people in their homes

Recent years have seen a resurgence of interest in prevention and early intervention. In relation to older people, a major priority is preventing the need for institutional care, whether in terms of helping people to maintain their independence, supporting those informal carers on whom some older people depend, or both. This reflects what older people want and coincides fortuitously with a fiscal need to minimize the use of more expensive services, such as acute hospital care. Prevention has always been a rather elastic concept, and has become more so in recent years where it has come to be used in relation to the prevention of social exclusion and the promotion of quality of life (ODPM, 2006). The continuum of preventive services is therefore long. They range from one-off home adaptations (such as grab rails on a bath, or a ramp), to very intensive home care or intermediate care. This, together with the variation in outcomes which these services are designed to achieve, complicates the evaluation of their effectiveness. We look first at low-level services.

Low-intensity services

Qualitative studies provide strong evidence that older people and carers view low-intensity services as an important factor in maintaining independence, improving quality of life and preventing (or delaying) admission to residential care (Clark *et al.*, 1998). These services typically encompass one or more of home care, day care and meals services. Following the NHS and Community Care Act 1990 it was this group that was sacrificed in order to focus services on those in greatest need, and who were at serious risk of institutional care (see Godfrey, 1999). In 1999, the Audit Commission concluded that prevention and rehabilitation could break the cycle of unplanned admissions of older people to hospital and, all too often thereafter, to long-term residential care (see also Audit Commission, 2004b). There has been no rigorous evaluation of the impact of low-intensity services (such as weekly shopping, gardening, cleaning) or, more importantly, of its ability to prevent or slow down factors that might result in the need for more intensive levels of services, hospitalization or admission to residential care. Certainly there have been no evaluations of the cost-effectiveness of such services. But Clarke *et al.*'s study (1998) and later work by the Joseph Rowntree Foundation illustrate a range of innovative ways in which councils and communities could make available low-level services that would make a significant difference to the quality of older people's lives and support their independence, and which may prove cost-effective:

> Older people are often seen as a problem to be solved. Many of the ideas from the Inquiry have come from, and are run by, older people. There is a need to engage locally with volunteers and like-minded organizations to tap the potential of local communities and community-development approaches.
>
> (Joseph Rowntree Foundation, 2005: 9)

In 2006 the Department of Health established 29 *Partnerships for Older People Projects* (POPPs) (Department of Health, 2007a) which are well placed to build on these experiences. These local authority-led partnerships were funded to deliver and evaluate local innovative schemes for older people. They were designed to help realize the government's intention to shift resources away from institutional and hospital-based crisis care and towards community-based interventions. The partnerships include health, voluntary, community and independent organizations, and range from low-level to high-level provision. The evaluation team reports that compared with non-POPP sites, POPP pilot sites appear to have a significant effect on hospital emergency bed-day use (the primary outcome indicator) and the results 'show reductions against trend that would produce a financially neutral outcome: for every £1 spent on POPP, £1 will be saved on hospital bed-days (DoH, 2007a). But, notably, in terms of process, the pilot sites report (1) improved multi-agency working; (2) development of shared procedures and protocols for cross-boundary services; (3) improved access for excluded groups through proactive case finding, greater publicity and links with the voluntary sector, and (4) a rebranding of services away from 'welfare' to health and well-being – an important factor for a group for whom the former can carry a certain stigma.

High-intensity services

High-intensity services have been the major focus of service development since the implementation of the NHS and Community Care Act, 1990. In this area there is more evidence about the impact of such packages of care (and care management itself) but mixed evidence of their cost-effectiveness. Our initial account draws on work by Godfrey and colleagues (Godfrey, 1999; Godfrey *et al.*, 2000a), which includes feedback from people who use home care services, and their carers. The authors point out that the focus on the prevention of institutional care is not always an appropriate outcome measure, as it does not always equate with high dependency needs. Other factors influence the admission of older people to care, including the relationship between the older person and those caring for them; the motivation and coping strategies or resilience of both, and external pressures (Godfrey *et al.*, 2000a). She also points out that most of the available evidence pre-dates policy changes in community care.

We concentrate here on the findings in relation to case-managed programmes of home care, aimed at maintaining frail older people who, owing to extreme difficulties in coping at home, were at risk of admission to residential or nursing care. The evidence comprises data from four randomized or quasi-experimental trials of case-managed programmes of care, three of which were undertaken in the UK by Challis and his colleagues (1986, 1989, 1990, 1991). The fourth was a programme in the United States (Brill and Horowitz, 1983). In the first two UK studies (East Kent and Gateshead Stage 1), case managers were provided with a budget valued at around two-thirds the cost of a residential home placement, which they could spend in ways not constrained by normal services (e.g. paying neighbours or friends to be helpers, providing care in the evenings and weekends). They could spend more with managerial approval. In the third project (Gateshead Stage 2) helpers were provided with training and support in relation to addressing health care needs. The fourth was designed to facilitate discharge of long-stay older patients from hospital. The main findings were:

1   Older people receiving case management in UK projects were less likely to be admitted to long-stay nursing homes, though it is possible that rates of institutionalization may have been delayed rather than prevented. After three years, between-group differences in the Kent scheme all but disappeared.
2   There was no evidence of improvement in physical functioning in the Kent study, and no evidence of a beneficial effect on survival rates.

3 There were significant positive effects of the subjective well-being of participants. People in the experimental groups reported better life satisfaction, a decline in depression, improved outcomes in relation to loneliness and morale, and improved perception about their capacity to cope with daily living.
4 There was a reduction in unmet needs across physical and mental health domain, types of services received, and the perception of the reliability, adequacy and effectiveness of care received.
5 These positive outcomes relating to subjective well-being (3) and unmet needs (4) were achieved without significant additional costs being incurred.
6 The UK demonstration projects seemed to benefit carers, though the sample sizes were small.

Since the publication of Godfrey's review, Davies and Fernandez have reported on a project, Evaluating Community Care for Elderly People (ECCEP). Results from this large before-and-after study suggest that changing the balance of services, with more emphasis on respite, day care and social work would improve outcomes within current resources (Davies and Fernandez, 2000).

These studies reinforce the need for well-organized, reliable home care, based on comprehensive assessments of need. They also point to a significant discrepancy between the emerging evidence of 'what works' in the 1980s (the Kent study) and the direction taken by policy. The decentralization of budgets and the flexibility it provided, for example, to buy meals from the local pub (which the older person would eat, unlike the meals on wheels), or to pay someone a modest sum for helping someone to bed when *they* wanted to go, rather than when the care assistant could call, was totally disregarded in the implementation of the community care reforms. Instead, case managers were constrained to use block purchased services; flexibility fell foul of 'health and safety' concerns, and generally the relational aspects of care management were lost. Current policy trends appear to be seeking to retrace the evidential steps to something more likely to chime with what older people want.

The projects highlight the importance of clear patterns of communication between service providers and different disciplines so that genuine collaboration occurs rather than a diffusion of responsibilities. They also point to the considerable project management skills needed by case managers in establishing complex, multidisciplinary packages of care: thousands of people requiring different services, but with the public and service users expecting *individual* care. This is a task for social services managers if there ever was one (see Lymbery 2006 – a wake-up call).

At the moment, the care market remains underdeveloped. This limits both availability and choice (see also Forder and Netten, 2000). When things go wrong, older people are often caught in the middle between purchasers (the care manager in the Social Services Department) and providers – who have limited contractual obligations. Further, poor commissioning results in short-termism, with the purchase of 'one-size-fits-all' packages of care that are unresponsive to the changing needs of older people – even if appropriate at the outset. Councils need to find ways to work with providers of services so that they have sufficient stability to be able to develop good-quality, flexible services (see CSCI, 2005).

Intermediate care

The concept of rehabilitation for older people has increasingly been incorporated as a key component of more recent schemes of 'intermediate care'. Intermediate care was promoted by the government as a means by which admission to hospital could be prevented or discharge from hospital facilitated (DoH, 2001b). Recent studies (Petch, 1993) however have raised important questions about the extent to which intermediate care is simply a way of freeing up hospital beds as opposed to being genuinely committed to supporting the independence of older people.

The *National Service Framework for Older People* refers to intermediate care as 'an opportunity to maximise people's physical functioning, build confidence, re-equip them with the skills they need to live safely and independently at home, and plan any on-going support needed' (Department of Health, 2001a). Again, the breadth of the definition makes assessing the effectiveness of what is, in effect, a varied group of interventions very difficult. Core features of intermediate care interventions are integrated health and social care provision which aim to promote independence, prevent admission or readmission to hospital and facilitate discharge. Intermediate care is a time-bound service of varying intensity, though it usually comprises high-intensity provision. We begin this section with a consideration of those services designed to help older people leave hospital at the earliest opportunities and to return to their own homes. These have traditionally been referred to as rehabilitation, though they are now also known as 'step-down' programmes (as opposed to 'step-up' – hospital avoidance). Godrey argues that the point at which people need or access intermediate care is not the defining issue, which is why the terminology has shifted from rehabilitation to intermediate care (Godfrey *et al.*, 2005).

Rehabilitation for older people

Nocon and Baldwin's policy review (1998) identifies a useful approach to thinking about rehabilitation work: 'The primary objective of rehabilitation invites restoration (to the maximum degree possible) either of function (physical or mental) or of role.' The word *restoration* occurs throughout dictionary definitions and research papers on rehabilitation. Although services sometimes have to be put in place following a slow decline in functions, more often they are needed to cope with the aftermath of a crisis, (e.g. the breakup of reliable family care; a stroke; a disabling cardiac condition; bereavement and associated depression; social withdrawal, where one partner has been dependent upon the other for care; a bad fall with both its physical and psychological effects; the increasingly acute effects of chronic diabetes; increasing physical disability). Therefore, rehabilitation work is often a form of post-acute medical and/or personal crisis intervention (or avoidance of the same) requiring a considerable sense of urgency and considerable logistical skills from staff: 'Rehabilitation will usually require a mixture of clinical, therapeutic and social interventions that also address issues relevant to a person's physical and social environment' (Nocon and Baldwin, 1998).

There are, however, best-practice recipes and experiences to report upon wherein multidisciplinary staff have collaborated early in the process of discharge, and meet regularly – reporting back on the progress of services so that lessons can be learned for the next series (see Henwood, 1994; Audit Commission, 2000; Herbert *et al.*,

2000; Evans *et al.*, 1995; Parker *et al.*, 2000; Trappes-Lomax *et al.*, 2002). Government target-setting, intended to strengthen the resolve of staff and managers, can however sometimes result in 'pass-the-parcel' services in rehabilitation.

There is perhaps a danger, given our need for more controlled studies, that we neglect the legacy of client-opinion studies in the research literature, including those featuring testimony as to what it is like to be on the receiving end of rehabilitative services, which for evidence-based practice means incorporating robust *qualitative* data into reviews of service effectiveness (see Trappes-Lomax *et al.*, 2003; SCIE, 2006). Here is a short list of prominent findings, many of which have already been cited in respect of other areas of practice:

1   When older people are sent home prematurely from hospital at short notice, without an opportunity for convalescence, and with a scramble to put basic care services in place, they know it, and are emotionally affected by it. Often they are precipitated into decisions they may later regret and find it difficult to unpick, such as agreement to residential care (see CSCI, 2004, 2005).

2   Outcomes (i.e. satisfaction rates relating to community services, lower readmission rates) are better where a multidisciplinary team provides the range of services required (i.e. nurses providing medical care; occupational therapists supplying home adaptations that might help; speech therapy services for recovering stroke patients; and a social worker/care manager to reconnect and coordinate the contribution of family, carers, friends and neighbours and help to deal with daunting forms).

3   Good assessments are crucial, and not to be side-stepped because of the time pressures often involved (see Chapter 5).

4   Older people value regular home visits that happen as planned, with a group of staff they can get to know well. This is not just a matter of technical efficiency, but of a reassuring familiarity that most older people value and rely upon.

5   Motivation is a key factor in recovery. Physical recovery is one thing, but a state of dependency and fearfulness about the future is quite another. Such factors rarely appear on assessment checklists, but work is needed sympathetically to urge clients towards small, restorative, optimistic steps. Low mood and depression are strongly associated with physical illness and loss of capacity in elderly people and in turn influence recovery in vicious circle fashion. The evidence is that small, carefully selected tasks, accompanied by reassurance and support – not things done *for* people, but *with* them – make a difference.

The reader will see that in this list of findings, we have steadily moved from physical provision to psychological and emotional factors. Key to the success of effective rehabilitation schemes is attention to such less readily visible influences as a sense of growing competency and well-being. The need to look beyond the home to the broader, local context in which people live, to facilitate a sense of connectness and reduce loneliness and isolation may also be important.

Effectiveness of intermediate care/rehabilitation

There are few methodologically robust UK evaluations of intermediate care. An RCT study showed that while intermediate care diverted people from hospital settings, the programme itself 'had no measureable impact upon survival rates, rates of admission to long-term residential or nursing home care or the proportion continuing to live at home' (Fleming *et al.*, 2004, quoted in Lymbery, 2005: 207). A national study on the impact of intermediate care on service systems and the costs of schemes (Barton *et al.*, 2006) found that patient satisfaction was generally high but overall the impact of such schemes on other services was generally limited (i.e. they did not impact significantly on admission rates to hospital or residential care). Importantly, the six-week time limit that usually operated within schemes was regarded as too little and elicited the lowest satisfaction scores from users (see also Manthorpe and Cornes, 2005). There is currently no consensus on whether or not intermediate care is cost-effective – again – because outcomes and measurements vary, as does the length of time over which the impact of the service is considered (Godfrey and Townsend, 2003).

A study by Trappes-Lomax *et al.* (2002), aptly entitled *Buying Time*, illustrates a number of common themes and provides some useful findings from which to learn. This matched comparison study exploited the fact that one of two neighbouring Social Services and community hospital catchment areas had a state-of-the-art multi-disciplinary rehabilitation unit, seen by most commentators as an example to be rolled out nationally. The other provided domiciliary care and brought in specialists as necessary. The researchers expected better outcomes for those who received the specialist programme. The study used a range of standardized outcome measures such as the Cope-ability and Daily Living measures (scales measuring what older people could now do that they couldn't before); measures of psychological reactions to the experience of rehabilitation, and some general pre-post quality-of-life measures. Each was administered at six and twelve months. The authors also gathered individual reactions to the experience and advice on how to improve such schemes. The results of this study of 206 clients, with an average age of 81 years, may be summarized as: *both* groups did well and much better than more limited interventions, but well-organized home care did as well as the residential alternative with reduced costs.

Telecare

Telecare equipment and services are beginning to make their mark in community care (Audit Commission, 2004). They include: information (on health, local services including shopping options); electronic aids and adaptations (automatic doors, stair lifts, aids that support self-medication, intelligent controls for heating and water); devices that monitor safety and security; devices that monitor people's safety and security (e.g. fall alarms or systems that monitor 'abnormal' patterns of behaviour); and devices that monitor personal well-being (such as vital signs monitoring). Given the role that anxiety and a sense of vulnerability can play in someone's perceived inability to cope alone, some of these products have much to offer (see Bowes and McColgan, 2005).

While unlikely ever to be a panacea, and certainly not a substitute for personal care, developments in this field will very likely change the profile of care packages and, at their best, offer considerable potential for maintaining people in their own homes. Many come at modest cost, and government guidance for the Preventive Technology Grant states that when provided after a community care assessment, such aids should be provided free of charge, with means-tested benefits applying to the weekly service charge. Pilot studies indicate that though these are often minimal they none the less deter people, and, for example, uptake of telecare packages in West Lothian increased considerably when this was abolished (Poole 2006). Telecare is likely to be a significant plank in any plans to extend the provision of community care services to those with lower levels of need. This is because (1) this is the group on whom it is likely to have the largest impact, (2) the early signs are that it is potentially very cost-effective, and (3) contrary to stereotype, older people appear generally enthusiastic (Poole, 2006a, 2006b, 2006c).

Carers

The 1995 Carers (Recognition and Services) Act gave carers providing a substantial amount of care an entitlement to an assessment of their needs and ability to care. Over ten years later, carers are often unaware of this entitlement (CSCI, 2008). The 2004 Carers (Equal Opportunities) Act now places a duty on councils to inform carers about their entitlements. The right to have their needs assessed recognizes the extent to which the care of older people is dependent on informal care. In England in 2000 there were between 3.4 and 4 million carers providing care to people aged 65 and over. Many carers are themselves over 65 and the evidence suggests that the availability of informal carers will not keep pace with demand. There have been a range of initiatives to impress upon councils and practitioners the importance of attending to carers' needs, but only recently have resources been made available, via the Carers Specific Grant (Department of Health, 1999). We cannot engage in an extensive discussion of carers' needs in this chapter, but would wish to emphasize the importance of attending to their situation, assessing their needs and not assuming that someone able and willing to care *now* will be *always* able and willing. Their circumstances change, as do those of older people. Here is one area where timely and often very minimal help can make a significant difference. Often carers need not only practical support, but emotional support and support in managing the sometimes serious stresses of caring (see Zarit and Edwards, 1999). Again, this is an important aspect of monitoring and review (see Seddon *et al.* (2007) for a discussion of this and other issues relevant to work with carers). Stress is not confined to one sort of caring and we have not focused on particular conditions or circumstances in this chapter. Older people face the loss of independence due to a wide range of factors. However, those caring for people with cognitive impairments often face particular challenges, and therefore we include a section on the dementias.

The dementias

20/3/83 To see Mum at Weston, it's a beautiful day, and we walk on the sands. 'Has Gordon been to see you?' 'Oh yes,' she says happily, 'though I'm saying he has, I don't know who he is.' She peers at me. 'Who am I?' 'Oh yes, erm, you're my son aren't you?' 'My name?' 'Ah, now then'. She laughs as if this is not information that any reasonable person could expect her to have. But it doesn't distress me because it doesn't distress her. We have our sandwiches on a hill outside Weston with a vast view over Somerset. She wants to say, 'What a good view' but her words are going too. 'Oh,' she exclaims, 'what a big lot of ... about'. There are sheep in the field. 'I know what they are' she says, 'but I don't know what they're called'. Thus Wittgenstein is routed by my mother.

(*Alan Bennett Diaries*, 1980–1990)

Adjusting to physical impairment and the inability to continue to do things for oneself is difficult enough, but many find the challenges of cognitive impairment particularly distressing. Cognitive impairment also has a profound impact on family and friends, and carries particular concerns about risk and safety. In this section, we consider the prevalence of the dementias and what is known about their causes and development. Social workers often lump together various conditions under the general heading of dementia, but there are various sets of (admittedly overlapping) symptoms with different aetiologies, different effects and different prognoses (see DSM IV TR, 2000: 147–180), knowledge of which can help us to adapt our services to their needs. Here are the main features of this group of disorders:

1   Multiple cognitive deficits, memory impairment and, in particular, short-term memory losses. In advanced cases it is quite common for people not to be able to remember what they had for breakfast but to remember the details of their earlier lives. In very severe cases both sets of memories fade. The composer Maurice Ravel (who suffered from Picks Disease – a particularly disabling form of dementia since it attacks the central cortex more strongly than most) used to be taken by friends to concerts of his own music as a restorative measure. He would applaud enthusiastically and then ask who the composer was. This contrast between previous competencies (in his case delicate artistry) and current mental state is particularly disheartening in the early stages of such conditions and should not be backed away from by staff.

2   The primary requirement for a diagnosis of dementia is that it is a recognizable brain disorder with a physical cause. Yet, as we have indicated, diagnoses are often complicated by environmental factors such as self-neglect, poor nutrition or growing sensory impairment (Iliffe, 1997).

3   In more severe cases – which are the ones likely to be represented in social care case loads – very profound lapses of cognitive ability, personal distress, and memory lapses, even regarding the names of close relatives, or of everyday objects, are common. In these troubling conditions, even remembering what one's last sentence was leads to long repetitions of the same idea. This can lead to severe anxiety and sometimes even to aggressive behaviour because, unlike some psychotic conditions, clients retain – in the earlier stages – a background knowledge of fading capabilities, and blame themselves or others for the problems.

4   Depression and agitation are associated with dementia but should not automatically be attributed to the physical condition: an easy option. Often, they are jointly caused or strongly exacerbated by living circumstances and by a sense of loss of control (see Marshall and Tibbs, 2006).

Most dementias occur at the age of 85 and beyond (though exceptionally, similar-looking conditions may be found in younger people, even children who have contracted AIDS or who have suffered severe head injury). Their prevalence doubles for every five years after the age of 65. The prevalence rate is 16 to 25 per cent for those over 85. The disorders are steadily progressive, and presently incurable – though their worst effects can be ameliorated by medical and psychosocial interventions and sympathetic care schemes (see below). Having summarized the effects of dementia in general, we now turn our attention to specific conditions.

Alzheimer's Syndrome

This is the commonest form of dementia, accounting for around 70 per cent of all diagnoses. It is named after Dr Alois Alzheimer (1864–1915) who was a professor of psychology. He collaborated with the neurologist Dr Frank Nissl on a six-volume work on the disorder, identifying both its symptoms and the underlying histology. They noticed from post-mortem samples 'a paucity of cells in the cerebral cortex and clumps of filaments between the nerve cells'. Microscope slide illustrations give the impression of a kind of cerebral 'eczema', which disrupts complex neural connections. However, we have to be careful here, since medications which reduce these *signs* have so far proved ineffectual in restoring mental functioning:

The DSM IV TR criteria for a diagnosis of dementia of the Alzheimer's type are (1) memory impairment (an inability to retain new information or to recall previously learned information); (2) one or more of the following cognitive deteriorations: (a) aphasia (language disturbances), (b) apraxia (impaired inability to carry out motor activities despite intact physical functions), (c) agnosia (failure to recognize or identify objects despite intact sensory functions); (d) disturbance in executive functioning (i.e. planning, organizing, sequencing, abstracting). All the above must present as significant impairments over previous capabilities, and must be differentiable by doctors from other disorders such as delirium, self-neglect, subdural haematoma, Huntingdon's Disease, or brain tumours.

Social care interventions, which look to practical needs, holding understanding dialogues which help keep people's fears at bay in circumstances which are increasingly troubling, are at present the mainstay of palliative care in the middle to final stages of this illness. In such circumstances support for carers is vital (Evers, 2007). Carers not only bear heavy personal costs, but also the psychological burden of witnessing the deterioration of a loved one's personality (Woods, 1997). Research suggests that we carry out our obligations to these beleaguered people only tolerably well, and that small measures of earlier support will often prevent the emergence of crises in care – the very opposite of the current policies of 'targeting' respite care only on the near exhausted (see Godfrey *et al.*, 2000a).

Dementia due to Parkinson's Disease

Dr James Parkinson (1755–1828) was an eighteenth-century physician who studied and gave his name to this condition, bringing his earlier researches together in an 'Essay on the Shaking Palsy' in 1817. Parkinson was also a social reformer, seeing a clear link between illness and social conditions, and was no mean psychologist when discussing the effects of the disease on the individual and the family. Later histological slides showed the intrusion of degenerated tissue between nerve cells ('Lewry bodies') plus overlapping effects with the other dementias.

Most of the early symptoms of this progressive disorder are physical, such as ambulatory difficulties (walking on splayed legs), waxy complexion, intention tremor (shaking hands when trying to grasp something) and micrographia – increasingly tiny handwriting. Later manifestations include a slowing down of cognition. There is also a noteworthy association with depression. Whether this is due to an alteration in brain functions, a reaction to increasing loss of control and diminished functioning in the face of, in the early to middle stages, retained insight, or a mixture of all, is not clear.

Other dementias

These are much rarer but produce even more disturbing symptoms. Table 15.1 summarizes key characteristics.

Table 15.1 Key characteristics of certain dementias

Dementia	Aetiology, symptoms and diagnosis
Huntingdon's Disease	A strongly inherited (50 per cent risk if you carry the genetic defect) progressive condition. Severe tremor and lack of motor control ('St Vitus dance') + severe cognitive impairment and negative personality changes. There is a diagnostic test, which some prefer not to take since they would rather not know.
Creutzfedlt–Jakobs Disease	Rare, but devastating. Typically develops between ages 40 to 65 years. Brain develops 'spongiform' lesions due to the effects of slow-acting, tiny, virus-like prions. The expected epidemic from Bovine Spongiform Encephalopathy (BSE) has, mercifully, not manifested itself, but some cases involving older people are turning up in nursing homes and hospices and they are associated with very distressing symptoms such as chronic fatigue, immune system damage, anxiety, sleeping disorders, rapid memory loss and severe physical incapacity.
Dementia linked to HIV/AIDS	Dementia resulting from HIV infection is designated by a specific test – but the consequences for the patient/client, partners and relatives are roughly the same. Symptoms may be apathy, social disconnection and, of course, a ready vulnerability to infections since this virus parasitizes the immune system. In addition to these problems comes prejudice against sufferers, particularly against gay and lesbian people and those who have used drugs (though this infection is by no means confined to these groups).
Dementia due to other medical conditions	Dementia may be caused by a range of other physiological conditions, notably (1) arteriosclerosis (furring of the arteries, reducing the blood supply to the brain, leading to infarctions – dead tissue); (2) severe or multiple, smaller strokes. In the latter case, the messages from research are clear: specialist physicians, backed up by specialist nurses, physiotherapists, occupational therapists and social workers, tangibly improve the prospects of rehabilitation.

Interventions in cases of dementia

Most cases of suspected, and then developing, dementia go through primary care, then on to specialist services, then on to community support services, then many on to residential care and/or to nursing homes. This is not an invariable pattern, rather an average progression, but one with many opportunities for creatively designed combinations of treatment and support at each stage.

Pharmaceutical treatments

One can well understand the desire on the part of carers and of patients themselves for a chemical solution to the signs of cognitive dysfunction, inexplicable anxiety, social disconnection and reduced standards of self-care. Indeed, early intervention with appropriate medications does slow down the progress of such symptoms, the danger being (and here is where social care staff come in) that environmental causes of dysfunction (e.g. chronic loneliness), which can in some cases lead to depression and self-neglect, are seen as secondary *symptoms*, not as secondary *causes*.

Symptomatic treatments

As we have seen, the dementias, particularly in advanced cases, can cause very considerable stress to sufferers and to their carers – who have to view the condition through the lens of the past. Memory loss plays a major role in these cases as reassurances and explanations are quickly forgotten. There is thus a case for medication to be prescribed such as anti-anxiety drugs. These can make a difference but they have a bad reputation because, without doubt, they are sometimes used in nursing homes and residential homes to quieten clients more for the comfort of the staff than for those older people with dementia. Nevertheless, carefully prescribed medication, regularly reviewed as a result of feedback from carers, nurses and social care staff, can be helpful and should not be casually opposed on vague ideological grounds from a safe distance (see Benbow, 1997).

Psychosocial interventions

Psychosocial approaches can make *some* worthwhile differences in cases of dementia, but mainly in respect of helping to slow down mental, social and physical decline, and through support for carers (see Palmer (1999) for a good systematic review). The main findings from this research follow.

We must bear in mind that the majority of clients with early/mid-course dementia are now living at home which, client-opinion research constantly tells us, is where they wish to remain. In order that this can happen the need is for well-organized, practical assistance. That is, help with cleaning, edible meals on wheels, advice on benefits, housing repairs, dealing with what may seem to be threatening letters from official bodies, and support for carers. Well-organized, practical social care should therefore be our first priority, for without it nothing else succeeds.

These general points aside, the available research evidence on the effectiveness of psychosocial interventions may be summarized as follows:

1   Whether provided at home, in sheltered accommodation, or in residential or nursing care homes, the most powerful effect on the well-being of clients is

patient, mildly stimulating, choice-affirming, respectful, identity-confirming care which supports the dignity of the person, and recognizes past and present achievements. Easy to say, but the approach requires great attention to detail, considerable logistical prowess on the part of staff, well-adapted physical facilities, and, in the face of demanding symptoms, stamina from helpers. Where these elements of good care *are* brought together, they probably account for the high levels of satisfaction reported.

The White Paper *Our Health, Our Care, Our Say* (Department of Health, 2006) sets out what is required, but such initiatives come 'flat-packed' and staff have to assemble them as best they can. The benefits of instruction booklets aside, such guidelines are a tall order for care staff on low pay rates, with too many people to look after. Sometimes, endless 'must-do' lists can generate the pressures which lead to emotional disconnection or, unforgivably, to abuse. Age Concern estimates that around 10 per cent of older people within the care system suffer physical abuse and bullying during their stay; they become deindividualized; they become 'the job'. Good leadership, staff support, respite breaks when necessary and good multidisciplinary training are therefore important (see Chapman, 1997). But all this is pious in the face of high staff turnover (changing faces and having to start all over again are significant problems identified by empirical research on the quality of care) and some structural problems – lack of time, feasibility, aids, over-demanding regulations and, again, money are formidable obstacles.

2   Given the damage done – particularly to short-term memory – by dementias, a perfectly reasonable proposition is that we should try to amplify and simplify the environmental cues as to time, place, identity, and what to expect next. Reality reorientation programmes based on this principle were tested in trials conducted from the 1980s onward (see Palmer, 1999). Measurable improvements were recorded both on cognitive skills, behaviour, and apparent sense of connectedness to circumstances (see Bandolier, 1998). However, there are two problems with this approach: (1) it is very labour-intensive and therefore expensive, and (2) it carries the risk of producing high-expressed emotion effects (see Chapter 5). The best solution appears to be to incorporate not over-directive and not endlessly repetitive reminders into social contacts, which are as natural as possible.

3   Brooker has proposed a person-centred dementia care model (2007), building on Tom Kitwood's work on personhood and psychosocial approaches to dementia care. This model emphasizes four key elements of person-centred care: (V) a value base that asserts the absolute value of all human lives regardless of age or cognitive ability; (I) an individualized approach, recognizing uniqueness; (P) understanding the world from the perspective of the service user, and (S) providing a social environment that supports psychological needs (Brooker, 2007: 13). The 'VIPS' model should provide professionals and care organizations with clear guidance on applying the principles of person-centred dementia care to practice (but guidance is one thing and face-to-face practice quite another).

4   Another plausible idea to hold back the psychosocial effects of dementia is to exploit the fact that short-term memory goes first, and that longer term memory remains more intact. Reminiscence and life story work (Bornat, 1994; Gibson,

1997) attempt to bolster a sense of identify by helping clients to recall what they can – about their schooldays, about World War II, about their marriages, about their children when they were young and so on. Clients who have the opportunity to discuss these reminiscences tend to retain cognitive and social skills for longer. The systematic review by Woods *et al.* (2005) concluded that the evidence for reminiscence therapy suggested that it was able to make a positive difference to cognition and mood (at follow-up, on a general measure of function) and provided carers with relief from strain (see also Webster and Haight, 2002). From a more therapeutic perspective, reminiscence and life history work with a person with dementia can provide a sense of continuity between the past and the present as well as valuing and respecting them (see Gibson, 1997).

5   The effectiveness of applied behavioural analysis has been established by a very large research literature across a wide range of problems (see Chapter 7). Findings have only recently been used successfully with clients suffering from dementia. This approach is based upon identifying the cues for agitated behaviour (remember that in advanced cases we do not always have the option of sitting down for a rational discussion about what is wrong); then looking at the reinforcement contingencies.

6   Where residential or sheltered care are required, the messages from research are clear and practical, i.e. the design layout and organization of the facilities should:

- compensate for impairment, whether physical or mental;
- maximize independence;
- enhance self-esteem and self-confidence;
- pay attention to individual needs;
- be orientating and understandable;
- reinforce personal identity;
- welcome relatives and encourage contact with the local community;
- encourage residents to help plan the service and regularly evaluate it;
- be of a small size;
- be familiar, domestic and homely in style;
- provide space for ordinary, non-regimented activities (e.g. kitchens and gardening facilities);
- have different rooms for different functions, including individual rooms with space for personal possessions;
- contain furniture appropriate to age and physical capabilities;
- recognize that choice and risk often compete in designing living environments and regimes. A very careful, individual assessment needs to be conducted, otherwise we get a very safe, but boring, individuality-depressing *milieu*, or more freedom but at the cost of unwarrantable physical risk. There are findings to guide us in these difficult matters (see Prime Minister's Strategy Unit, 2002; CSCI, 2006a; Marshall and Tibbs, 2006). The involvement of relatives in taking *considered* risks 'lays off the bet' a little, but they are often very risk-averse – however, not as averse as politicians, service providers, inspectors or politicians operating with the benefit of hindsight.

Case example

Mrs B, a widow, was only 74 years old but had rapidly advancing Alzheimer's Disease which robbed her of most of her short-term memory. She had spent a year in sheltered, warden-controlled accommodation but often pressed alarm bells when she was in an agitated state and wandered off on several occasions. Medication was prescribed, but due to another (slightly paranoid) view that people were trying to poison her, she would usually resist taking it. Many textbooks would take a rather romantic view of this troubled lady. 'Why not sit her down and explain that her husband had died four years earlier and so searching for him was in vain?' 'Why not take her to his grave in the nearby churchyard?' 'Why not get the remaining family to come in to explain matters to her, rather than just seek a solution via mood-altering pills?' Well, all of these things were done and made only very short-term differences, because Mrs B had no memory of what had passed between herself and these would-be helpers an hour later.

An analysis of Mrs B's behaviour showed that for around 50 per cent of her day she was not agitated or upset. The reaction of staff to these quiet periods was to leave her alone. A simple reversal of these reinforcement contingencies (i.e. engaging with her when she was *not* asking repetitive questions or wandering) produced useful results for two years.

(From Sheldon, 1995: 240)

Conclusions

1   Social workers in particular, and social care staff generally, are not good at making a case either to government or to the public at large for their effectiveness (see Lymbery, 2006). As we have argued this is partly due to the fact that professional association membership, independent of employing authorities, is so low (imagine the position of nursing without the RCN, or doctors casually forgoing representation by the BMA). This is an idle and indifferent response to current political realities and needs reversion.

2   Carers, whether family members or others, are central to the system of community care. However, since they would never withdraw their labour, they have little political clout, so much so that the recent Carers Bill allocates £33 million to local councils for 'Support Services', but mainly for training courses and (another) national Helpline. This amounts to a cool £4.16 per client.

3   Findings on the value of attempts to foster as much independence as is feasible – not in the eyes of the department only but in the eyes of clients and carers themselves – are ubiquitous; results from studies of home care and residential care show that regimes which encourage the retention of personal contact – a person-centred approach – even as a fighting retreat, and that gently emphasize choice in the way services are provided, are valued (see Lincoln *et al.*, 2002).

4   There is a growing literature on the value and effects of involving people who use services in the design and management of new projects. 'Nothing about us

without us' is a sound principle. There are circumstances when the testimony of service-users is decisive, but note that there are also others where their individual opinions are not a sufficient basis for generalization. Genuine partnerships require enough respect for each constituency of opinion, so that we are able, while recognizing the power imbalance, to come to an accord on current best evidence on what might be helpful. Where this happens, the results and the relevance of projects are significantly improved (see DOH, 2007a; CSCI, 2008).

Afterword

What is there left to say? Only that we would not like to leave you on whatever happens to be the last sentence in the last chapter. Between us, we have spoken at and organized about 500 conferences on evidence-based practice in social work over the past ten years. At the end of these lectures we are typically asked by participants to list just two or three measures to improve things. Here are our typical replies:

1   Social work has never had more intellectual riches than at present. These take the form of (1) empirically derived knowledge on the nature and development of personal and social problems, and (2) what is known from methodically robust research on what might ameliorate them. The problem, and the paradox, has not escaped us in writing this book, namely that students and front-line practitioners are rarely reading this material (see Sheldon and Chilvers, 2000; Sheldon *et al.*, 2004). This is not just an impression but an empirical fact. So read much more. If the 'corporate' demands of your employment discourage this, and you do not think that you can do anything about it (learned helplessness?), then you might just as well be working for a building society.

2   The teaching of scientific reasoning (see Gibbs, 1991); trends in effectiveness research, and basic statistics on social work curses is still a little sketchy. Teachers seem to favour emotion, ethics and 'inclusivity' over this essential knowledge. But, to repeat the point, what is the purpose of a social work scheme which provides 'equal access for all' to an ineffective service? Ethics, research and evidence-based practice are thus inextricably tied together. If you are not getting teaching on these issues then make a fuss.

3   The secondary aim of this book is to give social work a better sense of itself, the primary aim being to provide more effective services for needy people. However, the only known antidote to rampant bureaucracy and a distorting, politically convenient, target culture is professionalism and justifiable, expert opinion. We are not at all well organized in this regard, and therefore have a tiny voice in public discourse. By all means join a trade union to protect your employment conditions, but join also a professional association able to represent our wider aspirations for social justice – why we all joined, presumably.

Bibliography

Acheson, D. (1998) *Independent Inquiry into Inequalities in Health: Report.* London: HMSO.

Ainsworth, M., Biehar, M., Waters, E. and Wall, S. (1978) *Patterns of Attachment: A Psychological Study of the Strange Situation.* Hillsdale, NI: Lawrence Erlbaum.

The Albumin Reviewers (Alderson, P., Bunn, F., Li Wan Po, A., Li, L., Roberts, I. and Schierhout, G.) (2004) Human albumin solution for resuscitation and volume expansion in critically ill patients. *Cochrane Database of Systematic Reviews* 2004, Issue 4. Art. No.: CD001208. DOI: 10.1002/14651858.CD001208.pub2.

Aldgate, J. and Statham, J. (2001) *The Children Act Now.* London: The Stationery Office.

Aldgate, J. and Tunstill, J. (1996) *Making Sense of Section 17.* London: HMSO.

American Psychiatric Association (1988) *Diagnostic and Statistical Manual of Mental Disorders, Fourth Edition, Revised (DSM-IV-R).* Washington, DC: American Psychiatric Association.

Anglin, J.P. (2004) 'Creating "well-functioning" residential care and defining its place in a system of care', *Child and Youth Care Forum*, 33, 3, 175–192.

Anon. (late 1700s) Children's rhyme collected by *The Tickler Magazine*, 12, 1821.

Anthony, W.A. (1993) 'Recovery from mental illness; the guiding vision of mental health in the 1990s', *Psychosocial Rehabilitation Journal*, 14, 3, 10–17.

Appleby, L. (1997) *National Confidential Inquiry into Suicides and Homicides by People with Mental Illness.* London: Department of Health.

Appleton, P., Boll, V., Everett, J.M., Kelly, A.M., Meredith, K.H. and Payne, T.G. (1997) 'Beyond child development centres: care coordination for children with disabilities', *Child: Care, Health and Development*, 23, 29–40.

Arsenault, L., Cannon, M., Poulton, R., Murray, R., Laspi, A. and Moff, H.T.E. (2002) 'Cannabis use in adolescence and risk for adult psychosis: longitudinal prospective studies', *British Medical Journal*, 325: 1212–1213.

Arsenault, L., Moffitt, T.E., Caspi, A., Taylor, A., Rijsdijk, R.V., Jafee, S.R., Ablow, J.C. and Measelle, F.R. (2003) 'Strong genetic effects on cross-situational antisocial behaviour among 5-year-old children according to mothers, teachers, examiner-observers, and twins' self-reports', *Journal of Child Psychology and Psychiatry*, 44, 6, 832–848.

Asche, S.E. (1951) 'Opinions and social pressure', in S. Coopersmith (ed.), *Frontiers of Psychological Research.* London: Freeman.

Asdigan, N.L. and Finkelhor, D. (1995) 'What works for children in resisting assaults?', *Journal of Interpersonal Violence*, 10, 4, 402–418.

Asen, E. (2002) 'Outcome research in family therapy', *Advances in Psychiatric Treatment*, 8, 230–238.

Ashley, Lord (7th Earl of Shaftesbury) *Diaries* SHA/PD/3–6. National Register of Archives (after A. Scull, 1993).

Attlee, C. (1920) *The Social Worker.* London: Bell.

Aubrey, L.L. (1998) 'Motivational interviewing with adolescents presenting for outpatient substance abuse treatment'. *Dissertation Abstracts International*, Section B: *The Sciences and Engineering*, 59 (3-B), B.

Auden, W.H. (1994) 'The Shield of Achilles', in *Collected Poems*. London: Faber.

Audit Commission (1994) *Seen but not Heard: Coordinating Community Child Health and Social Services for Children in Need*. London: HMSO.

Audit Commission (2000) *The Way to go Home. Rehabilitation and Remedial Services for Older People*. London: Audit Commission.

Audit Commission (2001) *Changing Gear: Best Value Annual Statement 2001*. London: Audit Commission.

Audit Commission (2003) *Too Little, too Late: Services for Disabled Children and their Families*. London: Audit Commission.

Audit Commission (2004a) *Misspent Youth: Young People and Crime*. London: Audit Commission.

Audit Commission (2004b) *Older People: Implementing Telecare*. London: Audit Commission.

Audit Commission (2006) *Choosing Well: Analysing the Costs and Benefits of Choice in Local Public Services*. London: Audit Commission.

Audit Scotland (2008) *A Review of Free Personal and Nursing Care*. Edinburgh: Audit Scotland.

Audrey, R. (1966) *The Territorial Imperative*. New York: Atheneum.

Austin, A.M., Macgowan, M.J. and Wagner, E.F. (2005) 'Effective family-based interventions for adolescents with substance use problems: a systematic review'. *Research on Social Work Practice*, 15, 2, 67–83.

Babcock, J.C., Green, C.E. and Robie, C. (2004) 'Does batterers' treatment work? A meta-analytic review of domestic violence treatment', *Clinical Psychology Review*, 23, 1023–1053.

Bacon, F. (1605/1965) *The Advancement of Learning* ed. G. W. Kitchen. London: Dent.

Bacon, F. (1627/1974) 'Of Truth', in A. Johnson, *Essays*. London: Dent.

BADEN (2008) *Nutrition Screening Survey in the UK in 2007*. London: British Association for Parenteral and Enteral Nutrition.

Bakermans-Kranenburg, M. J., van IJzendoorn, M.H. and Juffer, F. (2003) 'Less is more: meta-analyses of sensitivity and attachment interventions in early childhood', *Psychological Bulletin*, 129, 2, 195–215.

Baldwin, S. and Carlisle, J. (1994) *Social Support for Disabled Children and their Families; A Review of the Literature*. London: National Children's Bureau.

Bamford, C. and Bruce, E. (2000) 'Defining the outcomes of community care: the perspectives of older people with dementia and their carers', *Ageing and Society*, 20, 5, 543–570.

Bandolier (1998) *Dementia, Diagnosis and Treatment*, 48, 5, 2–3, http://www.medicine.ox.ac.uk/bandolier/painres/download/Bando048.pdf

Bandura, A. (1969) *Principals of Behavioural Modification*. New York: Holt, Rinehart & Winston.

Bandura, A. (1977) *Social Learning Theory*. Englewood Cliffs, NJ: Prentice Hall.

Barclay Report (1982) *Social Workers: Their Role and Tasks*. London: Bedford Street Press/National Council for Voluntary Organizations.

Barker, P. (1992) *Regeneration*. Harmondsworth: Penguin.

Barker, W. (1988) *The Child Development Programme: An Evaluation of Process and Outcomes*. Bristol: Early Childhood Development Centre.

Barker, W. (1994) *Child Protection: The Impact of the Child Development Programme*. Bristol: Early Childhood Development Unit.

Barklay, R. (1990) *Attention Deficit Hyperactivity Disorder: A Handbook for Diagnosis and Treatment* (2nd edition). New York: Guilford Press.

Barlow, J. and Parsons, J. (2003) 'Group-based parent-training programmes for improving emotional and behavioural adjustment in 0–3 year old children', *Cochrane Database of Systematic Reviews*, Issue 2. Art. No.: CD003680. DOI: 10.1002/14651858.CD003680.

Barnard and McKeganey (2004) 'The impact of parental problem drug use on children: what is the problem and what can be done to help?', *Addiction*, 99, 5, 552–559.

Barnett, B., Blignault, I., Holmes, S., Payne, A. and Parker, G. (1987) 'Quality of attachment in a sample of 1-year old Australian children', *Journal of the American Academy of Child and Adolescent Psychiatry*, 26, 303–307.

Barnett, W.S. (1995) 'Long-term effects of early childhood programs on cognitive and school outcomes', *The Future of Children*, 5, 3, 25–30.

Barth, R.P. (1989) 'Evaluation of a task-centered child abuse prevention program', *Children and Youth Services Review*, 11, 117–132.

Barth, R.P. (2005) 'Residential care: from here to eternity', *International Journal of Social Welfare*, 14, 158–162.

Bartlett, K. (1950) *Remembering*. Cambridge: Cambridge Psychological Library.

Barton, P., Bryan, S., Glasby, J., Hewitt, G., Jagger, C., Kaambwa, B., Martin, G., Nancarrow, S., Parker, S., Regen, E. and Wilson, A. (2006). *A National Evaluation of the Costs and Outcomes of Intermediate Care for Older People*. Leicester: Leicester Nuffield Research Unit.

Bateson, G. (1973) *Steps to an Ecology of Mind*. London: Paladin.

Bateson, G., Jackson, D.P., Haley, J. and Weatland, J. (1956) 'Towards a theory of schizophrenia', *Behavioural Science*, 1, 251–264.

Battin, S.R. and Hill, K.G. (1998) 'The contribution of gang membership to delinquency beyond delinquent friends', *Criminology*, 36, 1, 93–116.

Baxter, C., Kamaljit, P., Ward, L. and Nadirshaw, Z. (1990) *Double Discrimination: Issues and Services for People with Learning Difficulties from Black and Ethnic Minority Communities*. London: King's Fund.

Bayes, Rev. T. (1958) 'An essay toward solving a problem in the doctrine of chances', *Biometrika*, 45, 293–315, and *Two Papers by Bayes*, with commentary by W. Deming, New York: Hafner, 1963.

Bayley, J. (2001) *Elegy for Iris*. London: Picador Books.

Bayliss, K. (2000) 'Social work values, anti-discriminatory practice and working with older lesbian service users', *Social Work Education*, 19, 1, 45–54.

Bazemore, G. and Elis, L. (2007) 'Evaluation of restorative justice', in G. Johnstone and D.W. Van Ness (eds), *Handbook of Restorative Justice*. Cullompton, Devon: Willan Publishing.

Bazemore, G. and Schiff, M. (2004) 'Paradigm muddle or paradigm paralysis? The wide and narrow roads to restorative justice reform (or a little confusion may be a good thing)', *Contemporary Justice Review*, 7, 1, 37–57.

Beamish, P., Lanello, L.L.P.F., Granello, D.H. and McSteen, P. (1996) 'Outcome studies in the treatment of panic disorder: a review', *Journal of Counselling and Development*, 74, 460–467.

Beattie, R. (1999) *Implementing Inclusiveness: Realising Potential*. Scottish Executive Report. Edinburgh: Scottish Executive.

Beck, A.T. (1976) *Cognitive Therapy and the Emotional Disorders*. New York: International Universities Press.

Becker, J.V., Alpert, J.L., Subia Bigfoot, D., Bonner, B.L., Geddie, L.F., Henggeler, S.W., Kaufmann, K.L. and Walker, C.E. (1995) 'Empirical research on child abuse treatment: report by the Child Abuse and Neglect Treatment Working Group, American Psychological Association', *Journal of Clinical Child Psychology* 24 (suppl), 23–46.

Beecher, W. (1998) *Having a Say! Disabled Children and Effective Partnership, Section 2:*

Practice Initiatives and Selected Annotated References. London: Council for Disabled Children.

Benbow, S. M. (1997) 'Therapies in old age psychiatry: reflections on recent changes', in M. Marshall (ed.), *State of the Art in Dementia Care*. London: Centre for Policy on Ageing.

Bennett, A. (1999) *Alan Bennett: Diaries (1980–1990)* London: BBC Audiobook Ltd.

Beresford, B. (1995) *Expert Opinions: A National Survey of Parents Caring for a Severely Disabled Child*. Bristol: The Policy Press.

Bergin, A.E. and Garfield, S.L. (1986) *Handbook of Psychotherapy and Behaviour*. Chichester: John Wiley & Sons.

Berglund, M., Andreasson, S., Franck, J., Fridell, M., Hakanson, I. and Johansson, B-A. (2001) *Treatment of Alcohol and Drug Abuse – An Evidence-based Review*. Sweden: Swedish Council on Technology Assessment in Health Dare, Report No. 156/1 (Vol. I); 156/2 (Vol. II).

Berk, L.E. (ed.) (2005) *Child Development*. London: Allyn & Bacon.

Berleman, W.C., Seaburg, J.R. and Steinburn, T.W. (1972) 'The delinquency prevention experiment of the Seattle Atlantic Center: a final evaluation', *Social Service Review*, 46, 323–346.

Berlin, I. (1996) *The Sense of Reality: Studies in Ideas and their History*. London: Chatto & Windus.

Bernazzani, O. and Tremblay, R.E. (2006) 'Early parent training', in B.C. Welsh and D.P. Farrington (eds), *Preventing Crime: What Works for Children, Offenders, Victims, and Places*. Dordrecht: Springer.

Bernstein, L. and Sondheim, S. (1961) *West Side Story*. United Artists.

Bernstein, P.L. (1996) *Against the Gods: The Remarkable Story of Risk*. Chichester: John Wiley.

Berridge, D. (2002) 'Residential care', in D. McNeish, T. Newman and J. Roberts (eds), *What Works for Children?* Buckingham: Open University Press.

Berridge, D. and Brodie, I. (1998) *Children's Homes Revisited*. London: Jessica Kinglsey.

Bertalanffy, L. von (1968) *General System Theory: Foundations, Development, Applications* (Revised edition). New York: George Braziller.

Beveridge, W. (1942) *Social Insurance and Allied Services* (known as The Beveridge Report). London; HMSO.

Bhugra, D., Leff, J., Mallett, R., Dev, G., Corridon, B. and Rudge, S. (1997) 'Incidence of schizophrenia in whites, African–Caribbeans and Asians in London', *Psychological Medicine*, 27, 791–798.

Biehal, N., Clayden, J., Stein, M. and Wade, J. (1994) *Moving On: Young People and Leaving Care Schemes*. London: HMSO.

Biestek, F. (1960) *A Casework Relationship*. London: George Allen & Unwin.

Bifulco, A., Brown, G.W., Moran, P., Ball, C. and Campbell, C. (1998) 'Predicting depression in women: the role of past and present vulnerability', *Psychological Medicine*, 28, 39–50.

Biggs, S. (1993) *Understanding Ageing*. Buckingham: Open University Press.

Billari, F.C., Philipov, D. and Baizán, P. (2001) 'Leaving home in Europe: the experience of cohorts born around 1980', *International Journal of Population Geography*, 7, 339–356.

Bilton, K. (1998) 'Child and family social work: organizational context and identity', *Child and Family Social Work*, 3, 197–203.

Birchall, E. and Hallett, S. (1998) *Working Together in Child Protection*. London: HMSO.

Birchwood, M. and Tarrier, N. (eds) (1992) *Innovations in the Psychological Management of Schizophrenia: Assessment, Treatment and Services*. Chichester: John Wiley & Sons.

Birchwood, M., Hallett, S. and Preston, M. (1988) *Schizophrenia: An Integrated Approach to Research and Treatment*. Harlow: Longman.

Bird, L. (1999) *The Fundamental Facts*. London: Mental Health Foundation.

Black, D., Morris, J., Smith, C. and Townsend, P. (1980) *Inequalities in Health*. London: BMJ.

Black, M.M. and Teti, L.O. (1997) 'Promoting mealtime communication between adolescent mothers and their infants through videotape', *Pediatrics*, 99, 3, 432–437.

Blackburn, C., Read, J. and Hughes, N. (2005) 'Carers and the digital divide: factors affecting Internet use among carers', *Health and Social Care in the Community*, B13, 3, 201–210.

Blackburn, I.M., Bishop, S., Glen, I., Whalley, L.J. and Christie, J.E. (1981) 'The efficacy of cognitive therapy in depression', *British Journal of Psychiatry*, 137, 181–189.

Blom-Cooper, L. (1985) *A Child in Trust*. London Borough of Brent.

Blom-Cooper, L. (1987) *A Child in Mind: Protection of Children in a Responsible Society*. Report of the Committee of Inquiry into the Circumstances Surrounding the Death of Tyra Henry. London: London Borough of Greenwich.

Blythe, R. (1964) *The Age of Illusion*. Harmondsworth: Penguin.

Bodanis, D. (2006) *Passionate Minds*. London: Little Brown.

Bohman, J. and Sigvardsson, S. (1990) 'Outcome in adoption: lessons from longitudinal studies', in D.M. Brodzinsky and M.D. Schecter (eds) *The Psychology of Adoption*. New York: Oxford University Press.

Bolt, R. (1996) *A Man of all Seasons*. London: Gardener/Methuen.

Bolton, A. and Hill, G. (1996) *Mind, Meaning and Mental Disorder*. Oxford: Oxford University Press.

Bonhoffer, D. (1967) *Letters and Papers from Prison*, ed. E. Bethge, trans. R. Fuller. London: SCM Press, Ltd (a more accessible edition with the same title is published by Folio (2000)).

Bornat, J. (ed.) (1994) *Reminiscence Reviewed: Evaluations, Achievements, Perspectives*. Buckingham: Open University Press.

Bould, L., Chesterman, J., Davies, B., Judge, K. and Mangalore, R. (2000) *Caring for Older People: An Assessment of Community Care in the 1990s*. Aldershot: Ashgate.

Bowes, A. and McColgan, G. (2005). *Smart Technology at Home: Users' and Carers' Perspectives, Interim Report*. Stirling: West Lothian Council and the University of Stirling.

Bowlby, J. (1951) *Attachment and Loss. Volume 1: Attachment*. London: Hogarth Press and the Institute of Psychoanalysis.

Bowlby, J. and Salter-Ainsworth, M. (1963) *Child Care and the Growth of Love*. Harmondsworth: Penguin.

Bowling, B. and Phillips, C. (2002) *Racism, Crime and Justice*. London: Longman.

Boydell, J., Van Os, J., McKenzie, K., Allerdyce, J., Goel, R., McCreadie, R. and Murray, R. (2001) 'Incidence of schizophrenia in ethnic minorities in London: an ecological study into interactions with the environment', *British Medical Journal*, 323, 1536.

Boyle, D. (2000) *The Tyranny of Numbers*. London: HarperCollins.

Boyle, M. (2002) *Schizophrenia: A Scientific Delusion*. London: Routledge.

Braithwaite, R. (2001) *Managing Aggression*. London: Routledge.

Brent, D., Holden, D. and Kolko, D. (1997) 'A clinical psychotherapy trial for adolescent depression comparing cognitive, family and supportive treatments', *Archives of General Psychiatry*, 54, 877–885.

Brewer, C. and Lait, J.C. (1980) *Can Social Work Survive?* London: Temple Smith.

Briggs, A. (1959) *The Age of Improvement*. London: Longman.

Briggs, A. and Macartney, A. (1984) *Toynbee Hall: The First Hundred Years*. London: Routledge & Kegan Paul.

Brill Roberts, S. and Horowitz, A (1983) 'The New York city home care project: a demonstration in coordination of health and social services', *Home Health Care Services Quarterly* 4, 3–4, 91–96.

British Association for Behavioural and Cognitive Psychotherapies (BABCP) (1993) *Behavioural & Cognitive Psychotherapy*, Supplement 1. Cambridge: Cambridge University Press.

British Association of Social Workers (1975) *A Code of Ethics for Social Work*. Birmingham: BASW.

Broad, B. (1998) *Young People Leaving Care: Life After the Children Act 1989*. London: Jessica Kingsley.

Broad, B. (2004) 'Kinship care for children in the UK: messages from research, lessons for policy and practice', *European Journal of Social Work*, 7, 2, 2111–2227.

Bronfenbrenner, U. (1979) *The Experimental Ecology of Human Development*. Cambridge, MA: Harvard University Press.

Brooker, D. (2007) *Person Centred Dementia Care: Making Services Better*. London: Jessica Kingsley.

Brown, G.W. and Birley, J.L.T. (1968) 'Crises and life changes and the onset of schizophrenia', *Journal of Health and Social Behaviour*, 9, 203–214.

Brown, G.W. and Harris, T. (1979) *Social Origins of Depression*. London: Tavistock Publications.

Brown, G.W., Birley, J.L.T. and Wing, J.K. (1972) 'Influence of family life on the cause of schizophrenia disorders: a replication', *British Journal of Psychiatry*. 121, 241–258.

Brown, M. and McCulloch, I. (1975) *Social Workers Use of Research, Clearing House for Social Services Research*. Birmingham: University of Birmingham.

Brown, R. (1965) *Social Psychology*. London: Collier, Macmillan.

Brown, R. (1986) *Social Psychology* (2nd edn). New York: Free Press.

Brown, T.G., Seraganian, P., Tremblay, J. and Annis, H. (2002) 'Process and outcome changes with relapse prevention versus Twelve Steps aftercare programmes for substance abusers', *Addiction*, 97, 677–689.

Brunk, M., Henggeler, S.W. and Whelan, J.P. (1987) 'Comparison of multisystemic therapy and parent training in the brief treatment of child abuse and neglect', *Journal of Consulting and Clinical Psychology*, 55, 2, 171–178.

Budd, T., Sharp, C. and Mayhew, P. (2005a) *Offending in England and Wales: First Results from the 2003 Crime and Justice Survey*. London: Home Office.

Budd, T., Weir, G., Wilson, D. and Owen, N. (2005b) *Findings from the 2004 Offending, Crime and Justice Survey*. London: Home Office.

Bullock, R. (1999) *Work with Children in Residential Care*. Research Highlights in Social Work 35. London: Jessica Kingsley.

Bullock, R. and Little, M. (1998) *Children Going Home: The Reunification of Families* (Dartington Social Research Series). Aldershot: Ashgate.

Burchardt, T. (2003) *Being and Becoming: Social Exclusion and the Onset of Disability*. ESRC Case Report 21, November.

Burleigh, M. (1995) *Death and Deliverance: 'Euthanasia' in Germany 1900–1945*. Cambridge: Cambridge University Press.

Burns, J. (1943) *Oral Traditions*. Oxford: Oxford University Press.

Butler, S. (1912/1951) *Samuel Butler's Notebooks*. London: Jonathan Care.

Byford, S., Harrington, R., Torgeson, D., Kerfoot, M., Dyer, E., Harrington, V., Woodham, A., Gill, J. and McNiven, F. (1999) 'Cost-effectiveness analysis of a home-based social work intervention for children and adolescents who have deliberately poisoned themselves: results of a randomised controlled trial', *British Journal of Psychiatry*, 174, 56–62.

Cabinet Office (2000) *Adoption: A New Approach* (White Paper). London: Department of Health.

Cabot, R.C. (1931) 'Treatment in social casework and the need for tests of its success and failure', *Proceedings of the National Conference of Social Work*. New York.

Cameron, A. *et al.* (2000) *Factors Promoting and Obstacles Hindering Joint Working: A Systematic Review.* Bristol: School for Policy Studies, University of Bristol.

Cameron, A., Macdonald, G., Turner, W. and Lloyd, L. (2007) *The Challenges of Joint Working: Lessons from the Supporting People Health Pilot Evaluation.* London: Department of Communities and Local Government.

Campbell, A.P. (1984) *Moderated Love: A Theology of Professional Care.* London: SPCK.

Campbell, D., Draper, R. and Crutchley, E. (1991) 'The Milan systemic approach to family therapy', in A. Gurman and D. Kniskern (eds) *Handbook of Family Therapy Vol II.* New York: Brunner Mazel.

Campbell, F.A. and Taylor, K. (1996) 'Early childhood programmes that work for children from economically disadvantaged families', *Young Children*, 51, 4, 74–80.

Cann, J., Falshaw, L., Nugent, F. and Friendship, C. (2003) *Understanding What Works: Accredited Cognitive Skills Programmes for Adult Men and Young Offenders.* London: Home Office Research Findings 226.

Carlile (1987) *A Child in Mind: The Report of the Commission of Inquiry into the Circumstances surrounding the death of Kimberley Carlile.* London: Borough of Greenwich.

Carr, A. (2000a) 'Evidence-based practice in family therapy and systemic consultation I Child-focused problems', *Journal of Family Therapy*, 22, 29–60.

Carr, A. (2000b) 'Evidence-based practice in family therapy and systemic consultation II Adult-focused problems', *Journal of Family Therapy*, 22, 273–295.

Carr, A. (ed.) (2000c) *What Works with Children and Adolescents?* London: Routledge.

Carr, A. (2006) *Family Therapy: Concepts, Process and Practice* (2nd edition). Chichester: John Wiley.

Carr-Hill, R., Dixon, P., Mannion, R., Rice, N., Rudat, K., Sinclair, R. and Smith, P.C. (1997) *A Model of the Determinants of Expenditure on Children's Personal Social Services.* York: University of York, Centre for Health Economics.

Carroll, L. (1865/1974) *Through the Looking Glass.* London: The Bodley Head.

Carroll, L.A., Miltenberger, R.G. and O'Neill, H.K. (1992) 'A review and critique of research evaluating child sexual abuse prevention programs', *Education and Treatment of Children*, 15, 335–354.

Caspi, A., Henry, B., McGee, R.O., Moffitt, T.E. and Silva, P.A. (1995) 'Temperamental origins of child and adolescent behavior problems: from age 3 to age 15', *Child Development*, 66, 55–68.

Caspi, A., McLay, J., Moffitt, T.E., Mill, J., Marin, J. and Craig, I.W. (2002) 'Role of genotype in the cycle of violence in maltreated children', *Science*, 297, 851–854.

Causley, C. (1992) *Collected Poems.* Basingstoke: Macmillan

Cavet, J. and Sloper, P. (2004) 'Participation of disabled chidren in individual decisions about their lives and in public decisions about service development', *Children and Society*, 18, 278–290.

Cecchin, G., Lane, G. and Ray, W. (1993) 'From strategising to non-intervention: toward irreverence in systemic practice', *Journal of Marital and Family Therapy*, 2, 125–136.

Central Council for Education, Training and Social Work (2001) *Annual Report.* London: CCETSW.

Centre for Evidence-based Social Services (CEBSS) (2001) *Annual Report.* Exeter: University of Exeter, Centre for Evidence-based Social Services.

Centre for Evidence-based Social Services (CEBSS) (2002) *Annual Report.* Exeter: University of Exeter, Centre for Evidence-based Social Services

Centre for Evidence-based Social Services (CEBSS) (2003) *Evidence-based Social Care*, Issue 13. Exeter: University of Exeter, Centre for Evidence-based Social Services

Centre for Reviews and Dissemination (CRD) (1999) 'Getting evidence into practice', *Effective Healthcare Bulletin*, 5(1), 1–16.

Chadwick, E. (1842) *Report into the Sanitary Conditions of the Labouring Population of Great Britain*. London: HMSO.

Chadwick, P., Birchwood, M. and Trower, P. (1996) *Cognitive-therapy for Delusions, Voices and Paranoia*. Chichester: John Wiley & Sons.

Chakrabarty, A. and McKenzie, K. (2002) 'Does racial bias cause mental illness?', *British Journal of Psychiatry*, 180, 475–477.

Challis, D. (1991) 'An evaluation of an alternative to long-stay hospital care for frail elderly patients: I. The model of care', *Age and Ageing*, 20, 4, 236–244.

Challis, D. and Davies, B. (1980) 'A new approach to community care for the elderly', *British Journal of Social Work*, 10, 1–18.

Challis, D. and Davies, B. (1986) *Case Management in Community Care*. Aldershot: Gower.

Challis, D., Chessum, R., Chesterman, J., Luckett, R. and Transke, K. (1990) *Case Management in Social and Health Care: The Gateshead Community Care Scheme*. Personal Social Services Research Unit, University of Kent.

Challis, D., Darton, R. and Stewart, K. (1998a) *Community Care, Secondary Health Care and Care Management*. Aldershot: Ashgate.

Challis, D., Darton, R., Hughes, J., Stewart, K. and Weiner, K. (1998b) *Care Management Study: Report on National Data*. Social Services Inspectorate. London: Department of Health.

Chalmers, I. (1989) 'Evaluating the effects of care during pregnancy and childbirth', in I. Chalmers, M. Enkin and M.J.N.C. Keirse (eds), *Effective Care in Pregnancy and Childbirth*. Oxford: Oxford University Press.

Chalmers, R., Matta, R.G., Smith, H. Jr. and Kunzler, A.M. (1977) 'Evidence favouring the use of anticoagulants in the hospital phase of acute myocardial infarction', *New England Journal of Medicine*, 297, 1091–1096.

Chamberlain, P. and Rosicky, J. (1995) 'The effectiveness of family therapy in the treatment of adolescents with conduct disorders and delinquency', *Journal of Marital and Family Therapy*, 21, 441–459.

Channel 4 Films, Close Call Films, Mad George Films and Samuel Goldwyn Company (1994) *The Madness of King George*.

Chapman, A. (1997) 'Is multidisciplinary training possible?', in M. Marshall (ed.), *State of the Art in Dementia Care*. London: Centre for Policy on Ageing.

Charlton, D.G. (1959) *Positivist Thought in France During the Second Empire*. Oxford: Oxford University Press.

Cheung, S.Y. and Heath, A. (1994) 'After care: the education and occupation of adults of who have been in care', *Oxford Review of Education*, 20, 3, 361–374.

Childs, D.J. (2001) *Modernism and Eugenics*. Cambridge: Cambridge University Press.

Churchill, R., Hunot, V., Corney, R., Knapp, M. and McGuire, H. (2001) 'A systematic review of controlled trials of the effectiveness of cost-effectiveness of brief psychological treatments for depression', *Health Technology Assessment*, 5, 35, http://www.hta.ac.uk/project/1003.asp.

Cicchetti, D. and Rizley, R. (1981) 'Developmental perspectives on the etiology, inter-generational transmission, and sequelae of child maltreatment', *New Directions for Child Development*, 11, 31–55.

Cicchetti, D. and Schneider-Rosen, K. (1986) 'An organizational approach to childhood depression', in M. Rutter, C.E. Izard and P.B. Read (eds), *Depression in Young People: Developmental and Clinical Perspectives* (pp. 71–134). New York: Guilford Press.

Cicchetti, D. and Toth, S.L. (1997) 'Transactional ecological systems in developmental psycho-pathology', in S.S. Luthar, J.A. Burack, D. Cicchetti and J.R. Weisz (eds), *Developmental Psychopathology: Perspectives on Adjustment, Risk, and Disorder*. New York: Cambridge University Press.

Cicchetti, D. and Valentino, K. (2006) 'An ecological-transactional perspective on child maltreatment: failure of the average expectable environment and its influence on child development', in D. Cicchetti and D.J. Cohen (eds), *Developmental Psychopathology*. Vol. 3: *Risk, Disorder and Adaptation*. New York: John Wiley.

Cicchetti, D., Rogosch, F.A. and Toth, S.L. (2000) 'The efficacy of toddler-parent psychotherapy for fostering cognitive development in offspring of depressed mothers', *Journal of Abnormal Child Psychology*, 28, 2, 135–148.

Cicourel, A. (1968) *The Social Organization of Juvenile Justice*. London: Heinemann.

Cigno, K. and Bourne, D. (eds) (2000) *Cognitive Behavioural Social Work in Practice*. Aldershot: Ashgate/Arena.

Clare, J. (1065) *John Clare: selected poems edited by J. W. Tibble and Anne Tibble*. London: Dent.

Claridge, G. (1985) *Origins of Mental Illness*. Oxford: Blackwell.

Clark, H., Dyer, S. and Horwood, J. (1998) *'That Bit of Help': The High Value of Low Level Preventative Services for Older People*. London: The Policy Press.

Clark, H., Gough, H. and McFarlane, A. (2004). *Making Direct Payments Work for Older People: Findings*. York: Joseph Rowntree Foundation.

Clark, R.W. (1980) *Freud*. London: Jonathan Cape and Weidenfeld & Nicolson.

Clarke-Stewart, A. (1983) 'Exploring the assumptions of parent education', in R. Haskins and D. Adams (eds) *Parent Education and Public Policy*. Norwood, NJ: Ablex Publishing.

Cleary, M., Hunt, G., Matheson, S., Siegfried, N. and Walter, G. (2008) 'Psychosocial interventions for people with both severe mental illness and substance misuse', *Cochrane Database of Systematic Reviews*, Issue 1. Art. No. CD001088. DOI: 10.1002/14651858. CD001088.pub2. page 1.

Cleaver, H. (2000) *Fostering Family Contact*. London: The Stationery Office.

Clémant, M-E. and Tourginy, M. (1997) 'A review of the literature on the prevention of child abuse and neglect: characteristics and effectiveness of home visiting programs', *International Journal of Child and Family Welfare*, 1, 6–20.

Clough, R., Bullock, R. and Ward, A. (2006) *What Works in Residential Child Care: A Review of Research Evidence and the Practical Considerations*. London: National Children's Bureau.

Clout, H. and Wood, P. (1986) *London: Problems of Change*. Harlow: Longman.

Clyde, J. J. (1992) *Report of the Inquiry into the Removal of Children from Orkney in February 1991*. Edinburgh: HMSO.

Cobb, R. (1997) *The End of the Line*. London: John Murray.

Cochrane, A.L. (1973) *Effectiveness & Efficiency: Random Reflections on Health Services*. London: Nuffield Provincial Hospitals Trust.

Cocker, C. and Allain, L. (2007) *Social Work with Looked After Children*. Exeter: Learning Matters.

Cohen, A. R. (1964) *Attitude Change and Social Influence*, New York: Basic Books.

Cohen, A. R. (1985) *The Symbolic Confirmation of Communities*. London: Tavistock.

Cohen, J. (1999) 'Does voluntary association make democracy work?', in S. Smelser and J. Alexander (eds), *Diversity and its Discontents: Cultural Conflict and Common Ground in Contemporary American Society*. New Haven, CT: Yale University Press.

Cohen, J.A. and Mannarino, A.P. (1996) 'A treatment outcome study for sexually abused pre-school children: initial findings', *Journal of American Academy of Child and Adolescent Psychiatry*, 35, 42–50.

Cohn, A.H. (1986) 'Preventing adults from becoming sexual molesters', *Child Abuse and Neglect*, 10, 559–562.

Cole, G.D.H. and Postgate, R. (1966) *The Common People*. London: University Paperbacks.

Coleman, P. (1993) 'Psychological ageing', in J. Bond, P. Coleman and S. Peace (eds), *Ageing in Society* (2nd edn). London: Sage/Open University.

Collinshaw, S., Maughan, B. and Pickles, A. (1998) 'Infant adoption: psycho-social outcomes in adulthood', *Social Psychiatry and Psychiatric Epidemiology*, 33, 57–65.

Colton, M., Drury, C. and Williams, M. (1995a) 'Children in need: definition, identification and support', *British Journal of Social Work*, 25, 6, 711–728.

Colton, M., Drury, C. and Williams, M. (1995b) *Staying Together: Supporting Families under the Children Act.* Aldershot: Arena.

Commission for Social Care Inspection (2004) *Direct Payments. What are the Barriers?* London: CSCI.

Commission for Social Care Inspection (CSCI) (2005a) *Safeguarding Children: The Second Joint Chief Inspectors' Report on Arrangements to Safeguard Children* at www.safeguarding children.org.uk.

Commission for Social Care Inspection (2005b) *The State of Social Care in England 2004–2005.* London: CSCI.

Commission for Social Care Inspection (CSCI) (2006a) *Supporting Parents, Safeguarding Children: Meeting the Needs of Parents with Children on the Child Protection Register.* London: CSCI.

Commission for Social Care Inspection (CSCI) (2006b) *Time to Care? An Overview of Home Care Services for Older People in England.* London: CSCI.

Commission for Social Care Inspection (CSCI) (2006c) *Making Choices: Taking Risks.* London: CSCI.

Commission for Social Care Inspection (CSCI) (2008) *The State of Social Care in England (2006–2007).* London: CSCI.

Conte, J.R. and Schuerman, J.R. (1987) 'Factors associated with an increased impact of child sexual abuse', *Child Abuse and Neglect*, 11, 201–212.

Cook, W.L. (2001) 'Interpersonal influence in family systems: a social relations model analysis', *Child Development*, 72, 1179–1197.

Cooley, C.H. (1909) *Social Organization: A Study of the Larger Mind.* New York: Scribner's.

Cooper, B. and Picton, C. (2000) 'The long term effects of relocation on people with an intellectual disability: quality of life, behaviour, and environment', *Research on Social Work Practice*, 10, 2, 195–208.

Corcoran, J. (2006) 'Therapeutic interventions with children who have experienced sexual and physical abuse in the US', in C. McAuley, P.J. Pecora and W. Rose (eds) *Enhancing the Well-being of Children and Families through Effective Interventions: International Evidence for Practice.* London: Jessica Kingsley.

Corrigan, P. and Leonard, P. (1978) *Social Work Practice Under Capitalism: A Marxist Approach.* London: Macmillan.

Cottrell, D. and Boston, P. (2002) 'Practitioner review: the effectiveness of systemic family therapy for children and adolescents', *Journal of Child Psychology and Psychiatry and Allied Disciplines*, 43(5), 573–586.

Cover-Jones, M. (1924) 'A laboratory study of fear: the case of Peter', *Pedagogical Seminary*, 31, 308–375.

Cox, M.J. and Paley, B. (1997) 'Families as systems', *Annual Review of Psychology*, 48, 243–267.

Craighead, W.E., Craighead, L.W. and Llardi, S. (1998) 'Psycho-social treatments for major depressive disorder', in P.E. Nathan and J.M. Gorman (eds) *Treatments that Work.* Oxford: Oxford University Press.

Crawford, A. and Newburn, T. (2003) *Youth Offending and Restorative Justice: Implementing Reform in Youth Justice.* Cullompton, Devon: Willan.

Crimmins, D.B., Bradlyn, A.S., St Lawrence, J.S. and Kelly, J.A. (1984) 'A training technique for improving the parent–child interaction skills of an abusive-neglectful mother', *Child Abuse and Neglect*, 8, 533–539.

Crisp, A.H., Norton, K., Gowers, S., Halek, C., Bowyer, C., Yeldham, D., Levett, G. and Bhat, H. (1991) 'A controlled study of the effect of therapies aimed at adolescent and family psychopathology in anorexia nervosa', *British Journal of Psychiatry*, 159, 325–333.

Crittenden, P.M. (1981) 'Abusing, neglecting, problematic, and adequate dyads: differentiating by patterns of interaction', *Merrill-Palmer Quarterly*, 27, 201–218.

Cronin, A.J. (1932) *The Stars Look Down and The Citadel*. London: Orion.

Culp, R.E., Little, V., Letts, D. and Lawrence, H. (1991) 'Maltreated children's self-concept: effects of a comprehensive treatment program', *American Journal of Orthopsychiatry*, 61, 114–121.

Culp, R.E., Richardson, M.P. and Heide, J. (1987) 'Differential developmental progress of maltreated children in day treatment', *Social Work*, November–December, 497–499.

Curtis, N.M., Ronan, K.R. and Borduin, C.M. (2004) 'Multisystemic treatment: a meta-analysis of outcome studies', *Journal of Family Psychology*, 18, 3, 411–419.

D'Onofrio, B.M., Slutske, W.S., Turkheimer, E., Emery, R.E., Harden, K.P., Heath, A.C., Madden, P.A.F. and Martin, N.G. (2007) 'Intergenerational transmission of childhood conduct problems: a children of twins study', *Archives of General Psychiatry*, 64, 7, 820–829.

Dalley, G. (1989) 'Professional ideology or organisational tribalism? The health service–social work divide', in R. Taylor and J. Ford (eds) *Social Work and Health Care*, 102–117. London: Jessica Kingsley.

Dalley, G. (1993) 'Professional ideology or organisational tribalism? The health service-social work divide', in J. Walmsley, J. Reynolds, P. Shakespeare and R. Woolfe (eds), *Health, Welfare and Practice: Reflecting on Roles and Relationships*, 32–39. Buckingham: Open University Press.

Dalrymple, J. (1994) 'Devils Island: what really happened on the Orkneys', London: *Sunday Times*, 27 February.

Dangerfield, G. (1935) *The Strange Death of Liberal England*. New York: H. Smith & R. Hass.

Daniels, M. and Hill, H.B. (1952) 'Chemotherapy of pulmonary tuberculosis in young adults: an analysis of three Medical Research Council trials', *British Medical Journal*, 1, 1162.

Darley, J.M. and Batson, C.D. (1973) '"From Jerusalem to Jericho": a study of situational and dispositional variables in helping behaviour', *Journal of Personality and Social Psychology*, 27, 1, 100–108.

Darlington, Y., Feeney, J.A. and Rixon, K. (2005) 'Practice challenges at the intersection of child protection and mental health', *Child and Family Social Work*, 10, 239–247.

Daro, D. (1988) *Confronting Child Abuse*. New York: New York Free Press.

Davey-Smith, G. and Egger, M. (1986) 'Commentary: Understanding it all – health meta-theories and mortality trends', *British Medical Journal*, 313, 1584–1585.

Davies, B., Fernández, J-L., with Nomer, B. (2000). *Equity and Efficiency Policy in Community Care*. Aldershot: Ashgate.

Davies, M. (2000) *The Blackwell Encyclopaedia of Social Work*. Oxford: Blackwell.

Davies, M. (2008) *The Blackwell Companion to Social Work*. Oxford: Wiley-Blackwell.

Davies, S., Thornicroft, G., Leese, M., Higginbottom, H. and Phelan, M. (1996) 'Ethnic differences in compulsory psychiatric admission among representative cases of psychosis in London', *British Medical Journal*, 312, 533–537.

Dawkins, R. (1976) *The Selfish Gene*. Oxford: Oxford University Press.

Dawkins, R. (2003). *A Devil's Chaplain*. London: Weidenfeld & Nicolson.

Day Lewis, C. (1963) *Collected Poems of Wilfred Owen*. London: Chatto & Windus.

Deblinger, E., Lippman, J.T. and Steer, R. (1996) 'Sexually abused children suffering post-traumatic stress symptoms: initial treatment outcomes findings', *Child Maltreatment*, 4, 1, 13–20.

Deegan, P.E. (1992) 'The independent living movement and people with psychiatric disabilities: taking back control over own lives', *Psychosocial Rehabilitation Journal*, 15, 3, 3–19.

Dennett, D.C. (1991) *Consciousness Explained*. London: Allen Lane.

Dennett, D.C. (1996) *Kinds of Minds: Towards an Understanding of Consciousness*. London: Weidenfeld & Nicolson.

Dennett, D.C. (2003) *Freedom Evolves*. London: Allen Lane.

Dennett, D.C. (2006) *Breaking the Shell*. London: Allen Lane.

Department of Children, Families and Skills (2006) *Care Matters: Transforming the Lives of Children and Young People in Care*. London: The Stationery Office.

Department of Health (1989a) *An Introduction to the Children Act 1989*. London: HMSO.

Department of Health (1989b) *Caring for People: Community Care in the Next Decade and Beyond*. Cmnd 849. London: Department of Health.

Department of Health (1998a) *Modernising Social Services: Promoting Independence, Improving Protection, Raising Standards*. London: The Stationery Office.

Department of Health (1998b) *The Quality Protects Programme: Transforming Children's Services*. Local Authority Circular, 98, 28.

Department of Health (1999) *Caring about Carers: A National Strategy for Carers*. London: Department of Health. Available online at: www.dh.gov.uk/assetRoot/04/04/93/23/04049323.pdf (accessed 4 November 2005).

Department of Health (2000a) *Framework for the Assessment of Children in Need and their Families*. London: Department of Health, Department for Education and Employment, Home Office.

Department of Health (2000b) *Assessing Children in Need and their Families: Practice Guidance*. London: The Stationery Office.

Department of Health (2001a) *Treatment Choice in Psychological Therapies and Counselling*. London: Department of Health. www.doh.gov.uk/mentalhealth/treatmentguideline.

Department of Health (2001b) *The National Service Framework for Older People*. London: HMSO.

Department of Health (2001c) *Valuing People: A New Strategy for Learning Disability for the 21st Century*. London: HSMO.

Department of Health (2001d) *Intermediate Care*, HSC2001/01: LAC (2001). London: Department of Health.

Department of Health (2002) *Fair Access to Care Services: Guidance on Eligibility for Adult Social Care*. Local Authority Circular, LAC, 13.

Department of Health (2003a) *Choice Protects: Improving Placement Quality and Choice*. London: Department of Health.

Department of Health (2003b) *The Community Care (Delayed Discharges etc) Act 2003: Guidance for Implementation*, HSC2003/009: LAC (2003) 21. London: Department of Health.

Department of Health (2004) *National Service Framework for Children, Young People and Maternity Services*. London: Department of Health.

Department of Health (2005) *Independence, Well-being and Choice: Our Vision for the Future of Social Care for Adults in England*. London: The Stationery Office.

Department of Health (2006) *Our Health, Our Care, Our Say: A New Direction for Community Services*. London: Department of Health.

Department of Health (2007a) *National Evaluation of Partnerships for Older People Projects: Interim report of progress*. London: Department of Health.

Department of Heath (2007b) *Modernising Adult Social Care – What's working*. London: Department of Health.

Department of Health Act (1999) Partnership arrangements. Available online at: www. dh.gov.uk/PolicyAndGuidance/OrganisationPolicy/IntegratedCare/HealthAct1999Part nershipArrangements/fs/en (accessed June 2008).

Department of Health, Home Office, Department for Education and Skills and Department for Culture, Media and Sport (2007) *Safe, Sensible, Social: The Next Steps for the National Alcohol Strategy*. London: Department of Health and Home Office.

Department of Health, Social Services and Public Safety (2008) *Looked After Children*. http://www.dhsspsni.gov.uk/statistics_and_research-cib_looked-after-children (accessed June 2008).

DfES (2005a) *Every Child Matters – Change for Children and 4 Sector Specific Guides*. London: Department for Education and Skills.

DfES (2005b) *Statutory Guidance on the Role and Responsibilities of the Director of Children's Services and the Lead Member for Children's Services*. London: Department for Education and Skills.

DfES (2005c) *Statutory Guidance on Inter-Agency Co-operation to Improve the Wellbeing of Children: Children's Trust Arrangements*. London: Department for Education and Skills.

DfES (2005d) *Guidance on Children and Young People's Plan*. London: Department for Education and Skills.

DfES (2005e) *Lead Professional Good Practice Guidance*. London: Department for Education and Skills.

DfES (2005f) *Common Assessment Framework: Implementation Guidance*. London: Department for Education and Skills.

DfES (2005g) *Multi-agency Working Toolkit*. London: Department for Education and Skills.

DfES (2005h) *The Children's Workforce Strategy*. London: Department for Education and Skills.

DfES (2006) *Information Sharing: Practitioners' Guide*. London: Department of Education and Skills.

DfES (2007) *Statutory Guidance on Making Arrangements to Safeguard and Promote the Welfare of Children under Section 11 of the Children Act 2004*. London: Department of Education and Skills.

Déscartes, R. (1637) 'Optics', in P.J. Olscamp (trans.) (1965), *Discourse on Methods, Optics, Geography and Meteorology*. Indianapolis: Library of Liberal Arts, Bobbs-Merril.

Déscartes, R. (1664) *Traitè de L'Homme*, trans. T.S. Holt. Cambridge: Cambridge University Press.

Déscartes, R. (1667) *The Passions of the Soul*. Cambridge: Cambridge University Press (1985 edn).

Dickens, C. (1852/1971) *Bleak House*. Harmondsworth: Penguin.

Dix, T. (1991) 'The affective organization of parenting: adaptive and maladaptive processes', *Psychological Bulletin*, 110, 1, 3–25.

Dixon, J., Lee, J., Wade, J., Byford, S. and Weatherly, H. (2004) *Young People Leaving Care: An Evaluation of Costs and Outcomes*. Report to Department for Education and Skills. York: University of York.

Dixon, N. (1976) *On the Psychology of Military Incompetence*. London: Macmillan.

Dobson, B. and Middleton, S. (1998) *Paying to Care: The Cost of Childhood Disability*. York: Joseph Rowntree Foundation.

Dobson, K. (1989) 'A meta-analysis of the efficacy of cognitive therapy for depression', *Journal of Consulting and Clinical Psychology*, 57, 414–419.

Dodge, K.A. (1991) 'The structure and function of reactive and proactive aggression', in D.J. Pepler and K.H. Rubin (eds) *The Development and Treatment of Childhood Aggression*. Hillsdale, NJ: Lawrence Erlbaum.

Dodge, K.A. and Coie, J.D. (1987) 'Social information processing factors in reactive and proactive aggression in children's peer groups', *Journal of Personality and Social Psychology*, 53, 1146–1158.

Dodge, K.A. and Schwartz, D. (1997) 'Social information processing mechanisms in aggressive behavior', in D.M. Stoff, J. Breiling and J.D. Maser (eds) *Handbook of Antisocial Behavior*. New York: Wiley.

Doel, M. and March, P. (1992) *Task-centered Social Work*. London: Ashgate.

Domassio, A.R. (1995) *Déscartes' Error*. London; Picador.

Donaldson, M. (1978) *Children's Minds*. London: Fontana Press. New York: Dover Publications.

Dorrell, S. (1997) Secretary of State for Health and Social Services in *The Times*, 14 June.

Dowling, M. (1998) *Poverty*. Birmingham: Venture Press.

Dowson, J.H. and Grounds, A.T. (1995) *Personality Disorders: Recognition and Clinical Management*. Cambridge: Cambridge University Press.

Draaisma, D. (2004) *Why Life Speeds Up When you Get Older*. Cambridge: Cambridge University Press.

DSM IV TR (2000) *Diagnostic and Statistical Manual of Mental Disorders*, Fourth Edition. Washington DC: American Psychiatric Association.

Durkheim, E. (1893/1933) *The Division of Labour in Society*. New York: Free Press.

Egan, K. (1983) 'Stress management with abusive parents', *Journal of Clinical Child Psychology*, 12, 292–299.

Egeland, B., Sroufe, L.A. and Erickson, M. (1983) 'The developmental consequences of different patterns of maltreatment', *Child Abuse and Neglect*, 7, 459–469.

Emerson, E., Barrett, S., Bell, C., Cummings, R., McCool, C., Toogood, A. and Mansell, J. (1987) *Developing Services for People with Severe Learning Difficulties and Challenging Behaviours*. Canterbury: Institute of Social and Applied Psychology.

Engels, F. (1844) *The Condition of the Working Class in England*. Rheinische Zeitunung, No. 359 (in German), trans. F.K. Wischenewetzkj (1892). London: Allen & Unwin.

England, H. (1986) *Social Work as Art: Making Sense of Good Practice*. London: Routledge.

Esbensen, F-A. and Weerman, F. (2005) 'Youth gangs and troublesome youth groups in the United States and the Netherlands', *European Journal of Criminology*, 2, 1, 5–37.

Etzioni, A. (1964) *Modern Organizations*. London: Prentice Hall.

Evans, R.J. (1976) 'Some implications of an integrated model of social work for theory and practice', *British Journal of Social Work*, 6, 2, 177–200.

Evers, C. (2007) 'Carer support and empowerment', *Psychiatry*, 7, 2, 80–83.

Everson, M.D., Hunter, W.M., Runyan, D.K., Edelsohn, G.A. and Coulter, M.L. (1989) 'Maternal support following disclosure of incest', *American Journal of Orthopsychiatry*, 59, 197–207.

Eysenck, H.J. (1965) *Fact and Fiction in Psychology*. Harmondsworth: Penguin.

Eysenck, H.J. (1976) *Experimental Studies of Freudian Theories*. London: Methuen.

Eysenck, H.J. (1985) *The Decline and Fall of the Freudian Empire*. Harmondsworth: Penguin.

Eysenck, H.J. (1991) *The Decline and Fall of the Freudian Empire*. New York: Penguin.

Eysenck, M. and Keane, M.T. (1990) *Cognitive Psychology*. London: Lawrence Erlbaum Associates.

Falloon, I.R.H. and Coverdale, J.H. (1994) 'Cognitive-behavioural interventions for major mental disorders', *Behavioural Change*, II, 213–222.

Falloon, I.R.H., Boyd, J.L. and McGill, C.W. (1984) *Family Care of Schizophrenia*. New York: The Guilford Press.

Falloon, I.R.H., Krekorian, H., Shanahan, W.J., Laporta, M. and McLees, S. (1990) 'The Buckingham Project: a comprehensive mental health service based upon behavioural psychotherapy', *Behaviour Change*, 7, 51–57.

Fantuzzo, J.W. (1990) 'Behavioral treatment of the victims of child abuse and neglect', *Behavior Modification*, 14, 316–339.

Fantuzzo, J.W., Jurecic, L., Stovall, A., Hightower, A.D., Goins, C. and Schachtel, D. (1988) 'Effects of adult and peer social initiations on the social behavior of withdrawn, maltreated preschoolers', *Journal of Consulting and Clinical Psychology*, 56, 34–39.

Fantuzzo, J.W., Stovall, A., Schachtel, D., Coins, C. and Hall, R. (1987) 'The effects of peer social initiations on the social behavior of withdrawn maltreated preschool children', *Journal of Behavior Therapy and Experimental Psychology*, 18, 357–363.

Fantuzzo, J., Sutton-Smith, B., Meyers, R., Atkins, M., Stevenson, H., Cooolahan, K., Weiss, A. and Manz, P. (1996) 'Community based resilient peer treatment of withdrawn maltreated preschool children', *Journal of Consulting and Clinical Psychology*, 64, 6, 1377–1386.

Farmer, E. and Pollock, S. (1998) *Sexually Abused and Abusing Children in Substitute Care.* Chichester: Wiley.

Farmer, E., Moyers, S. and Lipscombe, J. (2004) *Fostering Adolescents.* Chichester: John Wiley.

Farrington, D.P. (1992) 'Juvenile delinquency', in J.C. Coleman (ed.) *The School Years* (2nd edition). London: Routledge.

Farrington, D.P. (2001) *Child Delinquents: Development, Intervention and Service Needs.* London: Sage.

Farrington, D.P. and Welsh, B.C. (2007) *Saving Children from a Life of Crime: Early Risk Factors and Effective Intervention.* Oxford: Oxford University Press.

Farrington, D.P. and West, D.J. (1993) 'Criminal, penal and life histories of chronic offenders: risk and protective factors and early identification', *Criminal Behaviour and Mental Health*, 3, 492–523.

Farrington, D.P., Barnes, G.C. and Lambert, S. (1996) 'The concentration of offending in families', *Legal and Criminological Psychology*, 1, 47–63.

Feilzer, M. and Hood, R. (2004) *Differences of Discrimination?* London: Youth Justice Board.

Feilzer, M., Appleton, C., Roberts, C. and Hoyle, C. (2002) *Cognitive Behavioural Projects in Youth Justice.* Oxford: Centre for Criminological Research, University of Oxford.

Feilzer, M., Appleton, C., Roberts, C. and Hoyle, C. (2004) *Cognitive Behaviour Projects: The National Evaluation Of The Youth Justice Board's Cognitive Behaviour Projects.* Oxford: Centre for Criminological Research.

Felce, D. (2000) *Quality of Life for People with Learning Disabilities in Supported Housing in the Community: A Review of the Research.* Centre for Evidence-based Social Services. Exeter: Exeter University.

Felce, D., Lowe, K., Perry, J., Baxter, H., Jones, E., Hallam, A. and Beecham, J. (1998) 'Service support to people in Wales with severe intellectual disability and the most severe challenging behaviours: processes, outcomes and costs', *Journal of Intellectual Disability Research*, 42, 5, 390–408.

Feldman, M.A. (1998) 'Parents with intellectual disabilities: implications and interventions', in J.R. Lutzker (ed.), *Handbook of Child Abuse Research and Treatment.* New York: Plenum Press.

Feldman, M. and Walton-Allen, N, (1997) 'Effects of maternal mental retardation and poverty on intellectual, academic, and behavioral status of school-age children', *American Journal On Mental Retardation*, 101, 352–364.

Feldman, M.A., Case, L. and Sparks, B. (1992a) 'Effectiveness of a child-care training program for parents at-risk for child neglect', *Canadian Journal of Behavioral Science*, 24, 14–28.

Feldman, M.A., Case, L., Garrick, M., MacIntyre-Grande, W., Carnwell, J. and Sparks, B. (1992b) 'Teaching child care skills to parents with developmental disabilities', *Journal of Applied Behavior Analysis*, 25, 205–215.

Feldman, M.A., Case, L., Rincover, A., Towns, F. and Betel, J. (1989) 'Parent education project 111. Increasing affection and responsivity in developmentally handicapped mothers: Component analysis, generalisation, and effects on child language', *Journal of Applied Behavior Analysis*, 22, 211–222.

Feldman, M.A., Léger, M. and Walton-Allen, N. (1998) 'Stress in mothers with intellectual disabilities', *Journal of Child and Family Studies*, 6, 471–485.

Feldman, M.A., Sparks, B. and Case, L. (1993) 'Effectiveness of home-based early intervention on the language development of children of mothers with mental retardation', *Research in Developmental Disabilities*, 14, 387–408.

Ferguson, N. (2003) *Empire: How Britain Made the Modern World*. London: Channel Four Books.

Fergusson, D.M. and Horwood, J. (2000) 'Alcohol abuse and crime: a fixed effects regression analysis', *Addiction*, 85, 10, 1525–1536.

Fernando, S. (2002) *Mental Health, Race and Culture*. London: Palgrave.

Ferster, C.B. and Skinner, B.F. (1957) *Schedules of Reinforcement*. New York: Appleton-Century Crofts.

Feske, U. and Chambers, D. (1995) 'Cognitive-behavioural versus exposure-only treatment for social phobia: a meta-analysis', *Behavioural Therapy*, 26, 695–720.

Festinger, L. (1957) *A Theory of Cognitive Dissonance*. Evanston, IL: Row Peterson.

Field, J. (2003) *Social Capital*. London: Routledge.

Finkelhor, D. and Strapko, N. (1992) 'Sexual abuse prevention education: a review of evaluation studies', in D.J. Willis, E.W. Holden and M. Rosenberg (eds), *Prevention of Child Maltreatment*. New York: Wiley.

Finkelstein, N. (1994) 'Treatment issues for alcohol- and drug-dependent pregnant and parenting women', *Health and Social Work*, 19, 7–15.

Fiorentine, R. (1999) 'After drug treatment: are Twelve-Step programs effective in maintaining abstinence?', *American Journal of Alcohol Abuse*, 25, 617–131.

Fiorentine, R. and Hillhouse, M.P. (2000) 'Exploring the additive effects of drug misuse treatment and Twelve-step involvement: does Twelve-step ideology matter?', *Substance use Misuse*, 35, 3, 367–397.

Fischer, J. (1973) 'Is casework effective?: A review', *Social Work*, 1, 107–110.

Fischer, J. (1976) *The Effectiveness of Social Casework*, Springfield, IL: Charles C. Thomas.

Fischer, J. (1993) 'Evidence-based practice: the end of ideology', *Journal of Social Science Research*, 18, 1, 19–64.

Fischer, J. and Corcoran, K. (1994) *Measures for Clinical Practice*, Vol. I. London: Free Press.

Fischer, J. and Corcoran, K. (1995) *Measures for Clinical Practice: A Sourcebook*, Vol. 2. London: Free Press.

Fisher, H., Montgomery, P. and Gardner, F. (2008) 'Opportunities provision for preventing youth gang involvement for children and young people aged 7–16'. *Cochrane Database of Systematic Reviews 2008*, Issue 2, Art. No. CD007002.

Fisher, M., Newton, C. and Sainsbury, E. (1984) *Mental Health Social Work Observed*. London: George Allen & Unwin.

Flemons, D.G., Green, S.K. and Rambo, A.H. (1995) 'Evaluating therapists' practices in a post-modern world: a discussion and a scheme', *Family Process*, 35, 1, 43–56.

Flood-Page, C., Campbell, S., Harrington, V. and Miller, J. (2000) *Youth Crime: Findings From the 1998/99 Youth Lifestyle Survey*. Home Office Research Study 209. London: Home Office.

Folkard, M.S., Smith, D.D. and Smith, D.E. (1976) *IMPACT, Home Office Research Studies II*. London: HMSO, No. 36.

Foot, M. (1962) *Aneurin Bevan*. London: MacGibbon & Kee.

Ford, J. (1976) *Paradigms and Fairy Tales*, Vol. 1. London: Routledge & Kegan Paul.

Ford, P. and Postle, K. (2000) 'Task-centered practice and care management', in P. Stepney and P. Ford, *Social Work Models, Methods and Theories.* Lyme Regis: Russell House.

Forder, J. and Netten, A. (2000) 'The price of placements in residential and nursing home care', *Health Economics*, 9, 7, 643–657.

Foucault, M. (1967) *Madness and Civilization: A History of Insanity in the Age of Reason.* London: Tavistock Publications

Frankl, V. E. (1963) *Man's Search for Meaning.* New York: Washington Square Press, Simon & Schuster.

Franklin, A. and Sloper, P. (2005) 'Listening and responding? Children's participation in health care within England', *International Journal of Children's Rights*, 13, 11–29.

Franklin, M.E. and Foa, E.B. (1998) 'Cognitive-behavioural treatments for obsessive compulsive disorder', in P.E. Nathan and J.M. Gorman, *A Guide to Treatments that Work.* Oxford: Oxford University Press.

Fraser, M.W., Pecora, D.A. and Haapala, D.A. (1991) *Families in Crisis: The Impact of Intensive Family Preservation Services.* New York: Aldine de Gruyter.

Freedman, J. and Combs, G. (1996) *Narrative Therapy: The Social Construction of Preferred Realities.* New York: Norton.

Freire, P. (1973) *Education for Critical Consciousness.* London: Sheed & Ward.

Freud, A. (1937) *The Ego and the Mechanisms of Defence*, London: Tavistock.

Freud, S. (1940/1949) *The Structure of Unconsciousness, An Outline of Psychoanalysis*, trans. J. Strachey. London and New York: Hogarth Press.

Friedman, A. S., Terras, A. and Glassman, K. (2002) 'Multimodel substance use intervention programme for male delinquents', *Journal of Child & Adolescent Substance Abuse*, 11, 4, 43–65.

Froggett, L. and Sapey, B. (1997) 'Communication, culture and competence in social work education', *Social Work Education*, 16, 1, 41–53.

Galassi, M.D. and Galassi, J.P. (1977) *Assert Yourself.* New York: Human Sciences Press.

Gambrill, E. (1994) What's in a name? Task-centered, empirical and behavioural practice', *Social Services Review*, December, 578–599.

Gambrill E.D. (1997) *Social Work Practice: A Critical Thinker's Guide.* New York: Oxford University Press.

Gambrill, E.P. (1997) *Controversial Issues in Social Work, Ethics, Values and Obligations.* London: Allyn & Baker.

Gambrill, E. and Schlonsky, A. (2001) 'The need for comprehensive risk management systems in child welfare', *Children and Youth Services Review*, 23, 1, 79–107.

Garbarino, J. (ed.) (1992) *Children and Families in the Social Environment*, 2nd edn. New York: Aldine de Gruyter.

Garcia Coll, C., Ackerman, A. and Cicchetti, D. (2000) 'Cultural influences on developmental processes and outcomes. Implications for the study of developmental psychology and psychopathology', *Development and Psychopathology*, 12, 333–356.

Garland, J.E. (2004) 'Facing the evidence: antidepressant treatment in children and adolescents', *Canadian Medical Journal*, 489–491.

Garvin, C. (1987) 'Developmental work for task-centered groupwork with chronic mental patients', *Social Work with Cramps*, 19, 3, 31–42.

Gaudin, J. (1993) 'Effective interventions with neglectful families', *Criminal Justice and Behavior*, 20, 66–89.

Gaudin, J., Wodarski, J.S., Arkinson, M.K. and Avery, L.S. (1990–1991) 'Remedying child neglect: effectiveness of social network interventions', *Journal of Applied Social Sciences*, 15, 97–123.

Geary, D.C. and Bjorklund, D.F. (2000) 'Evolutionary developmental psychology', *Child Development*, 71, 1, 55–65.

Gelder, M.G., Lopez-Ibor, J.J. and Andreasen, N. (2001) *New Oxford Textbook of Psychiatry.* Oxford: Oxford University Press.

Gelles, R.J. (1992) 'Poverty and violence toward children', *American Behavioural Scientists,* 35, 258–264.

Gendreau, P. and Ross, R. (1987) 'Revivication of rehabilitation: evidence from the 1980s', *Justice Quarterly,* 4, 3, 349–407.

General Social Care Council (2002) *Annual Report.* London: GSCC.

Geraedts, M., Heller, G. and Harrington, C. (2000). 'Germany's long-term care insurance: putting a social insurance model into practice', *The Millbank Quarterly,* 78, 3, 375–401.

Gershater-Molko, Ronit M., Lutzker, J.R. and Sherman, J.A. (2002) 'Intervention in child neglect: an applied behavioral perspective', *Aggression and Violent Behavior,* 7, 103–124.

Ghake. D. and Hazel, N. (2004) *Parenting in Poor Environments.* London: Jessica Kingsley.

Gibbs, L.E (1991) *Scientific Reasoning for Social Workers: Bridging the Gap between Research and Practice.* New York: Macmillan.

Gibson, F. (1997) 'Owning the past in dementia care: creative engagement with others in the present', in M. Marshall (ed.), *State of the Art in Dementia Care.* London: Centre for Policy on Ageing.

Gibson, M., Gregory, S. and Pandya, S. (2003) *Long-term Care in Developed Nations: A Brief Overview.* Washington, DC: AARP.

Gigerenzer, G. (2007) *Gut Feelings: The Intelligence of the Unconscious.* London: Allen Love.

Gilbert, P. (1992) *Depression: The Evolution of Powerlessness.* London: Lawrence Erlbaum.

Gilbert, P. (2003) *The Value of Everything: Social Work and its Importance in the Field of Mental Health.* Lyme Regis: Russell House Publishing.

Gilovich, T. (1991) *How We Know What Isn't So: The Fallibility of Human Reason in Everyday Life.* New York: The Free Press.

Ginzberg, K., Solomon, Z. and Bleich, A. (2002) 'Repressive coping style, acute stress disorder, and post traumatic stress disorder after myocardial infarction', *Psychosomatic Medicine,* 65, 95, 748.

Glasby, J. and Littlechild, R. (2002) *Social Work and Direct Payments.* Bristol: The Policy Press.

Glaser, D. (2000) 'Child abuse and neglect and the brain: a review', *Journal of Child Psychology and Psychiatry and Allied Professions,* 41, 1, 97–116.

Glendinning, C. (1986) *A Single Door.* London: Allen & Unwin.

Goddard, E. (1996) *Teenage Drinking in 1994.* London: HMSO.

Godfrey, M. (1999) *Preventive Strategies for Older People: Mapping the Literature on Effectiveness and Outcomes.* York: Joseph Rowntree Trust.

Godfrey, M. and Townsend, J. (2008) 'Older people in transition from illness to health: trajectories of recovery', *Qualitative Health Research,* 218, 7, 939–951.

Godfrey, M., Keen, J., Townsend, J., Moore, J., Ware, P., Hardy, B., West, R., Weatherley, H. and Henderson, K. (2005) *An Evaluation of Intermediate Care for Older People.* Leeds: Institute of Health Sciences and Public Research, University of Leeds.

Godfrey, M., Randall, T., Long, A. and Grant, M. (2000a) *Home Care: Review of Effectiveness and Outcomes.* CEBSS/Nuffield Institute for Health, University of Leeds/Health Care Practice R&D Unit, University of Salford.

Godfrey, M., Randall, T., Long, A. and Grant, M. (2000b) *Review of Effectiveness and Outcomes: Home Care.* Centre for Evidence-Based Social Services, University of Exeter,

Goldberg, D. and Huxley, P. (1992) *Common Mental Disorders: A Bio-social Model.* London and New York: Routledge.

Goldberg, E.M. (1970) *Helping the Aged.* London: George Allen & Unwin.

Goldstein, H. (1973) *Social Work Practice: A Unitary Approach.* Illinois: F.E. Peacock.

Goodman, G.S., Taub, E.P., Jones, D.P.H., England, P, Port, L.K., Ruby, L. and Prado, L.

(1992) 'Testifying in criminal courts: emotional effects of criminal court in child sexual assault', in *Monograph of the Society for Research in Child Development*, 57. Chicago, IL: University of Chicago Press.

Goodson, B.D., Layzer, J.I., St Pierre, R.G., Bernstien, L.S. and Lopez, M. (2000) 'Effectiveness of a comprehensive, five-year family support program for low-income children and their families: findings from the comprehensive child development program', *Early Childhood Research Quarterly*, 15, 1, 5–39.

Goodwin, D.W. (1981) *Alcoholism: The Facts*. Oxford: Oxford University Press.

Goodwin, F.K. and Redfield Jamison, K. (2004) *Manic Depressive Illness*. Oxford: Oxford University Press.

Gordon, D., Adelman, L., Ashworth, K., Bradshaw, J., Levitas, R., Middleton, S., Pantazis, C., Patsios, D., Payne, S., Townsend, P. and Williams, J. (2000) *Poverty and Social Exclusion in Britain*. York: Joseph Rowntree Foundation.

Gossop, M. (2006) *Treating Drug Misuse Problems: Evidence of Effectiveness*. London: National Treatment Agency for Substance Misuse.

Gossop, M., Marsden, J., Stewart, D. and Rolfe, A. (1999) 'Treatment retention and one-year outcomes for residential programmes in England', *Drug and Alcohol Dependence*, 57, 89–98.

Gossop, M., Marsden, J., Stewart, D., Lehman, P., Edwards, C., Wilson, A. and Segar, G. (1998) 'Substance use, health and social problems of clients at 54 drug treatment agencies: intake data from the National Treatment Outcome Study (NTORS)', *British Journal of Psychiatry*, 173, 166–171.

Gottesman, I.I. (1991) *Schizophrenia Genesis: The Origins Of Madness*. New York: Freeman.

Gottman, J.M., Katz, L.F., Swanson, C.C., Tyson, R. and Swanson, K.R. (2002) *The Mathematics of Marriage*. Cambridge, MA: MIT Press.

Gough, D.A. (1993) *Child Abuse Interventions: A Review of the Research Literature*. London: HMSO, University of Glasgow Public Health Research Unit.

Goulden, C. and Sondhi, A. (2001) *At the Margins: Drug Use by Vulnerable Young People in the 1998/99 Youth Lifestyles Survey*. Home Office Research Study 228. London: Home Office.

Grady, K.E. and Wallston, B.S. (1988) 'Research in health care settings', *Applied Social Research Methods Series*, Vol. 14. London: Sage.

Graham, J. and Bowling, B. (1995) *Young People and Crime*. London: Home Office.

Graham, P.J. (ed.) (2004) *Cognitive Behaviour Therapy for Children and Families*. Cambridge: Cambridge University Press.

Greco, V., Sloper, P., Webb, R. and Beecham, J. (2005) *An Exploration of Different Models of Multi-agency Partnerships in Key Worker Services for Disabled Children: Effectiveness and Costs*. DfES Research Report 656. DfES Publications, Nottingham.

Greene, J. and D'Oliveira, M. (1989) *Learning to Use Statistical Tests in Psychology*. Milton Keynes: Open University Press.

Greer, G. (1970) *The Female Eunuch*. London: MacGibbon & Kee.

Gregory, R.L. (1970) *The Intelligent Eye*. London: Weidenfeld & Nicolson.

Gregory, R.L. (1988) *Odd Perceptions*. New York: Routledge.

Griest, D.L. and Wells, K.C. (1983) 'Behavioral family therapy with conduct disorders in children', *Behavior Therapy*, 14, 38–43.

Griffiths, R. (1988) *Community Care: Agenda for Action: A Report to the Secretary of State for Social Services by Sir Roy Griffiths*. London: HMSO.

Grinnell, R.M. (1981) *Social Work Research and Evaluation*. Illinois: FE Peacock Publishers.

Grotevant, H. and McRoy, R. (1998) *Openness in Adoption: Exploring Family Connections*. Thousand Oaks, CA: Sage.

Gustaffson, P., Kjellman, N. and Cederbald, M. (1986) 'Family therapy in the treatment of severe childhood asthma', *Journal of Psychosomatic Research*, 30, 369–374.

Haapasalo, J. and Pokela, E. (1999) 'Child-rearing and child abuse antecedents of criminality', *Aggression and Violent Behavior*, 1, 107–127.

Hague, G. (2001) 'Multi-agency initiatives', in J. Taylor-Browne (ed.) *What Works in Reducing Domestic Violence*. London: Whiting and Birch.

Haley, J. (1976) *Problem Solving Therapy*. San Francisco, CA: Jossey Bass.

Hall, J.A., Schlesinger, D.J. and Dinees, J.P. (1997) 'Social skills training in groups with developmentally disabled adults', *Research on Social Work Practice*, 7, 187–201.

Halmos, P. (1965) *The Faith of Counselors*. London: Constable.

Halsey, A.H. and Webb, J. (eds) (2000) *Twentieth-century British Social Trends*, 3rd edition. Houdminlls, Basingstoke: Palgrave Macmillan.

Hammersley, R., Marsland, L. and Reid, M. (2003) *Substance Use by Young Offenders: The Impact Of The Normalisation Of Drug Use In The Early Years Of The 21st Century*. Home Office Research Study 261. London: Home Office Research and Statistics Directorate.

Hanifan, L.J. (1916) 'The rural school community centre', *The Annals of the American Academy of Political and Social Science*, 67, 1, 130–138.

Hardy, J.B. and Street, R. (1989) 'Family support and parenting education in the home: an effective extension of clinic-based preventive health care services for poor children', *Journal of Pediatrics*, 115, 927–931.

Hardy, T. (1906) *Far from the Madding Crowd*. London: Macmillan.

Harrington, R., Whittaker, J. and Shoebridge, P (1998) 'Psychological treatment of depression in children and adolescents. A review of treatment research', *British Journal of Psychiatry*, 173, 291–298.

Harrington, V. (2000) *Underage Drinking: Findings from the 1998/99 Youth Lifestyles Survey, Home Office Research Findings 125*. London: Home Office.

Harris, E.G. and Lindsay, C. (2002) 'How professionals think about contact between children and their birth parents', *Clinical Child Psychology and Psychiatry*, 7, 2, 147–161.

Harris, P. (1972) in K. Connolly (ed.), *Psychology Survey*. London: George Allen & Unwin.

Harrison, G., Holton, A., Neilson, D., Amas, D., Boot, D. and Cooper, J. (1989) 'Severe mental disorder in Afro-Caribbean patients: social, demographic and service factors', *Psychological Medicine*, 19, 683–696.

Hasler, F. (1993) Developments in the disabled people's movement, in J. Swain *et al. Disabling Barriers – Enabling Environments*. London: Sage.

Hasler, F., Campbell, J. and Zarb, G. (1999) *Direct Routes to Independence: A Guide to Local Authority Implementation and Management of Direct Payments*. London: Policy Studies Institute.

Hawton, K. and van Heerington, K. (eds) (2002) *The International Handbook of Suicide and Attempted Suicide*. Chichester: John Wiley.

Hayden, C. (2004) 'Parental substance misuse and child care social work: research in a city social work department in England', *Child Abuse Review*, 13, 18–30.

Hayes, H. (2007) 'Reoffending and restorative justice', in G. Johnstone and D.W. Van Ness (eds) *Handbook of Restorative Justice*. Cullompton: Willan Publishing.

Heatherington, E.M. and Park, R.D. (1986) *Child Psychology* (3rd edn). London: McGraw Hill International.

Heffernan, J., Shuttlesworth, G. and Ambrosino, R. (1992) *Social Work and Social Welfare: An Introduction*. St Paul, MS: West Publishing.

Hegel, G.W.F. (1956) *Lectures on the Philosophy of History*, trans. J. Sibtree. New York: Dover.

Hendrick, H. (2006) 'Histories of youth crime and justice', in B. Goldson and J. Muncie (eds), *Youth Crime and Justice*. London: Sage.

Henggeler, S.W. and Borduin, C.M. (1995) 'Multisystemic treatment of serious juvenile offenders and their families', in I.M. Schwartz and P. AuClaire (eds) *Home-based Services for Troubled Children*. Lincoln: University of Nebraska Press.

Henggeler, S.W., Borduin, C.M. and Melton, G.B. (1991) 'Effects of multisystemic therapy on drug use and abuse in serious juvenile offenders: a progress report from two outcome studies', *Family Dynamics of Addiction Quarterly*, 1, 3, 51.

Henggeler, S.W., Clingempeel, W.G., Brondino, M. J. and Pickrel, S.G. (2002) 'Four-year follow-up of multisystemic therapy with substance abusing and dependent juvenile offenders', *Journal of the American Academy of Child & Adolescent Psychiatry*, 41, 868–874.

Henggeler, S.W., Schoenwald, S.K., Borduin, C.M., Rowland, M.D. and Cunningham, P.B. (1998) *Multisystemic Treatment of Anti-social Behavior in Children and Adolescents.* New York: Guilford Press.

Henwood, M. (ed.) (1994) *Hospital Discharge Workbook: A Manual on Hospital Discharge Practice.* London: Department of Health.

Henwood, M. (2001) *Future Imperfect?: Report of the King's Fund Inquiry into Care and Support Workers.* London: King's Fund.

Henwood, M. (2006) 'Effective partnership working: a case study of hospital discharge', *Health and Social Care in the Community*, 14, 5, 400–407.

Herbert, G., Townsend, J., Ryan, J., Wright, D., Ferguson, B. and Wishaw, G. (2000) *Rehabilitation Pathways for Older People: A Study of the Impacts of Rehabilitation Services and Social Care Networks on the Aftercare of Older People with Rehabilitation Needs.* Leeds: Nuffield Institute for Health.

Herbert, M. (1990) *Planning a Research Project: A Guide for Practitioners and Trainers in the Helping Professions.* London: Gaskell.

Hersen, N. and Barlow, P. (1976) *Single Case Experiment Designs.* New York: Pergamon.

Hester, M., Pearson, C. and Harwin, N. (2007) *Making an Impact: Children and Domestic Violence. A Reader* (2nd edn). London: Jessica Kingsley.

Hetterna, J., Steele, J. and Miller, W.R. (2005) 'Motivational interviewing', *Annual Review of Clinical Psychology*, April, 1, 91–111.

Hewitt, D. (2004) 'Human rights and mental health', in T. Ryan and J. Pritchard, *Good Practice in Adult Mental Health.* London: Jessica Kingsley.

Hiddum, D.C. and Brown, R.W. (1956) 'Verbal reinforcement and interview bias', *Abnormal and Social Psychology* 50, 3, 108–111.

Hinshaw, S., Klein, R. and Abikoff, H. (1998) 'Childhood attention deficit hyperactivity disorder; nonpharmacological and combination approaches', in P. Nathan and J. Gorman (eds) *A Guide to Treatments that Work.* New York: Oxford University Press.

Hirschi, T. (1969) *Causes of Delinquency.* Berkeley, CA: University of California Press.

Hirst, M. and Baldwin, S. (1994) *Unequal Opportunities; Growing Up Disabled.* London: HMSO.

HM Treasury, Department of Health (2002) *Tackling Health Inequalities: 2002 Cross-cutting Review.* London: Stationery Office.

Hogg, J. (2005) 'Assessment method and professional directions', in N. Malin (ed.), *Services for People with Learning Disabilities.* London: Routledge.

Hollis, F. (1964) *Casework, A Psycho-social Therapy.* New York: Random House.

Hollon, D., Shelton, R.C. and Loosen, P.T. (1991) 'Cognitive therapy and pharmacotherapy for depression', *Journal of Consulting and Clinical Psychology*, 59, 88–89.

Holman, R. (1987) 'Research from the underside', *British Journal of Social Work*, 17, 669–683.

Holman, R. (1992) *Family Centres, Highlight, III.* London: National Children's Bureau.

Holman, R. (1995) *The Evacuation: A Very British Revolution.* Oxford: Lion.

Holman, R. (1999) *The New Welfare. Ending Child Poverty*, ed. R.E. Walker. Bristol: The Policy Press.

Homans, G. (1967) *The Nature of Social Science.* New York: Harcourt, Brace & World.

Home Office (2004) *Developing Domestic Violence Strategies – A Guide for Partnerships.* London: Violent Crime Unit.

Home Office (2005) *Juvenile Reconviction: Results from the 2003 Cohort*. London: Home Office Online report, July.

Home Office (2007) *Out of Crime, Into Treatment*. London: Home Office.

Hough, M., Clancy, A., McSweeney, T. and Turnbull, P.J. (2003) *The Impact of Drug Treatment and Testing Orders on Offending: Two-year Reconviction Results*. London: Home Office.

Housman, A.E. (1896) 'A Shropshire Lad', in *The Collected Poems of A.E. Housman*. London: Jonathan Cape.

Houts, A., Berman, J. and Abramson, H. (1994) 'Effectiveness of psychological and pharmacological treatments for nocturnal enuresis', *Journal of Consulting and Clinical Psychology*, 62, 737–745.

Howard, K.I., Kkapka, S.M., Krause, M.S. and Orlinsky, D.A. (1986) 'The dose-effect relationship in psychotherapy', *American Psychologist*, 41, 159–164.

Howe, D. (1995) *Attachment Theory for Social Work Practice*. Basingstoke: Macmillan.

Howe, D. (2006) *Child Abuse and Neglect: Attachment, Development and Intervention*. Basingstoke: Palgrave Macmillan.

Howell, E.M., Heiser, N. and Harrington, M. (1999) 'A review of recent findings on substance abuse treatment for pregnant women', *Journal of Substance Misuse Treatment*, 16, 3, 195–219.

Howitt, D. (1992) *Child Abuse Errors: When Good Intentions Go Wrong*. Hertfordshire: Harvester Wheatsheaf.

Huber, J. and Skidmore, P. (2003) *The New Old: Why Baby Boomers won't be Pensioned Off*. London: Demos.

Hudson, B. (2007) 'Diversity, crime and criminal justice', in M. Maguire, R. Morgan and R. Reinger (eds) *The Oxford Handbook of Criminology*. Oxford: Oxford University Press.

Hughes, B. (2007) Interview on the *Today* Programme, 28 August.

Human Psychiatric Association (1997) 'Practice guidelines for the treatment of patients with Alzheimer's Disease and other dementias of later life', *American Journal of Psychiatry*, 154, 1–39.

Humphries, C. and Stanley, N. (eds) (2006) *Domestic Violence and Child Protection*. London: Jessica Kingsley.

Hunt, J. (2003) *Family and Friends Care; Scoping Paper Prepared for the Department of Health*. London: Department of Health.

Hunt, J. and Macleod, A. (1999) *The Best-laid Plans: Outcomes of Judicial Decisions in Child Protection Cases*. London: The Stationery Office.

Hunt, P. (1966) *Stigma; The Experience of Disability*. London: Geoffrey Chapman.

Hutton, W. (1995) *The State We're In*. London: Vintage.

Iliffe, S. (1997) 'Problems in recognizing dementia in general practice: how can they be overcome?', in M. Marshall (ed.), *State of the Art in Dementia Care*. London: Centre for Policy on Ageing.

Information Centre (2005) Drug use, smoking and drinking among young people in England in 2005. http://www.ic.nhs.uk/pubs/youngpeopledruguse-smoking-drinking 2005.

Information Centre (2007) Statistics on drug misuse: England 2007. http://www.ic.nhs.uk/.

Iveson, C. (2002) 'Solution-focused brief therapy', *Advances in Psychiatric Treatement*, 8, 149–156.

Jack, G. (1997) 'An ecological approach to social work with children and families', *Child and Family Social Work*, 2, 109–120.

Jack, G. and Jack, D. (2000) 'Ecological social work: the application of a systems model of development in context', in P. Stepney and D. Ford (eds), *Social Work Models and Theories*. Lyme Regis: Russell House Publishers.

Jaffe, P., Wolfe, D.A. and Wilson, S. (1990) *Children of Battered Women*. Newbury Park, CA: Sage.

James, H. (2004) 'Promoting effective working with parents with learning disabilities', *Child Abuse Review*, 13, 31–41.

Jenkins, J., Felce, D., Toogood, A., Mansell, J. and de Kock, U. (1988) *Individual Programme Planning*. Kidderminster: British Institute of Mental Handicap.

Jenkins, S. and Rigg, J. (2003) 'Disability and disadvantage: selection, onset, and duration effects'. Working Papers of the Institute for Social and Economic Research, paper 2004–18. Colchester: University of Essex.

Joanning, H. (1992) 'Treating adolescent drug abuse: a comparison of family systems therapy, group therapy, and family drug education', *Journal of Marital and Family Therapy*, 18, 4, 345–356.

Johnson, M. (ed.) (2005) *The Cambridge Handbook of Age and Ageing*. Cambridge: Cambridge University Press.

Johnson, Z., Howell, F. and Molloy, B. (1993) 'Community mothers' programme: randomised controlled trial of non-professional intervention in parenting', *British Medical Journal*, 306, 1449–1452.

Johnstone, E.C., Deakin, J.F.W., Frith, C.D., Lawter, P., McPherson, K., Stevens, M. and Crow, T.J. (1980) 'The Northwick Park electro-convulsive therapy trial', *Lancet*, 20/27 December.

Johri, M., Beland, F. and Bergman, H. (2003). 'International experiments in integrated care for the elderly: A synthesis of the evidence', *International Journal of Geriatric Psychiatry*, 18, 3, 222–235.

Jones, L., Sumnall, J., Witty, K., Wareing, M., McVeigh, J. and Bellis, M.A. (2006) *A Review of Community-based Interventions to Reduce Substance Misuse Among Vulnerable and Disadvantaged Young People*. Liverpool: Collaborating Centre for Drug Prevention, Centre for Public Health, Liverpool John Moores University.

Jones, W.C. and Borgatta, E.F. (1972) 'Methodology of evaluation', in E.J. Mullen and J.R. Dumpson (eds), *Evaluation of Social Intervention*. San Francisco, CA: Jossey-Bass.

Jordan, B. (1995) 'Beyond offending behaviour', in M. Drakeford and M. Vasnstone (eds), *Poverty*. Aldershot: Ashgate Publishing.

Jordan, B. (1997) 'Social work and society', in M. Davies (ed.), *The Blackwell Companion to Social Work*. Oxford: Blackwell.

Jordan, B. (2004) *Sex, Money and Power: The Transformation of Collective Life*. Cambridge: Polity Press.

Jordan, W. (1996) 'Social work and society', in M. Davies (ed.), *The Blackwell Companion to Social Work*. Oxford: Blackwell.

Joseph Rowntree Foundation (2005) *That Bit of Help – Conference and Handouts*. York: JRF.

Joseph, S., Williams, R. and Yule, W. (1995) 'Psycho-social perspectives on post-traumatic stress', *Clinical Psychology Review*, 15, 515–544.

Juby, H. and Farrington, D.P. (2001) 'Disentangling the link between disrupted families and delinquency', *British Journal of Criminology*, 41, 22–40.

Julie, H. (2006) 'Labour child policies is flawed', *Sunday Times*, 17 September, p.12.

Kahneman, D. and Tversky, A. (1972) 'Subjective probability: a judgement of representativeness', *Cognitive Psychology*, 3, 237–251.

Katz, L., Robinson, C. and Spoonemore, N. (1994) 'Concurrent planning: from permanency planning to permanency action'. Seattle, WA7 Lutheran Social Services of Washington and Idaho.

Kavanagh, D.J. (1992) 'Recent developments in expressed emotion and schizophrenia', *British Journal of Psychiatry*, 160, 601–620.

Kazdin, A.E. (1994) 'Anti-social behaviour and conduct disorder', in L.W. Craighead,

E.W. Craighead, A.E. Kazdin and M.K. Mahoney (eds), *Cognitive and Behavioural Intervention: An Empirical Approach to Mental Health Problems*, A Longwood Professional Book. Massachusetts: Allyn & Bacon.

Kazdin, A.E (1998) 'Psychological treatments for conduct disorder in children', in P. Nathan and J. Gorman (eds) *A Guide to Treatments that Work*. New York: Oxford University Press.

Kazdin, A.E (2003) 'Psychotherapy for children and adolescents', *Annual Review of Psychology*, 54, 253–276.

Kazi, M. and Wilson, J.T. (1996) 'Applying single-case evaluation methodology in a British social work agency', *Research on Social Work Practice*, 6, 5–226.

Kenny L. and Kenny, B. (2000) 'Psychodynamic theory in social work. A view from practice', in P. Stepney and D. Ford (eds), *Social Work Models, Methods and Theories*. Lyme Regis: Russell House Publishing.

Kershaw, C., Chivite-Matthews. N., Thomas, C. and Aust, R. (2001) *The British Crime Survey*. London; Home Office.

Kick, P.E. and McElroy, S.L. (1998) 'Pharmacological treatment of Bipolar Disorder', in P.E. Nathan and J.M. Gorman, *Treatments that Work*. Oxford: Oxford University Press.

Kingsley, C. (1848) 'Letters to the Chartists No.2', *Politics for the People*, 3.

Kingsley, C. (1863) *The Water Babies*. London: Macmillan.

Kinship Care Alliance (2007) *The Role of the State in Supporting Relatives Raising Children who Cannot Live with their Parents*. A policy response from the Kinship Care Alliance to the *Care Matters* Green Paper: *Transforming the Lives of Children and Young People in care*. May. At http://www.frg.org.uk/pdfs/FINAL%20070520%20_2.pdf.

Kipling, R. (1885) *'If': The Definitive Edition of Rudyard Kipling's Verse*. London: Hodder & Stoughton.

Kirk, S.A. and Reid, W.J. (2002) *Science and Social Work: A Critical Appraisal*. New York: Columbia University Press.

Knight, S.H. (1921) *Uncertainty and Profit*. New York: Essential Reprints.

Koch, H.W. (ed.) (1972) *The Origins of the First World War: Great Power Rivalry + German War Aims*. London; Basingstoke: Macmillan.

Koenen, K.C., Caspi, A., Moffit, T.E., Rijsdijk, F. and Taylor, A. (2006) 'Genetic influences on the overlap between low IQ and antisocial behavior in young children', *Journal of Abnormal Psychology*, Nov, 115, 4, 787–797.

Kopelowicz, A. and Liberman, R.P. (1995) 'Behavioural treatment and rehabilitation of schizophrenia', *Harvard Review of Psychiatry*, 3, 55–64.

Kopelowicz, A. and Liberman, R.P. (1998) 'Pychosocial treatments of schizophrenia', in P.E. Nathan and J.M. Gorman, *A Guide to Treatments that Work*. Oxford: Oxford University Press.

Kownacki, R.J. and Shadish, W.R. (1999) 'Does Alcoholics Anonymous work: the results from a meta-analysis of controlled experiments', *Substance Use and Misuse*, 34, 13, 1897–1916.

Krol, N., Morton, J. and De Bruyn, E. (2004) 'Theories of conduct disorder: a causal modelling analysis', *Journal of Child Psychology and Psychiatry*, 45, 4, 727–742.

Kuhn, T. (1970) *Structure of Scientific Revolutions*. Chicago, IL: University of Chicago Press.

Lahey, B.B., Waldman, I.S. and McBurnett, K. (1999) 'Annotation: the development of antisocial behavior: an integrative causal model', *Journal of Child Psychology and Psychiatry*, 40, 5, 669–682.

Laing, R.D. (1960) *The Divided Self*. Harmondsworth: Penguin.

Laing, R.D. (1972) *Knots*. Harmondsworth: Penguin.

Laing, R.D. and Esterson, H. (1979) *Sanity, Madness and the Family*. London: Tavistock.

Laming, Lord (2003) *The Victoria Climbié Inquiry: Report of an Enquiry*. London: HMSO.

Langan, M. and Lee, P. (1989) *Social Work Today*. London: Unwin Hyman.

Langley, J. (2001) 'Developing anti-oppressive empowering social work practice with older lesbian women and gay men', *British Journal of Social Work*, 31, 917–932.

Larkin, P. (1974) 'Annus Mirabillis', in *Collected Poems*. London: Faber.

Larkin, P. (2003) 'The Old Fools', in *Collected Poems*. London Faber.

Laub, J.H. and Sampson, R.J. (2001) 'Understanding desistance from crime', in M. Tonry (ed.), *Crime and Justice: A Review of Research*, 28, 1–70.

Lazarus, R.S. and Folkman, S. (1984) *Stress, Appraisal and Coping*. New York: Springer.

Ledwith, M. (2003) *Community Development, A Critical Approach*. Birmingham: Venture Press.

Lee, D.T.F., Woo, J. and Mackenzie, A.E. (2002) 'A review of older people's experiences with residential care placement', *Journal of Advanced Nursing*, 37, 19–27.

Leece, D. and Leece, J. (2006) 'Direct payments: creating a two-tiered system in social care?', *British Journal of Social Work*, 36, 1379–1393.

Leece, J. (2004) 'Money talks, but what does it say? Direct payments and the commodification of care', *Practice: The Journal of the British Association of Social Workers*, 16, 3, 211–21.

Leff, J. (ed.) (1997) *Care in the Community: Illusion or Reality?* Chichester: Wiley.

Leff, J. and Trieman, N. (2000) 'Long stay patients discharged from psychiatric hospitals', *British Journal of Psychiatry*, 176, 217–223.

Leff, J., Kuipers, L., Bertowitz, R., Erberleien-Vries, R. and Sturgeon, D. (1982) 'A controlled trial of social intervention with schizophrenia patients', *British Journal of Psychiatry*, 141, 121–134.

Lehrman, L.J. (1949) *Success and Failure of Treatment of Children in Child Guidance Clinic of the Jewish Board of Guardians*. Research Monographs, I, New York: Jewish Board of Guardians.

Leonard, H.L. and Bernstein, A. (1960) *The Anatomy of Psychotherapy*. New York: Colombia University Press.

Lester, D. (2000) *Why People Kill Themselves: A 2000 Summary of Research on Suicide*. London: Charles C. Thomas.

Levy, P. (1987) *If This is a Man*. London: Abacus.

Lewinsohn, P. and Gotliz, I.H. (1995) 'Behavioural theory and the treatment of depression', in E.E. Becker and W. Leber (eds), *Handbook of Depression*. New York: The Guilford Press.

Lewinsohn, P., Clarke, G. and Hops, H. (1990) 'Cognitive behavioural treatment for depressed adolescents', *Behaviour Therapy*, 21: 385–401.

Lewinsohn, P., Clarke, G. and Rohde, T. (1996) 'A course in coping: a cognitive behavioural approach to the treatment for depression', in E. Hibbs and P. Jensen (eds) *Psychosocial Treatments for Child and Adolescent Disorders*. Washington, DC: American Psychiatric Association (APA).

Lewinsohn, P.M., Steinmetz, J.L., Larson, D.W. and Franklin, J.L. (1981) 'Depression-related cognitions: antecedent or consequence?', *Journal of Abnormal Psychology*, 90, 213–219.

Lewis, J. and Glennerster, H. (1996) *Implementing the New Community Care*. Philadelphia, PA: Open University Press.

Lewis, R.A., Piercy, F.P. and Sprenkle, D.H. (1990) 'Family-based interventions for helping drug-abusing adolescents', *Journal of Adolescent Research*, 5, 1, 95.

Liabo, K., Newman, T., Stephens, J. and Lowe, K. (2001) *A Review of Key Worker Systems for Disabled Children and the Development of Information Guides for Parents, Children and Professionals*. Cardiff: Office of R&D for Health and Social Care.

Liddle, H. and Dakof, G. (1995) 'Efficacy of family therapy for drug abuse: promising but not definitive', *Journal of Marital and Family Therapy*, 21, 511–543.

Liddle, H.A., Dakof, G.A. and Parker, K. (2001) 'Multidimensional family therapy for adolescent drug abuse: results of a randomized clinical trial', *American Journal of Drug and Alcohol Abuse*, 27, 4, 651–688.

Liddle, H.A., Rowe, C.L. and Dakof, G.A. (2004) 'Early intervention for adolescent substance abuse: pretreatment to posttreatment outcomes of a randomized clinical trial comparing multidimensional family therapy and peer group treatment', *Journal of Psychoactive Drugs*, 36, 1, 49–63.

Lipsey, M.W. and Landenberger, N.A. (2006) 'Cognitive-behavioural interventions', in B.C. Welsh and D.P. Farrington (eds), *Preventing Crime: What Works for Children, Offenders, Victims, and Places*. Dordrecht: Springer.

Littell, J.H., Popa, M. and Forsythe, B. (2005) 'Multisystemic therapy for social, emotional, and behavioral problems in youth aged 10–17', *Cochrane Database of Systematic Reviews*, Issue 4. Art. No.: CD004797. DOI: 10.1002/14651858.CD004797.pub4.

Lloyd, L. (2006) 'A caring profession? The ethics of care and social work with older people', *British Journal of Social Work*, 36, 7, 1171–1185.

Local Government Management Board (LGMB)/Central Council for Education and Training in Social Work (CCETSW) (1997) *Human Resources for Personal Social Services: From Personnel Administration to Human Resources Management*. London: LGMB.

Loch, C.S. (1883) *The Friendly Visitor*. New York: Russell Sage.

Loeber, R. and Hay, D.F. (1994) 'Developmental approaches to aggression and conduct problems', in M. Rutter and D.F. Hay (eds), *Development Through Life: A Handbook for Clinicians*. Oxford: Blackwell Scientific.

Logan, J. and Smith, C. (1999) 'Adoption and direct post adoption contact', *Adoption and Fostering*, 23, 4, 48–59.

Lomax, T. and Ellis, A. (2002) *Buying Time: Study of the Effectiveness of a Rehabilitation Service for Elderly People*. Centre for Evidence-based Social Services, University of Exeter.

Lösel, F. and Beelmann, A. (2003) 'Effects of child skills training in preventing antisocial behaviour. A systematic review of randomized evaluations', *Annals of the American Society of Political and Social Science*, 587, 84–109.

Lösel, F. and Beelmann, A. (2006) 'Child social skills training', in B.C. Welsh and D.P. Farrington (eds), *Preventing Crime: What Works for Children, Offenders, Victims, and Places*. Dordrecht: Springer.

Lovering, K., Frampton, I., Crowe, B., Moseley, A. and Broadhead, M. (2006) *Emotional and Behavioural Difficulties*, 11, 2, 83–104.

Lucas, P.J., Dowling, S.F., Joughin, C., Laing, G., Mackintosh, K., Newbury, J., Logan, S., Petticrew, M., Shiell. A. and Roberts, H. (2007) 'Financial benefits to low income or socially disadvantaged families for child health outcomes in the developed world', *Cochrane Database of Systematic Reviews* 2008. Issue 2, Art. No. CD006358.

Lutzker, J.R. and Rice, J.M. (1984) 'Project 12-ways: measuring outcome of a large-scale in-home service for the treatment and prevention of child abuse and neglect', *Child Abuse and Neglect*, 8, 519–524.

Lymbery, M. (2005) *Social Work with Older People: Context, Policy and Practice*, London: Sage.

Lymbery, M. (2006) 'United we stand? Partnership working in health and social care and the role of social work in services for older people', *British Journal of Social Work*, 36, 1119–1134.

Macdonald, G.M. (1996) 'Evaluating the effectiveness of social intervention', in A. Oakley and H. Roberts (eds), *Evaluating Social Intervention*. Barkingside: SSRU/Barnardos.

Macdonald, G.M. (2001) *Effective Interventions for Child Abuse and Neglect, An Evidence-Based Approach to Assessment, Planning and Evaluation*. Chichester: John Wiley.

Macdonald, G.M. (2003) *Using Systematic Reviews to Improve Social Care*. London: SCIE.

Macdonald, G.M. and Kakavelakis, I. (2004) *Helping Foster Carers to Manage Challenging Behaviour. Evaluation of a Cognitive-Behavioural Training Programme for Foster Carers*. University of Exeter: Centre for Evidence-based Social Services.

Macdonald, G.M. and Macdonald, K.I. (1999a) 'Perceptions of risk', in P. Parsloe (ed.), *Risk Assessment in Social Care and Social Work*. London: Jessica Kingsley.

Macdonald, G.M. and Macdonald K.I. (1999b) 'Empowerment: a critical view', 50–78, in W. Shera and L.M. Wells (eds) *Empowerment Practice in Social Work: Developing Richer Conceptual Foundations*, Toronto: Canadian Scholars' Press.

Macdonald, G.M. and Roberts, H.H. (1995) *What Works in the Early Years?* Barkingside: Barnardos.

Macdonald, G.M. and Sheldon, B. (1992) 'Contemporary studies of the effectiveness of Social Work', *British Journal of Social Work*, 22, 615–643.

Macdonald, G.M. and Sheldon, B. (1997) 'Community services for the mentally ill: consumers' views', *International Journal of Social Psychiatry*, 43, 1, 35–55.

Macdonald, G.M. and Sheldon, B. (1998) 'Changing one's mind: the final frontier?', *Issues in Social Work Education*, 18, 1, 3–25.

Macdonald, G.M. with Winkley, A. (1999) *What Works in Child Protection?* Barkingside: Barnardos.

Macdonald, G.M., Bennett, C., Dennis, J., Coren, E., Patterson, J., Astin, M. and Abbott, J. (2007) 'Home-based support for disadvantaged teenage mothers'. *Cochrane Database of Systematic Reviews*, Issue 3. Art. No.: CD006723. DOI: 10.1002/14651858.CD006723.

Mackaskill, C. (2002) *Safe Contact/Children in Permanent Placements and Contact with their Birth Relatives*. Lyme Regis, UK: Russell House.

MacMillan, H.L., MacMillan, J.H., Offord, D.R., Griffith, L. and MacMillan, A. (1994a) 'Primary prevention of child physical abuse and neglect: a critical review. Part 1', *Journal of Child Psychology and Psychiatry and Allied Professions*, 35, 5, 835–856.

MacMillan, H.L., MacMillan, J.H., Offord, D.R., Griffith, L. and MacMillan, A. (1994b) 'Primary prevention of child sexual abuse: a critical review. Part 2', *Journal of Child Psychology and Psychiatry and Allied Professions*, 35, 5, 857–876.

MacMillan, H.L., Thomas, B.H., Jamieson, E., Walsh, C.A., Boyle, M.H., Shannon, H.S. and Gafini, A. (2005) 'Effectiveness of home visitation by public-health nurses in prevention of child physical abuse and neglect : a randomized controlled trial', *Lancet*, 1786–1793.

Madame de Stael (1807) *Coreenne, Book 18*, ch. 5.

Maguin, E. and Loeber, R. (1996) 'Academic performance and delinquency', in M. Tonry and D.P. Farrington (eds), *Crime and Justice*, Vol. 20. Chicago, IL: University of Chicago Press.

Maguire, M. (2007) 'Crime data and statistics', in M. Maguire, R. Morgan and R. Reiner *The Oxford Handbook of Criminology* (4th edition). Oxford: Oxford University Press.

Malcolm, J.L. (1984) *In the Freud Archives*. London: Jonathan Cape.

Malepa, N.J. and Reid, W.J. (2000) *Integrating Case Management and Grief-treatment Strategies: A Hospital Based Geriatic Programme Social Work and Healthcare*, 31, 4, 1–23.

Maluccio, A. (1979) *Book-learning from Clients*. New York: Free Press.

Man, L. and Roe, S. (2006) *Drug Misuse Declared: Findings from the 2005/6 British Crime Survey Home Office Statistical Bulletin 15/06*. London: Home Office.

Mansell, J. and Beadle-Brown, J. (2004) 'Person-centred planning or person-centred action? Policy and practice in intellectual disability services', *Journal of Applied Research in Intellectual Disabilities*, 17, 1–9.

Manthorpe, J. and Cornes, M. (2005) 'Something to expect each day', *Community Care*, 8–14 December, 36–37.

Mao Zedong (1957) in *Quotations of Chairman Mao*, 1966.

Maria Colwell Report (1974) *Report of the Committee of Inquiry into the Care and Supervision Provided in Relation to Maria Colwell*. London: HMSO.

Marsh, P. (1997) 'Task centered work', in M. Davies (ed.), *The Blackwell Companion to Social Work*. Oxford: Blackwell.

Marsh, P. and Crow, G. (1998) *Family Group Conferences in Child Welfare*. Oxford: Blackwell Science.

Marsh, P. and Triseliotis, J. (1996) *Ready to Practise/Social Workers and Probation Officers: Their Training and Their First Year of Work*. Aldershot: Avebury.

Marshall, M. and Tibbs, M-A. (2006) *Social Work and People with Dementia: Partnerships, Practice and Persistence*. Bristol: B.A.S.W. Policy Press.

Marshall M, Gray A, Lockwood A, Green R. (1998) Case management for people with severe mental disorders. *Cochrane Database of Systematic Reviews* 1998, Issue 2. Art. No.: CD000050. DOI: 10.1002/14651858.CD000050.

Marx, K. (1887) *Das Kapital*, trans. F. Engels. Hamburg: Messner.

Masserman, J.H. (1943) *Behaviour and Neurosis*. Chicago, IL: University of Chicago Press.

Masson, J.M. (1985) *The Assault on Truth: Freud's Suppression of the Seduction Theory*. London: Penguin.

Mathers, C. (1999) 'International trends in health expectancies: do they provide evidence for expansion or compression of morbidity?', in *Compression of Morbidity (Department of Health and Aged Care Occasional Papers Series no 4)*. Canberra: Department of Health and Aged Care.

Mathias, J., Mertin, P. and Murray, A. (1995) 'The psychological functioning of children from backgrounds of domestic violence', *Australian Psychologist*, 30, 47–56.

Matrix Research and Consultancy and Institute for Criminal Policy Research (2007) *Evaluation of Drug Interventions Programme Pilots for Children and Young People: Arrest Referral, Drug Testing and Drug Treatment and Testing Requirements*. London: Home Office Research Development and Statistics Directorate. At http://www.homeoffice.gov.uk/rds.

Matthews, A.M., Gelder, G.G. and Johnson, D.W. (1981) *Agoraphobia: Nature and Treatment*. London: Tavistock.

Maughan, B. and Lindelow, M. (1997) 'Secular change in psychosocial risks: the case of teenage motherhood', *Psychological Medicine*, 27, 1129–1144.

Maughan, B., Collishaw, S. and Pickles, A. (1998) 'School achievement and adult qualifications among adoptees: a longitudinal study', *Journal of Child Psychology and Psychiatry*, 39, 5, 669–685.

Mayer, J.E. and Timms, N. (1970) *The Client Speaks: Working Class Impressions of Casework*. London: Routledge & Kegan Paul.

Maynard, A. and Chalmers, I. (1997) *Non-random Reflections on Health Services Research*. London: BMJ Publishing Group.

McCambridge, J. and Strang, J. (2004) 'The efficacy of single-session motivational interviewing in reducing drug consumption and perceptions of drug-related risk and harm among young people: results from a multi-site cluster randomized trial', *Addiction*, 99, 1, 39–52.

McCambridge, J. and Strang, J. (2005) 'Deterioration over time in effect of motivational interviewing in reducing drug consumption and related risk among young people', *Addiction*, 100, 4, 470–478.

McCord, J. (2000) 'Longitudinal analysis: an introduction to the special issue', *Journal of Quantitative Criminology*, 16, 2, 237–253.

McCord, J. (2003) 'Cures that harm. Unanticipated outcomes of crime prevention programs', *Annals of the American Society of Political and Social Science*, 587, 16–30.

McGillicuddy, N.B., Rychtarik, R.G. and Duquette, J.A. (2001) 'Development of a skill training programme for parents of substance-abusing adolescents', *Journal of Substance Abuse Treatment*, 20, 1, 59–68.

McGoldrick, M., Gerson, R. and Shellenberger, S. (1999) *Genograms: Assessment and Intervention* (2nd edition). New York: Norton.

McGuire, J. (ed.) (1995) *What Works in Reducing Reoffending*. London: Wiley.

McGuire, J. (2000) *Cognitive-behavioural Approaches. An Introduction to Theory and Research.* Liverpool: University of Liverpool.

McGuire, J. (2002) 'Integrating findings from research reviews', in J. McGuire (ed.), *Offender Rehabilitation and Treatment – Effective Programme and Policies to Reduce Offending.* Chichester: John Wiley.

McIvor, G. (1998) 'Pro-social modelling and legitimacy: lessons from a study of community service', in S. Rex and A. Matravers (eds), *Pro-social Modelling and Legitimacy: The Clark Hall Day Conference.* Cambridge: Institute of Criminology, University of Cambridge.

McIvor, G., Kemshall, H. and Levy, G. (2002) *Serious Violent And Sexual Offenders: The Use Of Risk Assessment Tools In Scotland.* Edinburgh: The Stationery Office.

McNeish, D., Newman, T. and Roberts, H. (eds) (2002) *What Works for Children?* Buckingham, PA: Oxford University Press.

Means, R. and Smith, R. (1998) *From Poor Law to Community Care* (2nd edition). Bristol: Policy Press.

Medewar, P. (1982) *Pluto's Republic.* London: Methuen.

Melechi, A. (2003) *Fugitive Minds: On Madness, Sleep and other Twilight Afflictions.* London: Heinemann.

Melton, G.B. (1992) 'The improbability of prevention of sexual abuse', in D. Willis, E.W. Holden and M. Rosenberg (eds), *Prevention of Child Maltreatment: Developmental Perspectives.* New York: John Wiley & Sons.

Merrell, C., Tymms, P. and Jones, P. (2007) *Changes in Children's Cognitive Development at the Start of School in England 2000-2006.* Durham: CEM Centre (http://www.cemcentre.org/).

Merrington, S. and Stanley, S. (2004) '"What works?": revisiting the evidence in England and Wales', *Probation Journal*, 51, 7, 7–20.

Mezey, G.C. and Bewley, S. (1997) 'Domestic violence and pregnancy', *British Medical Journal*, 314: 1295.

Middleton, L. (1995) *Making a Difference: Social Work with Disabled Children.* Birmingham: Venture Press.

Midgley, M. (1995) *Beastive Man.* London: Routledge.

Midgley, M. (2003) *The Myths We Live By.* London: Routledge.

Milford, H. (1913) *Prose and Poetry of William Morris (1865–1870).* Oxford: Oxford University Press.

Milgram, S. (1974) *Obedience to Authority.* London: Tavistock.

Milkowitz, D.J., Simoneau, T.C., Sachs-Erikson, N., Warner, R. and Suddarth, R. (1996) 'Family risk indicators in the course of bipolar affected disorder', in C. Mundt, M.J. Goldstein, K. Hahlweg and P. Fiedler (eds) *Interpersonal Factors in the Origin and Course of Affective Disorders*, 204–217. London: Gaskell Books.

Mill, J.S. (1859; 1971) *On Liberty.* London: Dent.

Miller, W.B. (1962) 'The impact of a total community control project', *Social Problems*, autumn, 168–191.

Mingay, G.E. (1976) *Rural Life in Victorian England.* London: Heinemann.

Minichiello, V., Browne, J. and Kendig, H. (2000) 'Perceptions and consequences of ageism: views of older people', *Ageing and Society*, 20, 3, 253–278.

Minuchin, P. (2002) 'Looking toward the horizon: present and future in the study of family systems', in J.P. McHale and W.S. Grolnick (eds), *Retrospect and Prospect in the Psychological Study of Families.* Mahwah, NJ: Erlbaum.

Mitchell, B. (2005) *The Boomerang Age: Transitions to Adulthood in Families.* London: Transaction Publishers.

Mitchell, M. and Jolley, J. (1988) *Research Design Explained.* London: Holt, Rinehart & Winston.

Modell, J. and Elder, G.H. (2002) 'Children develop in history: so what's new', in W.W. Hartup and R.A. Weinberg (eds), *Child Psychology in Retrospect and Prospect.* Mahwah, NJ: Erlbaum.

Moffitt, T.E. (1993) 'The neuropsychology of conduct disorder', *Development and Psychopathology,* 5, 135–152.

Moffitt, T.E., Lynam, D. and Sylva, P.A. (1994) 'Neuropsychological tests predict persistent male delinquency', *Criminology,* 32, 101–124.

Monck, E., Reynolds, J. and Wigfall, V. (2004) 'Using concurrent planning to establish permanency for looked after young children', *Child and Family Social Work,* 9, 4, 321–331.

Montgomery, B. (1948) *El Alemein to the River Sangro.* London: Hutchinson.

Moore, P. (1990) From Discovering Psychology Program 18 (PBS Video Series) Washington, DC: Annenberg/CPB program. See also, Zimbardo, P.G. Zimbardo, P. (2000) *Psychology and Life* (13th edition). New York: HarperCollins.

Morgan, R. (2005) *Children's Rights Report 2005 – What Inspectors Say About the Work of Services for Children Living Away from Home.* Newcastle: Office of the Children's Rights Director, Commission for Social Care Inspection.

Morgan, R. (2006). *About Social Workers: A Children's Views Report.* Newcastle: Office of the Children's Rights Director, Commission for Social Care Inspection.

Morris, J. (1998) *Don't Leave us Out: Involving Children and Young People with Communication Problems.* York: York Publishing Services.

Morris, J. (1999) *Hurtling into the Void. Transition to Adulthood for Young Disabled People with 'Complex Health and Support Needs'.* Brighton: Pavilion Publishing.

Morris, J. (2003) 'Including all children: finding out about the experiences of children with communication and/or cognitive impairments', *Children and Society,* 17, 337–348.

Morris, K. and Burford, G. (2007) 'Working with children's existing networks – building better opportunities?', *Social Policy and Society,* 6, 2, 209–217.

Mountain, G. (2000) *Occupational Therapy in Social Services Departments: A Review of the Literature.* London: CEBSS/College of Occupational Therapists.

Mullen, E.J. and Dumpson, J.R (eds) (1972) *The Evaluation of Social Intervention.* San Francisco, CA: Jossey-Bass.

Mullender, A. and Humphries, C. with Saunders, H. (1998) *Domestic Violence and Child Abuse: Policy and Practice Issues for Local Authorities and Other Agencies.* Local Government Association Briefing Paper from the Task Group on Domestic Violence and Child Abuse.

Müller-Oerlinghansen, Berghöfr, A. and Baner, M. (2002) 'Bi-polar disorder', *The Lancet,* 359, 19 January.

Muncie, J. (2004) *Youth and Crime: A Critical Introduction.* London: Sage.

Munro, E. (2005) 'What tools do we need to improve identification of child abuse?', *Child Abuse Review,* 14, 374–388.

Munroe, E. (2002) *Effective Child Protection.* London: Sage.

Nathan, P.E. and Gorman, J.M. (1998) *A Guide to Treatments that Work.* Oxford: Oxford University Press.

National Association of Social Workers (NASW) (2002) *Annual Report.* New York: NASW.

National Center for Health Statistics (NCHS) (2001) *International Classification of Diseases, Tenth Revision, Clinical Modification (ICD-10-CM).* Maryland: NCHS.

National Foster Care Association (NFCA) (2000a) *Family and Friends Carers' Handbook.* NFCA. London.

National Foster Care Association (NFCA) (2000b) *Family and Friends Carers: Social Workers' Training Guide.* NFCA. London.

National Institute for Clinical Exellence (NICE) (2002) *Appraisal Guidance No. 59:36.* Centre for Reviews and Dissemination, University of York.

National Institute for Clinical Excellence (NICE) (2007a) *Community-based Interventions to Reduce Substance Misuse among Vulnerable and Disadvantaged Children and Young People*: NICE Public Health Intervention Guidance No. 4. London: NICE.

National Institute for Clinical Excellence (NICE) (2007b) *Interventions to Reduce Substance Misuse among Vulnerable Young People. Costing Report*: Implementing NICE guidance. London: NICE.

National Probation Service (2004) *A Brief Introduction to Enhanced Community Punishment*. London: Home Office.

Neil, E. (2000) *Contact with Birth Relatives after Adoption: A Study of Young, Recently Placed Children*. Unpublished thesis, University of East Anglia.

Nelson, T.A. and Smock, S.A. (2005) 'Challenges of an outcome-based perspective for marriage and family therapy education', *Family Process*, 44, 3, 355–362.

Nelson-Zlupco, L., Kauffman, E. and Dore, M.M. (1995) 'Gender differences in drug addiction and treatment: implications for social work intervention with substance abusing women', *Social Work*, 40, 45–54.

Nemeroff, B. and Shatzberg, H.F. (1998) 'Pharmacological treatment of unipolar depression', in P.E. Nathan and J.M. Gorman (eds), *A Guide to Treatments that Work*. New York: Oxford University Press.

Newberger, C.M., Gremy, I.M., Waternaux, C.M. and Newberger, E.H. (1993) 'Mothers of sexually abused children: trauma and repair in longitudinal perspective', *American Journal of Orthopsychiatry*, 33, 92–102.

Newell, A. (1990) *Unified Theories of Cognition*. Cambridge, MA: Harvard University Press.

Nicol, A.R., Smith, J., Kay, B., Hall, D., Barlow, J. and Williams, B. (1988) 'A focused casework approach to the treatment of child abuse: a controlled comparison', *Journal of Child Psychology and Psychiatry*, 29, 5, 703–711.

Nixon, P. (2001) 'Making kinship partnerships work: examining family group conferences', in B. Broad (ed.), *Kinship Care: The Placement Choice for Children and Young People*. Lyme Regis: Russell House Publishing.

Nixon, P. (2007) *Seen but Not Heard? Children and Young People's Participation in Family Group Decision Making: Concepts and Practice issues*. At www.americanhumane.org/site/DocServer/PCNixon.pdf?docID=5721.

Nixon, P., Burford, G., Quinn, A. with Edelbaum, J. (2005) 'A survey of international practices, policy and research on family group conferencing and related practices', May. At www.americanhumane.org/site/DocServer/FGDM_www_survey.pdf?docID=2841.

Nocon, A. and Baldwin, S. (1998) *Trends in Rehabilitation Policy*. London: Audit Commission/King's Fund.

Northern Ireland Office (NIO) (2004) *Evaluation of Youth Justice Agency Community Services*. Northern Ireland: NIO Research and Statistical Series, Report No. 11.

O'Brien, J. and Lovett, H. (1992) *Finding a Way Towards Everyday Lives: The Contribution of Person Centered Planning*. Harrisburg, PA: Pennsylvania Office of Mental Retardation.

O'Neill, O. (2002) *A Question of Trust*. BBC Reith Lectures. Cambridge: Cambridge University Press.

O'Reilly, D. (2005) *Conduct Disorder and Behavioural Parent Training: Research and Practice*. London: Jessica Kingsley.

Oakley, A. (2000) *Experiments in Knowing: Gender and Method in the Social Sciences*. Cambridge: Polity Press.

Oates, R.K., Gray, J., Schweitzer, L., Kempe, R.S. and Harmon, R.J. (1995) 'A therapeutic preschool for abused children: The Keepsafe Project', *Child Abuse and Neglect*, 19, 11, 1379–1386.

Oates, R.K., O'Toole, N.I., Lynch, D.L., Stern, A. and Cooney, G (1994) 'Stability and change in outcomes for sexually abused children', *Journal of the American Academy of Child and Adolescent Psychiatry*, 33, 7, 945–953.

Office for National Statistics (2006) *Life Expectancy and Healthy Life Expectancy in Self-perceived Good or Fairly Good General Health 1981–2001*. Available online at: www.statistics.gov.uk/statbase/Expodata/Spreadsheets/D8486.xls (accessed June 2008).

Office of the Deputy Prime Minister (2006) *Making Life Better for Older People: An Economic Case for Preventative Services and Activities*. Wetherby: ODPM.

Office of the Deputy Prime Minister (ODPM) (2004) *Mental Health and Social Exclusions*. London: Social Exclusion Unit.

Olds, D. (1997) 'The Prenatal Early Infancy Project: preventing child abuse and neglect in the context of promoting child and maternal health', in D. A. Wolfe, R.J. McMahon and R. De V. Peters (eds) *Child Abuse: New Directions in Prevention and Treatment across the Lifespan*. Thousand Oaks, CA: Sage.

Olds, D. and Kitzman, H. (1990) 'Can home visiting improve the health of women and children at environmental risk?', *Pediatrics*, 86, 108–116.

Olds, D.L. and Kitzman, H. (1993) 'Review of research on home visiting', *The Future of Children*, 3, 4, 51–92.

Olds, D., Henderson, C., Chamberlain, R. and Tatelbaum, R. (1986) 'Preventing child abuse and neglect: a randomised trial of nurse home visitation', *Pediatrics*, 78, 65–78.

Olds, D., Henderson, C.R. and Kitzman, H. (1994) 'Does prenatal and infancy nurse home visitation have enduring effects on qualities of parental caregiving and child health and 25 to 50 months of life?', *Pediatrics*, 93, 89–98.

Olds, D., Henderson, C.R., Kitzman, H. and Cole, R. (1995) 'Effects of prenatal and infancy nurse home visitation on surveillance of child maltreatment', *Pediatrics*, 95, 365–372.

Olds, J. (1956) 'Pleasure centers in the brain', *Scientific American*, 195, 105–116.

Oliansky, D.M., Wildenhaus, K.J. and Manlove, K. (1997) 'Effectiveness of brief interventions in reducing substance use among at-risk primary care patients in three community-based clinics', *Substance Abuse*, 18, 3, 95–103.

Oliver, J. (1981) 'Behavioural treatment of obsessive-compulsive disorder', *International Journal of Behavioural Social Work*, 1, 1, 12–16.

Oliver, M. (1983) *Social Work with Disabled People*. Tavistock: Macmillan.

Oliver, M. (1996) *Understanding Disability: From Theory to Practice*. Basingstoke: Macmillan.

Oliver, M. and Barnes, C. (eds) (1998) *Disabled People and Social Policy: From Exclusion to Inclusion*. London: Longman.

Oliver, M. and Sapey, B. (2006) *Social Work with Disabled People* (3rd edition). London: Palgrave Macmillan.

Olsen, M.R. (ed.) (1984) *Social Work and Mental Health*. London: Tavistock.

Optimum Health Services NHS Trust (1999) *Young Adults Transitions Project*. London: Young Adults Transitions Project.

Osgood, D.W., Wilson, J.K., O'Malley, P.M., Bachman, J.G. and Jonston, L.D. (1996) 'Routine activities and individual deviant behavior', *American Sociological Review*, 61, 635–655.

Owen, W. (1916/1963) *Collected Poems of Wilfred Owen*. London: Chatto & Windus.

Oxman, N.D., Thompson, M.A., Davis, D.A. and Haynes, R.B. (1995) 'No magic bullets: a systematic review of 102 trials of interventions to improve professional practice', *Canadian Medical Association Journal*, 153, 10, 1123–1431.

Paine, T. (1791–1792) *The Rights of Man* (Parts 1 and II). Boston, MA: Thomas and Andrews. For a more accessible version see Paine, T. (1987) *The Rights of Man*. Harmondsworth: Penguin Classics.

Palazzoli, M.S., Boscolo, L., Cecchin, G. and Prata, G. (1978) *Paradox and Counter-paradox*. New York: Jason Aronson.

Palmer, C. (1999) *Evidence-based Briefing*. London: Royal College of Psychiatrists/Gaskel.

Pankhurst, C. (1959) *Unshackled: The Story of How We Won the Vote*. London: Hutchinson.

Parke, R.D. (2004) 'Development in the Family', *Annual Review of Psychology*, 55, 365–399.

Parke, R.D. and O'Neil, R. (1999) 'Social relationships across contexts: family–peer linkages', in W.A. Collins, B. Laursen (eds), *Minnesota Symposium on Child Psychology*. Hillsdae, NJ: Erlbaum.

Parker, G., Bhakta, P. and Karbamna, S. (2000) 'Best place of care for older people after acute, and during sub-acute illness: a systematic review', *Journal of Health Services Research and Policy*, 5, 3, 176–189.

Parker, H., Measham, F. and Aldridge, J. (1995) *Drugs Futures: Changing Patterns of Drug use Amongst English Youth*. London: Institute for the Study of Drug Dependence.

Parker, R. (1996) *Decision Making in Child Care: A Study of Prediction in Fostering*. London: Allen & Unwin.

Parkes, C.M. (1994) 'Bereavement as a psychosocial transition: processes of adaptation to change', in M.S. Stroebe and R.O. Hansson (eds), *Handbook of Bereavement: Theory, Research and Intervention*. Cambridge: Cambridge University Press.

Parsloe, P. (ed.) (2000) *Risk in Social Work and Social Care*. Basingstoke: Macmillan.

Parsons, M. and Starns, P. (1999) *The Evacuation: The True Story*, London: BBC Publications.

Parton, N. (1997) 'Child protection and family support: current debates and future prospects', in N. Parton (ed.), *Child Protection and Family Support: Tensions, Contradictions and Possibilities*. London: Routledge.

Parton, N. (1998) 'Risk, Advanced Liberalism and Child Welfare: The Need to Rediscover Uncertainty and Ambiguity', *British Journal of Social Work*, 28, 1, 5–28.

Patmore, C. (2002) *Towards Flexible, Person-centred Home Care Services: A Guide to Some Useful Literature for Planning, Managing or Evaluating Services for Older People*. York: SPRU.

Patterson, G.R. (1982) *A Social Learning Approach to Family Intervention: Coercive Family Process*. Eugene, OR: Castilia Publishing.

Patterson, G.R., Chamberlain, P. and Reid, J.B. (1982) 'A comparative evaluation of a parent training program', *Behavior Therapy*, 13, 638–650.

Pavlov, I.P. (1897/1928) *Lectures on Conditioned Reflexes*, trans. W.H. Gannt. New York: International.

Pavlov, I.P. (1927) *Conditioned Reflexes*, trans. G.V. Anrep. London: Oxford University Press.

Perlman, H.H. (1960) 'Are we creating dependancy?', *Social Service Review*, 34.

Pervin, L.A. (1989) *Personality: Theory and Research*. New York: John Wiley & Sons.

Petch, A. (1993) 'Intermediate care or integrated care: the Scottish perspective on support provision for older people', *Journal of Integrated Care*, 11, 6, 7–14.

Peterson, C., Maier, S.F. and Seligman, E.P. (1993) *Learned Helplessness: A Theory for the Age of Personal Control*. New York; Oxford: Oxford University Press.

Petrosino, A., Petrosino, C. and Finchenouer, J.O. (in press) 'Our well-meaning programs can have harmful effects! Lessons from the Scared Straight experiments', *Crime and Delinquency*. (Also via Campbell Collaboration's Social, Psychological, Educational and Criminological Trials Register C2-SPECTR.)

Petrosino, A., Turpin-Petrosino, C. and Buehler, J. (2002) 'The effect of Scared Straight and other "kids visit prisons" programmes on juvenile delinquency', *The Cochrane Database of Systematic Reviews*, Issue 2, Art No.: CD002796. DOI: 10.1002/14651858.CD002796.

Petrosino, A., Turpin-Petrosino, C. and Buehler, J. (2006) 'Scared Straight and other juvenile awareness programs', in B.C. Welsh and D.P. Farrington (eds), *Preventing Crime: What Works for Children, Offenders, Victims, and Places*. Dordrecht: Springer.

Pharoah, F., Mari, J., Rathbone, J. and Wong, W. (2006) Family intervention for schizophrenia. *Cochrane Database of Systematic Reviews* 2006, Issue 4. Art. No.: CD000088. DOI: 10.1002/ 14651858.CD000088.pub2.

Phillips, C. and Bowling, B. (2007) 'Ethnicities, racisms, crime and criminal justice', in M. Maguire, R. Morgan and R. Reiner (eds), *The Oxford Handbook of Criminal Justice* (4th edn). Oxford: Oxford University Press.

Piaget, J. (1929) *The Child's Conception of the World*, trans. J. Tomlinson and A. Tomlinson. London: Routledge & Kegan Paul.

Piaget, J. (1958) *The Child's Construction of the World*. London: Routledge & Kegan Paul.

Pilling, S., Bebbington, P., Kuipers, E., Garety, P., Geddes, J., Orbach, G. and Morgan, C. (2002a) 'Psychological treatments in schizophrenia: I. Meta-analysis of family interventions and cognitive behavioural therapy', *Psychological Medicine*, 32, 763–782.

Pilling, S., Bebbington, P., Kuipers, E., Garety, P., Geddes, J., Martindale, B. Orbach, G. and Morgan, C. (2002b) 'Psychological treatments in schizophrenia: I. Meta-analysis of social skills and cognitive remediation', *Psychological Medicine*, 32, 783–791.

Pincus, A. and Minahan, A. (1973) *Social Work Practice: Model and Method*. Illinois: F.E. Peacock.

Pinker, R. (1980) *Social Workers: Their Role and Tasks*. London: Bedford Square Press/National Institute for Social Work.

Pinker, R.A. (1982) 'Minority Report' (Appendix B), in Barclay Report, *Social Workers, Their Roles and Tasks*, London: Bedford Square Press.

Pinker, S. (2002) *The Blank Slate*. London: Allen Lane.

Piquero, A.R., Farrington, D.P. and Blumstein, A. (2007) *Key Issues in Criminal Career Research: New Analyses of the Cambridge Study in Delinquent Development*. Cambridge: Cambridge University Press.

Pirsig, R.M. (1974) *Zen and the Art of Motorcycle Maintenance*. London: Corgi.

Pitcher D. (1999a) *When Grandparents Care*. Plymouth: Plymouth City Council Social Services Department.

Pitcher D. (1999b): *Assessing Grandparents who Care: Plymouth's Framework for Assessing Grandparents who Care for their Grandchildren*. Plymouth: Plymouth City Council Social Services Department.

Plasse, B.R. (2000) 'Components of engagement: women in a psychoeducational parenting skills group in substance abuse treatment', *Social Work with Groups*, 22, 4, 33–50.

Plomin, R. (1994) 'The Emanuel Miller Memorial Lecture 1993: Genetic research and identification of environmental influences', *Journal of Child Psychology and Psychiatry*, 35, 5, 817–834.

Polster, R.A., Dangel, R.F. and Rasp, R. (1987) 'Research in behavioral parent training in social work: a review', *Behavior Modification*, 1, 323–350.

Poole, T. (2006a) *Direct Payments and Older People*. London: Kings Fund. Background paper: Wanless Social Care Review.

Poole, T. (2006b) *Dementia Care*. London: Kings Fund. Background paper: Wanless Social Care Review.

Poole, T. (2006c) *Telecare and Older People*. London: Kings Fund. Background paper: Wanless Social Care Review.

Popper, K. (1963) *Conjectures and Refutations*. London: Routledge & Kegan Paul.

Porter, R. (2000) *The Creation of the Modern World: The British Enlightenment*. New York: W.W. Norton.

Powers, E. and Witmer, H. (1951) *An Experiment in the Prevention of Delinquency – The Cambridge-Somerville Youth Study*. New York: Columbia University Press.

Powers, G.T., Meenagahn, T.M. and Toomey, B.G. (1985) *Practice Focused Research: Integrating Human Service Practice and Research*. Englewood Cliffs, NJ: Prentice-Hall.

Prendergast, M.L., Podus, D., Chang, E. and Urada, D. (2002) 'The effectiveness of drug abuse treatment: a meta-analysis of comparison group studies', *Drug and Alcohol Dependence*, 67, 53–72.

Preston, G. (2006) 'Families with disabled children, benefits and poverty', *Benefits*, 14, 1, 39–43.

Priestley, J.B. (1934) *An English Journey, Being a Rambling but Truthful Account of What One Man Saw and Heard and Felt and Thought During a Journey Through England During the Autumn of the Year 1933*. London: William Heinemann.

Prime Minister's Strategy Unit (2002) *Risks: Improving the Government's Capability to Handle Risk and Uncertainty*. London: Cabinet Office.

Prior, V. and Glaser, D. (2006) *Understanding Attachment and Attachment Disorders: Theory, Evidence and Practice*. London: Jessica Kingsley.

Pritchard, C. (2001) *A Family–Teacher–Social Work Alliance to Reduce Truancy and Delinquency – The Dorset Healthy Alliance Project*. RDS Occasional Paper No. 78. London: Home Office.

Proctor, H. (2003) 'Family therapy', in F. Fransella (ed.) *International Handbook of Personal Construct Psychology*. Chichester: John Wiley.

Putnam, R.P. (2000) *Bowling Alone: The Collapse and Revival of American Community*. New York: Simon & Schuster.

Quinton, D. (2004) *Supporting Parents: Messages from Research*. London: Jessica Kingsley.

Quinton, D. and Selwyn, J. (2006) 'Adoption in the UK: outcomes, influences and support', in C. McAuley, P. Pecora and W. Rose (eds) *Effective Interventions for Children and Families*. London: Jessica Kingsley.

Quinton, D., Rushton, A., Dance, C. and Mayes, D. (1997) 'Contact between children placed away from home and their birth parents: research issues and evidence', *Clinical Child Psychology and Psychiatry*, 2, 393–1045.

Quinton, D., Selwyn, J. Rushton, A. and Dance, C. (1999) 'Contact between children placed away from home and their birth parents: Ryburn's "Reanalysis" analysed', *Clinical Child Psychology and Psychiatry*, 4, 4, 519–532.

Rabbitt, P. (2005) 'Cognitive changes across the lifespan', in M. Johnson (ed.), *The Cambridge Handbook of Age and Ageing*. Cambridge: Cambridge University Press.

Rabiee, P., Sloper, P. and Beresford, B. (2005) 'Desired outcomes for children and young people with complex health care needs, and children who do not use speech for communication', *Health and Social Care in the Community*, 13, 5, 478–487.

Rachman, S.J. and Wilson, G.T. (1980) *The Effects of Psychological Therapy*. Oxford: Pergamon Press.

Radcliffe, R. and Hegarty, J.R. (2001) 'An audit approach to evaluating individual planning', *British Journal of Developmental Disabilities*, 47, 93, 87–97.

Ramsay, J., Rivas, C. and Feder, G. (2005) *Interventions to Reduce Violence and Promote the Physical and Psychosocial Well-being of Women who Experience Partner Violence: A Systematic Review of Controlled Evaluations*. London: Department of Health.

Raynor, P. and Vanstone, M. (1996) 'A reasoning and rehabilitation in Britain: the result of the straight thinking on probation (STOP) programme', *International Journal of Offender Therapy and Comparative Criminology*, 40, 279–291.

Read, J. (1996) *A Different Outlook: Service Users' Perspectives on Conductive Education*. Birmingham: Foundation for Conductive Education.

Read, J., Clements, L. and Ruebain, D. (2006) *Disabled Children and the Law: Research and Good Practice*. London: Jessica Kingsley.

Redfield Jamison, K. (1996) *Touched with Fire: Manic-depressive Illness and the Artistic Temperament*. Glasgow: Simon & Schuster.

Redfield Jamison, K. (1997) *An Unquiet Mind*. New York: Picador.

Reed, J. (1997) 'Risk assessment and clinical risk management: the lessons from recent inquiries', *British Journal of Psychiatry*, 170, suppl. 32, 4–7.

Reed, R. and Reed, S. (1965) *Mental Retardation: A Family Study*. New York: Saunders.

Rees, S. (1986) *Verdicts on Social Work* (2nd edn). London: Arnold.

Reid, W.J. (1978) *The Task-centered System*. New York: Columbia University Press.

Reid, W.J. (1992) *Task Strategies: An Empirical Approach to Clinical Social Work*. New York: Columbia University Press.

Reid, W.J. (1994) 'The Empiricial Practice Movement', *Social Service Review*, June, 65–184.

Reid, W.J. and Epstein, L. (1972) *Task-centered Casework*. New York: Columbia University Press.

Reid, W.J. and Hanraham, P. (1980) 'The effectiveness of social work: recent evidence', in E.M. Goldberg and N. Connolly (eds), *Evaluative Research in Social Care*. London: Heinemann Educational.

Reid, W.J. and Shyne, A.W. (1969) *Brief and Extended Casework*. New York: Columbia University Press.

Reiner, B. and Kaufmann, M. (1969) *Character Disorders in the Parents of Delinquents*. New York: Family Service Association of America.

Repetti, R. and Wood, J. (1997) 'Effects of daily stress at work on mothers' interaction with preschoolers', *Journal of Family Psychology*, 11, 90–108.

Reynolds, B. (1946) *An Uncharted Journey: Fifty Years Growth in Social Work*. New York: Citadel Press.

Rhee, S. and Waldman, I.D. (2002) 'Genetic and environmental influences on antisocial behavior: A meta-analysis of twin and adoption studies', *Psychologycal Bulletin*, 29, 490–529.

Richan, C. and Mendelsohn, A.R. (1973) *Social Work: The Unloved Profession*. New York: Franklin Watts.

Richardson, A., Budd, T., Engineer, R., Phillips, A., Thompson, J. and Nicholls, J. (2003) *Drinking, Crime and Disorder*. London: HMSO.

Richmond, M. (1917) *Social Diagnosis*. New York: Russell Sage Foundation.

Rispens, J., Aleman, A. and Goudena, P.P. (1997) 'Prevention of child sexual abuse victimzation: a meta-analysis of school programs', *Child Abuse and Neglect*, 21, 10, 975–987.

Rivers, W.H. (1922, Posthumous) *Conflict and Dreams*. London: Chatto & Windus.

Robbins, M.S., Szapocznik, J., Alexander, J.F., and Miller, J. (1998) 'Family systems therapy with children and adolescents', in M. Hersen and A.S. Bellack (series eds) and T.H. Ollendick, *Comprehensive Clinical Psychology: Vol. 5, Children and Adolescents: Clinical Formulation and Treatment*. Oxford: Elsevier Science, pp. 149–180.

Roberts, H. (1997) 'Children, inequalities and health', *British Medical Journal*, 314, 1122–1125.

Robertson, J., Emerson, E. and Hatton, C. (2005) *The Impact of Person-centred Planning*. Lancaster: Institute for Health Research, Lancaster University.

Robinson, J. and Banks, P. (2005) *The Business of Caring: King's Fund Inquiry into Care Services for Older People in London*. London: King's Fund.

Roe, S. and Man, L. (2006) *Drug Misuse Declared: Findings from the 2005/06 British Crime Survey*. London: Home Office.

Rogers, C.R. (1951) *Client-centred Therapy: Its Current Practice, Implications and Theory*. Boston, MA: Houghton Mifflin.

Rogers, C.R. (1961) *On Becoming a Person*. London: Constable.

Rogers, C.R. and Skinner, B.F. (1956) 'Some issues concerning the control of human behavior: a symposium', *Science*, 124, 3231, 1057–1066.

Rogers, L. (2006) 'Britons, the most stupid people in the Western world', *The Times*, 29 October, p. 13.

Rollinson, R., Smith, B., Steel. C., Jolley, S., Onwumere, J., Garety, P., Kuipers, E., Freeman, D., Bebbington, P., Dunn, G., Startup, M. and Fowler, D. (2008) 'Measuring adherence in

CBT for psychosis: a psychometric analysis of an adherence scale', *Behavioural and Cognitive Psychotherapy*, 36, 2, 163–178.

Rose, D., Fleischmann, P., Wykes, T., Leese, M. and Bindman, J. (2003) 'Patients' perspectives on electroconvulsive therapy: systematic review', *British Medical Journal*, 326, 1–5.

Rose, G. and Marshall T.M. (1975) *Counselling and Social Work: An Experimental Study.* London: John Wiley.

Rose, J. (2002) *Working with Young People in Secure Accommodation: From Chaos to Culture.* Hove: BrunerRoutledge.

Rosenhan, D.L. (1973) 'On being sane in insane places', *Science*, 179, 250–258.

Roth, A.D. and Pilling, S. (2008) 'Using an evidence-based methodology to identify the competencies required to deliver effective cognitive and behavioral treatment for depression and anxiety disorders', *Behavioral and Cognitive Psychology*, 36, 129–147.

Rowe, D.C. and Farrington, D.P. (1997) 'The family transmission of criminal convictions', *Criminology*, 35, 177–201.

Rowntree, B.S. (1901) *Poverty, A Study of Town Life.* London: Macmillan.

Royal College of Psychiatrists (1996) *Report of the Confidential Inquiry into Homicide and Suicide by Mentally Ill People.* London: Gaskell.

Royal College of Psychiatrists (2002) *Advice to Commissioners and Purchasers of Modern Substance Misuse Services.* London: Council Report CR100.

Royal College of Psychiatry (2003) *Employment Opportunities for People with Psychiatric Disability.* London: Royal College of Psychiatry.

Royal Commission on the Poor Laws Report (1909) London: UK Royal Commission.

Rushton, A. (2003) *The Adoption of Looked After Children: A Scoping Review.* London: Social Care Institute of Excellence.

Rushton, A. (2004) 'A scoping and scanning review of research on the adoption of children placed from public care', *Clinical Child Psychology and Psychiatry*, 9, 1, 89–106.

Rushton, A. and Dance, C. (2004) 'The outcomes of late permanent placements – the adolescent years', *Adoption and Fostering*, 28, 1, 49–58.

Rushton, A., Quinton, D., Dance, C. and Mayes, D. (1998) 'Preparation for permanent placement: evaluating direct work with older children', *Adoption and Fostering*, 21, 4, 41–48.

Russell, B. (1946) *History of Western Philosophy.* London: Unwin University Books.

Russell, G.F.M., Szmukler, G.I., Dare, C. and Eisler, I. (1987) 'An evaluation of family therapy in anorexia nervosa and bulimia nervosa', *Archives of General Psychiatry*, 44, 1047–1056.

Russell, P. (1991) 'Working with children with physical disabilities and their families – the social work role', in M. Oliver (ed.) *Social Work: Disabled People and Disabling Environments.* London: Jessica Kingsley.

Russell, P. (1998) *Having a Say: Disabled Children and Effective Partnership in Decision Making. Section 1: The Report.* London: Council for Disabled Children.

Russell, P. (2003) *Disabled Children, Their Families and Child Poverty.* London: Council for Disabled Children/End Child Poverty

Rutter, M. (1972) *Maternal Deprivation Reassessed.* Harmondsworth: Penguin.

Rutter, M. (2006) 'Is Sure Start an effective preventive intervention?', *Child and Adolescent Mental Health*, 11, 3, 135–141.

Rutter, M. (2007) 'Gene-environment interdependence', *Developmental Science*, 10, 1, 12–18.

Rutter, M. and Hersov, L. (eds) (1987) *Child and Adolescent Psychiatry: Modern Approaches.* Oxford: Blackwell Scientific.

Rutter, M. and Quinton, D.L. (1984) 'Parental psychiatric disorder; Effects on children', *Psychological Medicine*, 14, 853–880.

Rutter, M. and Sroufe, L.A. (2000) 'Developmental psychopathology: concepts and challenges', *Development and Psychopathology*, 12, 3, 265–296.

Rutter, M., Giller, H. and Hagell, A. (1998) *Antisocial Behaviour by Young People.* Cambridge: Cambridge University Press.

Rutter, M., Kim-Cohen, J. and Maughan, B. (2006a) 'Continuities and discontinuities in psychopathology between childhood and adult life', *Journal of Child Psychology and Psychiatry*, 44, 3/5, 276–295.

Rutter, M., Maughan, B., Meyer, J., Pickles, A., Silberg, J., Simonoff, E. and Taylor, E. (1997) 'Heterogeneity of antisocial behavior: causes, continuities and consequences', in R. Diensbier and D.W. Osgood (eds), Nebraska Symposium on Motivation, Vol. 44: *Motivation and Delinquency.* Lincoln: University of Nebraska.

Rutter, M., Moffitt, T.E. and Caspi, A. (2006b) 'Gene-environment interplay and psychopathology: multi varieties but real effects', *Journal of Child Psychology and Psychiatry*, 47, 3/4, 226–261.

Rutter, M., Taylor, E. and Hersov, L. (eds) (1994) *Child and Adolescent Psychiatry: Modern Approaches.* Oxford: Blackwell Scientific.

Ryburn, M. (1999) 'Contact between children placed away from home and their birth parents: a reanalysis of the evidence in relation to permanent placements', *Clinical Child Psychology and Psychiatry*, 4, 505–518.

Sackett, D.L., Rosenberg, W.M., Gray, J.H.M., Haynes, R.B. and Richardson, W.S. (1996) 'Evidence-based practice: what it is and what it isn't', *British Medical Journal*, 312, 7203, 71–72.

Salzberger-Wittenberg, I. (1970) *Psycho-analytic Insight and Relationships.* London: Routledge & Kegan Paul.

Sameroff, A.J. and Chandler, M.J. (1975) 'Reproductive risk and the continuum of caretaking casualty', in F.D. Horowitz (ed.), *Review of Child Development Research*, 4, 187, 244. Chicago, IL: University of Chicago Press.

Sanderson, H. (2000) *Person Centred Planning: Key Features and Processes.* York: Joseph Rowntree.

Sandifer, M.G., Pettus, C. and Quade, D. (1964) 'A study of psychiatric diagnosis', *Journal of Nervous and Mental Disease*, 139, 350–356.

Santisteban, D.A., Coatsworth, J.D. and Perez-Vidal, A. (2003) 'Efficacy of brief strategic family therapy in modifying Hispanic adolescent behavior problems and substance use', *Journal of Family Psychology:* Journal of the Division of Family Psychology of the American Psychological Association (Division 43), 17, 1, 121–133.

Scally, B.G. (1957) 'Marriage and mental handicap: some observations in Northern Ireland', in F.F. de la Cruz and G.D. La Veck (eds), *Human Sexuality and the Mentally Retarded.* New York: Brunner/Mazel.

Scheff, T.J. (1997) *Emotions, the Social Bond and Human Reality: Part/Whole Analysis.* Cambridge: Cambridge University Press.

Schofield, G. (2003) *Part of the Family: Pathways Through Foster Care.* London: BAAF.

Schutz, A. (1954) 'Concept and theory formation in the social sciences', *Journal of Philosophy*, 51, 9, 257–273.

Schwartz, W. (1969) *Private troubles versus public issues: one social work job or two?* The Social Welfare Forum, National Conference on Social Welfare (pp. 22–43). New York: Columbia University Press.

Schweinhart, L.J., Barnes, H.V. and Weikart, D.P. (1993) *The High/Scope Perry Preschool Study Through Age 27.* Ypsilanti, MI: The High/Scope Press.

Scott, M. (1989) *A Cognitive – Behavioural Approach to Client's Problems.* London: Tavistock.

Scott, S. (2001) 'Financial costs of social exclusion; follow up study of antisocial children into adulthood', *British Medical Journal*, July, 323, 191.

Scottish Executive (2006) *Looked After Children 2005–2006.* A Scottish Executive National Statistics Publication ISSN 1479-7569.

Scull, A. (1993) *The Most Solitary of Afflictions: Madness and Society in Britain, 1700–1900.* London: Yale University Press.

Seddon, D., Robinson, C., Reeves, C., Tommis, Y., Woods, B. and Russell, I. (2007) 'In their own right: translating the policy of carer assessment into practice', *British Journal of Social Work*, 37, 1335–1352.

Seebohm Report (1968) *Report of the Committee on Local Authority and Allied Personal Social Services*, Cmnd. 3703. London: HMSO.

Seed, P. (1973) *The Expansion of Social Work in Britain*. London: Routledge & Kegan Paul.

Seligman, M. (1975) *Helplessness*. San Francisco, CA: Freeman.

Seligman, M.E.P. (1971) 'Phobias and preparedness', *Behaviour Therapy*, 2, 1–22.

Selwyn, J., Frazer, L. And Quinton, D. (2006) 'Paved with good intentions: the pathway to adoption and the costs of delay', *British Journal of Social Work*, 36, 561–576.

Selwyn, J., Sturgess W., Quinton, D. and Baxter, K. (2003) *Costs and Outcomes of Non-infant Adoptions*. Report to the Department for Education and Skills/Department of Health.

Serketich, W.J. and Dumas, J.E. (1996) 'The effectiveness of behavioral parent training to modify antisocial behavior in children: a meta-analysis', *Behavior Therapy*, 27, 2, 171–186.

Shadish, W.R. and Baldwin, S.A. (2005) 'Effects of behavioral marital therapy: a meta-analysis of randomised controlled trials', *Journal of Consulting and Clinical Psychology*, B73, 1, 6–14.

Shadish, W.R., Montgomery, L.M., Wilson, P., Wilson, M.R., Bright, I. and Okwumabua, T. (1993) 'Effects of family and marital psychotherapies: a meta-analysis', *Journal of Consulting and Clinical Psychology*, 61, 992–1002.

Shakespeare, T. (2000) *Help*. Birmingham: Venture Press.

Shanks, D.R. (1995) *The Psychology of Associative Learning, Problems in the Behavioural Sciences*. Cambridge: Cambridge University Press.

Sharp, C. and Budd, T. (2005) Minority ethnic groups and crime: findings from the Offending, Crime and Justice Survey 2003. Home Office online report 33/05.

Sharma, A.R., McGue, M.K. and Benson, P. (1995) 'The emotional and behavioral adjustment of United States adopted adolescents – Part 11. Age at adoption', *Children and Youth Services Review*, 18, ½, 101–114.

Sheldon, B. (1977) 'Theory and practice in social work; a re-examination of a tenuous relationship', *British Journal of Social Work*, 8, 1, 1–22.

Sheldon, B. (1978) 'Social influence: social work's missing link', in M.R. Olsen (ed.), *The Unitary Model*. Birmingham: BASW Publications.

Sheldon, B. (1980) *The Use of Contracts in Social Work*. Birmingham: British Association of Social Work.

Sheldon, B. (1983a) 'The use of single case experimental designs in the evaluation of social work', *British Journal of Social Work*, 2, 1.

Sheldon, B. (1983b) 'Social workers: their role and tasks: a review', *British Journal of Social Work*, 16, 1, 590–595.

Sheldon, B. (1985) *Evaluation – Oriented Case – Recording, in Managing Information in Practice*. Edinburgh: Scottish Education Department/Social Work Services Group.

Sheldon, B. (1986) 'Social work effectiveness experiments: review and implications', *British Journal of Social Work*, 16, 223–242.

Sheldon, B. (1987a) 'The psychology of incompetence', in G. Drewry, B. Martin and B. Sheldon (eds), *After Beckford: Essays on Child Abuse*. Egham, Surrey: Royal Holloway and Bedford New College.

Sheldon, B. (1987b) 'Implementing the findings of social work effectiveness research', *British Journal of Social Work*, 17, 573–586.

Sheldon, B. (1989) *Studies of the Effectiveness of Social Work.* Ph.D. Thesis, University of Leicester.

Sheldon, B. (1994a) 'Biological and social factors in mental disorders: implications for services', *International Journal of Social Psychiatry*, 40, 87–105.

Sheldon, B. (1994b) 'Social work effeciveness research: implications for probation and juvenile justice services', The *Howard Journal of Criminal Justice*, Vol. 33, No. 3, August. Oxford: Blackwell Publishers for The Howard League

Sheldon, B. (1995) *Cognitive Behavioural Therapy: Research, Practice and Philosophy.* London: Routledge.

Sheldon, B. (2001) 'The validity of evidence-based practice in social work: a reply to Stephen Webb', *British Journal of Social Work*, 31, 801–809.

Sheldon, B. and Baird, P. (1978) 'The use of closed circuit television in the training of social workers', *Social Work Today.* 11, 18, 4–8.

Sheldon, B. and Baird, P. (1982) 'The use of closed circuit television in training social workers', *Social Work Today*, 14, 3.

Sheldon, B. and Chilvers, R. (2000) *Evidence-based Social Services: Prospects and Problems.* University of Exeter.

Sheldon, B. and Macdonald, G.M. (1996) *The Sutton Sponsored Day-care Project.* Centre for Evidence-based Social Service, University of Exeter.

Sheldon, B. and Macdonald, G.M. (1999) *Research and Practice in Social Care: Mind the Gap.* Centre for Evidence-based Social Services, University of Exeter.

Sheldon, B., Ellis, A., Moseley, A. and Tierney, S. (2004) *Evidence-based Social Care: An Update of Prospects and Problems.* A follow-up to the survey by Sheldon and Chilvers (2000).

Sheldon, B., Ellis, A., Moseley, A. and Tierney, S. (2005) 'A pre-post empirial study of opportunities for, and obstacles to, evidence-based practice in social care', in A. Bilson (ed.), *Evidence-based Practice in Social Care.* London: Whiting & Birch.

Shields, J. and Slater, E. (1967) 'Genetic aspects of schizophrenia', *Hospital Medicine*, 1967, 579–584.

Shenger-Kristovnikova, N.R. (1921) 'Contributions to the question of diffferentiation of visual stimuli and the limits of differentiation by the visual analyser of the dog', *Bulletin of the Institute of Science*, 3.

Simey, T.S. and Simey, M.B. (1960) *Charles Booth – Social Scientist.* Oxford: Oxford Univerity Press.

Simons, K. and Watson, D. (1999) *New Directions: Day Services for People with Learning Disabilities in the 1990s: A Review of the Research.* Centre for Evidence-based Social Services, University of Exeter.

Sinclair, I. (2006) 'Residential care in the UK', in C. McAuley, P. Pecora and W. Rose *Enhancing the Well-being of Children and Families through Effective Interventions.* London: Jessica Kingsley.

Sinclair, I. and Gibbs, I. (1998) *Children's Homes: A Study in Diversity.* Chichester: Wiley.

Sinclair, I., Gibbs, I. and Wilson, K. (2004) *Foster Carers: Why They Stay and Why They Leave.* London: Jessica Kingsley.

Skinner, B.F. (1953) *Science and Human Behaviour.* London: Collier Macmillan.

Skinner, B.F. (1973) *Beyond Freedom and Dignity.* Harmondsworth: Penguin.

Skinner, B.F. (1977) *About Behaviourism.* New York: Alfred A. Knopf.

Slater, E. & Cowie, V. (1971) *The Genetics of Mental Disorders.* London: Oxford University Press.

Slevin, M. (2003) *Resuscitating the NHS.* London: Centre for Policy Studies.

Sloan, J.J.I., Smykla, J.O. and Rush, J.P. (2004) 'Do juvenile drug courts reduce recidivism?: Outcomes of drug court and an adolescent substance abuse programme', *American Journal of Criminal Justice*, 29, 1, 95–115.

Sloper, P. (1999) 'Models of service support for parents of disabled children: what do we know? What do we need to know?', *Child Care, Health and Development*, 25, 85–99.

Sloper, P. and Turner, S. (1992) 'Service needs of families of children with severe physical disability', *Child Care, Health and Development*, 18, 259–282.

Sloper, P., Greco, V., Beecham, J. and Webb, R. (2006) 'Key worker services for disabled children: what characteristics of services lead to better outcomes for children and families?', *Child Care, Health and Development*, 32, 2, 147–157.

Smith, C. (1996) *Developing Parenting Programmes*. London: National Children's Bureau.

Smith, C.A. and Farrington, D.P. (2004) 'Continuities in antisocial behavior and parenting across three generations', *Journal of Child Psychology and Psychiatry*, 45, 2, 230–247.

Smith, J.E. and Rachman, S.J. (1984) 'Non-accidental injury to children 11: a controlled evaluation of a behavioural management programme', *Behaviour Research and Therapy*, 22, 4, 349–366.

Snow, C.P. (1933) *The Two Cultures*. Cambridge: Cambridge University Press.

Social Care Institute for Excellence (SCIE) (2002) *Annual Report*. SCIE. London.

Social Care Institute for Excellence (SCIE) (2006) *Using Qualitative Research in Systematic Reviews: Older People's Views of Hospital Discharge*. SCIE. London.

Social Services Inspectorate (SSI) (2002) *A Joint Chief Inspectors' Report on Safeguarding Children*. London: Social Services Inspectorate, Commission for Health Improvement, Her Majesty's Inspectorate of Constabulary, Her Majesty's Crown Prosecution Inspectorate, Her Majesty's Magistrates' Courts Inspectorate, Ofsted, Her Majesty's Inspectorate of Prisons, Her Majesty's Inspectorate of Probation.

Socialstyrelsen (2003) *Knowledge Development in Social Services – A Presentation of the Project for National Support*. Stockholm: The National Board of Health and Welfare.

Sokal, A. and Bricmont, J. (1998) *Intellectual Impostures*. London: Profile Books.

Soloman, S.D., Gerrity, E.T. and Muff, A.N. (1992) 'Efficacy of treatments for post-traumatic stress disorder: an empirical review', *JAMA*, 268, 6338.

Solzhenitsyn, A. (1974) *The Gulag Archipelago* (3 vols). New York: Harper & Row.

Spencer, N. (2000) *Poverty and Child Health* (2nd edn). Oxford: Radcliffe Medical Press.

St Pierre, R.G., Layzer, J.I., Goodson, B.D. and Bernstein, L.S. (1999) 'The effectiveness of comprehensive case management interventions. Evidence from the national evaluation of the Comprehensive Child Development Program', *American Journal of Evaluation*, 20, 1, 15–34.

Stallworthy, J. (1974) *Wilfred Owen, A Biography*. London: Oxford University Press/Chatto & Windus.

Stanton, M.D. and Shadish, W.R. (1997) 'Outcome, attrition, and family-couples treatment for drug abuse: a meta-analysis and review of the controlled, comparative studies', *Psychological Bulletin*, 122, 2, 170–191.

Statham, J. and Holtermann, S. (2004) 'Families on the brink: the effectiveness of family support services', *Child and Family Social Work*, 9, 153–166.

Stein, M. (2004) *What Works for Young People Leaving Care?* Ilford: Barnardos.

Stein, M. (2006) 'Research Review: Young people leaving care', *Child and Family Social Work*, 11, 3, 273–279.

Stein, S.L., Garcia, F., and Marler, B. (1992) 'A study of multiagency collaborative strategies: did juvenile delinquents change?', *Journal of Community Psychology*, 20, 88–105.

Stein, T.J. and Gambrill, E.D. (1976) 'Behavioural techniques in foster care', *Social Work*, 21, 1, 34–39.

Steinbeck, J. (1939) *The Grapes of Wrath*. New York: Viking.

Stepney, P. and Ford, D. (eds) (2000) *Social Work Models, Methods and Theories*. Lyme Regis: Russell House Publishing.

Strang, H. and Sherman, L. (2006) 'Restorative justice to reduce victimization', in B.C. Welsh and D.P. Farrington (eds), *Preventing Crime: What Works for Children, Offenders, Victims, and Places*. Dordrecht: Springer.

Stuart, S. and Bowers, W. (1995) 'Cognitive therapy with in patients: review and meta-analysis', *Journal of Cognitive Psychotherapy*, 9, 85–92.

Stuart, S. and Thase, N. (1994) 'In-patient aplications of cognitive-behavioural therapy: a review of recent developments', *Journal of Psychotherapy Practice and Research*, 3, 284–299.

Sutton, C. (1994) *Social Work, Community Work and Psychology*. Leicester: British Psychological Society Books.

Swain, J., Finkelstein, V., French, S. and Oliver, M. (eds) (1993) *Disabling Barriers – Enabling Environments* (2nd edition). London: Sage.

Swain, J., French, S. and Cameron, C. (2003) *Controversial Issues in a Disabling Society* Maidenhead: Open University Press.

Swenson, C.C. and Hanson, R.F. (1997) 'Sexual abuse of children: assessment, research, and treatment', in. J. Lutzker (ed.) *Handbook of Child Abuse Research and Treatment: Issues in Clinical Child Psychology*. New York: Plenum Press.

Sylva, K. (1994) 'School influences on children's development', *Journal of Child Psychology and Psychiatry and Allied Professions*, 35, 1, 135–170.

Szasz, T. (1961) *The Myth of Mental Illness*. New York: Harper & Row.

Szasz, T.S. (1971) *The Manufacture of Madness*. London: Routledge & Kegan Paul.

Taft, J. (1920) 'The relation of psychiatry to social work', *The Family*, 7, 199–201.

Tait, R.J. and Hulse, G.K. (2003) 'A systematic review of the effectiveness of brief interventions with substance using adolescents by type of drug' (DARE structured abstract)', *Drug and Alcohol Review*, 22, 337–346.

Tait, T., Beattie, A. and Dejnega, S. (2002) 'Service coordination: a successful model for the delivery of multi-professional services to children with complex needs', *Journal of Research in Nursing*, 8, 1, 19–32.

Tanner, D. (1998) 'Empowerment and care management: swimming against the tide', *Health and Social Care in the Community*, 6, 6, 447–457.

Tanner, D. and Harris, J. (2008) *Working with Older People*. London: Routledge.

Taylor-Browne, J. (2001) *What Works in Reducing Domestic Violence: A Comprehensive Guide for Professionals*. London: Whiting and Birch.

Tedeschi, J.T. (1972) *The Social Influence Processes*. London: Aldive.

Temerlin, M.K. (1968) 'Suggestive effects in psychiatric diagnoses', *Journal of Nervous and Mental Disease*, 147, 4, 16–27.

Thapar, A., Davies, G., Jones, T. and Rivett, M. (1992) 'Treatment of childhood encopresis: a review', *Child Care, Health and Development*, 8, 343–353.

Tharyan, P. and Adams, C.E. (2005) Electroconvulsive therapy for schizophrenia. *Cochrane Database of Systematic Reviews* 2005, Issue 2. Art. No.: CD000076. DOI: 10.1002/14651858.CD000076.pub2.

Thatcher, M. (2002) *Statecraft: Strategies for a Changing World*. London: HarperCollins.

Thiele, L.P. (2006) *The Heart of Judgement: Practical Wisdom, Neuroscience and Narrative*. Cambridge: Cambridge University Press.

Thoburn, J., Lewis, A. and Shemmings, D. (1995) 'Paternalism or partnership? Family involvement in the child protection process', *Studies in Child Protection*. London: HMSO.

Thomas, A. and Chess. S. (1982) 'Temperament and follow up to adulthood', in A.R. Porter and G.M. Collins (eds), *Temperamental Differences in Young Children*. London: Pitman.

Thomas, A., Chess, S. and Birch, H.G. (1968) *Temperament and Behaviour Disorder in Children*. New York: New York University Press.

Thomas, C.M. and Morris, M. (2003) 'Cost of depression among adults in England in 2000', *British Journal of Psychiatry*, 183, 514–519.

Thomas, M. (2005) *Social Work with Young People in Care*. Basingstoke: Palgrave Macmillan.

Thomas, N. and O'Kane, C. (1998) 'The ethics of participatory research with children', *Children and Society*, 12, 5, 336–348.

Thompson, N. (2001) *Anti-Discriminatory Practice* (3rd edition). Basingstoke: Palgrave.

Thorndike, E.L. (1898) 'Animal intelligence: an experimental study of the associative processess in animals', *Psychological Review*, Monograph 2.

Thornton, D.M., Curran, L., Grayson, D. and Holloway, V. (1984) *Tougher Regimes in Detention Centres: Report of an Evaluation by the Young Offenders Psychology Unit*. London: HMSO.

Thyer, B. (1989) *Behavioral Family Therapy*. Springfield, IL: Charles C. Thomas.

Tierney, S. (2004) *A Study of the Effectiveness of Interventions for Eating Disorders*. Ph.D. Thesis, University of Exeter.

Timmins, N. (2001) *The Five Giants: A Biography of the Welfare State*. London: HarperCollins.

Titmuss, R. (1957) *Essays on the Welfare State*. London: Allen & Unwin.

Townsley, R., Abbott, D. and Watson, D. (2004) *Making a Difference? Exploring the Impact of Multi-agency Working on Disabled Children with Complex Health Care Needs, Their Families and the Professionals Who Support Them*. Bristol: Policy Press.

Tracey, E.M. and Farkas, K.J. (1994) 'Preparing practitioners for child welfare practice with substance-abusing families', *Child Welfare*, 75, 57–68.

Training Organization for Personal Social Services (TOPSS) (2002) *Annual Report*. Leeds: TOPSS.

Trappes-Lomax, T., Ellis, A.J. and Fox, M (2002) *Buying Time: An Evaluation and Cost Effectiveness Analysis of a Joint Health/Social Care Residential Rehabilitation Unit for Older People on Discharge from Hospital*. Centre for Evidence-based Social Services, University of Exeter.

Trappes-Lomax, T., Ellis, A., Terry, R. and Stead, J. (2003) *The User Voice: Three Qualitative Studies of the Views of Older People Concerning Rehabilitation Services*. Centre for Evidence-based Social Services, University of Exeter.

Trevelyan, G.M. (1944) *English Social History*. London: Longmans, Green & Co.

Trinder, E. and Reynolds, S. (2000) *Evidence-based Practice: A Critical Appraisal*. Oxford. Blackwell Scientific.

Triseliotis, J. (2002) 'Long-term foster care or adoption? The evidence examined', *Child and Family Social Work*, 7, 23–33.

Triseliotis, J., Borland, M. and Hill, M. (1999) *Delivering Foster Care*. London; BAAF.

Triseliotis, J., Borland, M., Hill, M. and Lambert, L. (1995) *Teenagers and the Social Work Services*. London; HMSO.

Truax, C. and Carkhuff, R. (1966) *Towards Effective Counselling and Psychotherapy*. Chicago, IL: Aldine.

Tsogia, D., Copello, A. and Orford, J. (2001) 'Entering treatment for substance misuse: a review of the literature', *Journal of Mental Health*, 10, 5, 481–499.

Tsuang, M.T. and Vandermey, R. (1980) *Genes and the Mind: Inheritance of Mental Illness*, Oxford: Oxford University Press.

Tunstill, J. (1997) 'Implementing the family support clauses of the 1989 Children Act. Legislative, professional and organisational obstacles', in N. Parton (ed.), *Child Protection and Family Support. Tensions, Contradictions and Possibilities*. London: Routledge.

Tunstill, J., Meadows, P., Akhurst, S., Allnock D., Chrysanthou, J., Garbers, C., Morley, A. and the National Evaluation of Sure Start Team (2005) *Report 10: Implementing Sure Start Local Programmes: An Integrated Overview of the First Four Years*. London: HMSO.

Turner, L.C.F. (1970) *Origins of the First World War*. London: Edward Arnold.

Turner, W., Macdonald, G.M. and Dennis, J.A. (2007) 'Behavioural and cognitive behavioural training interventions for assisting foster carers in the management of difficult behaviour', *Cochrane Database of Systematic Reviews*, Issue 1. Art No. CD003760.

Tuvblad, C., Grann, M. and Lichtenstein, P. (2006) 'Heritability for adolescent antisocial behavior differs with socioeconomic status: gene-environment interaction', *Journal of Child Pscyhology and Psychiatry*, 47, 7, 34–43.

Twelvetrees, A. (2002) *Community Work*. Basingstoke: Palgrave.

Tymchuk, A. and Feldman, M. (1991) 'Parents with mental retardation and their children: review of research relevant to professional practice', *Canadian Psychology*, 32, 486–496.

Ullman, L.P. and Krasner, L. (1969) *A Psychological Approach to Abnormal Behaviour*. Englewood Cliffs, NJ: Prentice Hall International.

Unnithan, A., Glossop, M. and Strang, J. (1992) 'Factors associated with relapse among opiate addicts in an outpatient detoxification programme', *British Journal of Psychiatry*, 161, 654–657.

UPIAS (1976) *Fundamental Principles of Disability*. London: Union of Physically Impaired Against Segregation.

Utting, D. (1996) *Reducing Criminality Among Young People: A Sample of Relevant Programmes in the United Kingdom*. London: Home Office.

Utting, D. and Vennard, J. (2000) *What Works with Young Offenders in the Community?* Barkingside: Barnardos.

Utting, W. (1991) *Children in the Public Care*. London: HMSO.

Valenstein, E.S. (ed.) (1980) *The Psychology Debate*. New York: Freeman.

Vaughn, C.E. and Leff, J.P. (1976a) 'The influence of family and social factors on the cause of psychiatric illness: a comparison of schizophrenic and depressed neurotic patients', *British Journal of Psychiatry*, 129, 125–137.

Vaughn, C.E. and Leff, J.P. (1976b) 'The measurement of expressed emotion in families of psychiatric patients', *British Journal of Social and Clinical Psychology*, 15, 159–165.

Veblen, A. (1966) *The Leisure Class*. Harmondsworth: Penguin.

Wade, J. and Biehal, N. with Clayden, J. and Stein, M. (1998) *Going Missing: Young People Absent from Care*. Chichester: Wiley.

Wade, J. and Dixon, J. (2006) 'Making a home, finding a job: investigating early housing and employment outcomes for young people leaving care', *Child and Family Social Work*, 11, 3, 199–208.

Waldron, H.B. (1996) 'Adolescent substance abuse and family therapy outcome: a review of randomised trials', *Advances in Clinical Child Psychology*, 19, 199–234.

Walker, S. and Akister, J. (2004) *Applying Family Therapy: A Guide for Caring Professionals in the Community*. Lyme Regis: Russell House Publishing.

Wanigaratne, S., Davis, P., Pryce, K. and Brotchie, J. (2005) *The Effectiveness of Psychological Therapies on Drug Misusing Clients*. National Treatment Agency for Substance Misuse: Research Briefing 11. London: NHS.

Wanless, D. (2006) *Securing Good Care for Older People: Taking a Long-term View*. London: Kings Fund.

Watson, J.B. and Rayner, R. (1920) 'Conditioned emotional reactions', *Journal of Experimental Psychology*, 3, 1–14.

Webb, S.A. (2001) 'Some considerations on the validity of evidence-based practice in Social Work', *British Journal of Social Work*, 31, 57–79.

Webster, J.D. and Haight, B.K. (eds) (2002) *Critical Advances in Reminiscence Work: From Theory to Application*. New York: Springer.

Webster-Stratton, C. and Herbert, M. (1993) 'What really happens in parent-training?', *Behavior Modification*, 17, 407–456.

Webster-Stratton, C. and Herbert, M. (1994) *Troubled Families – Problem Children. Working with Parents: A Collaborative Process*. Chichester: John Wiley.

Weiner, N. (1948/1961) *Cybernetic, or Control and Communication in the Animal and Machine*. Cambridge, MA: MIT Press.

Welsh, B.C. and Farrington, D.P. (2001) 'A review of research on the monetary value of preventing crime', in B.C. Welsh, D.P. Farrington and L.W. Sherman (eds), *Costs and Benefits of Preventing Crime*. Oxford: Westview Press.

West, D.J. and Farrington, D.P. (1973) *Who Becomes Delinquent?* London: Heinemann.

Whitaker, D.S. and Archer, J.L. (1989) *Research by Social Workers: Capitalising on Experience*, CCETSW Study 9. London: CCETSW.

White, A. (1933/1978) *Frost in May*. London: Virago Classics.

White, M. (2000) *Reflections on Narrative Practice: Essays and Interviews*. Adelaide: Dulwich Centre Publications.

White, M. and Epston, D. (1989) *Literate Means to Therapeutic Ends*. Adelaide: Dulwich Centre Publications (republished in 1990 as *Narrative Means to Therapeutic Ends*. New York: Norton).

Whiteman, M., Fanshel, D. and Grundy, J.F. (1987) 'Cognitive-behavioral interventions aimed at anger of parents at risk of child abuse', *Social Work*, November-December, 469–474.

Whittaker, D., Archer, L. and Hicks, L. (1998) *Working in Children's Homes: Challenges and Complexities*. Chichester: John Wiley

Who Cares Trust (1993) *Not Just a Name: The Views of Young People in Foster and Residential Care*. London: National Consumer Council.

Widom, C. (1997) 'Child abuse, neglect and witnessing violence', in D.M. Stoff, J. Breiling and J.D. Master (eds), *Handbook of Antisocial Behavior*, New York: Wiley.

Wikström, P-O.H. and Butterworth, D.A. (2006) *Adolescent Crime: Individual Differences and Lifestyles*. Cullompton: Willen Publishing.

Wikström, P-O.H. and Sampson, R.J. (2003) 'Social mechanisms of community influences on crime and pathways in criminality', in B.B. Lahey, T.E. Moffitt and A. Caspi (eds), *Causes of Conduct Disorder and Juvenile Delinquency*. New York: The Guilford Press.

Wilber, G.T. and Fairburn, C.G. (2002) 'Treatments for eating disorders', in P.E. Nathan and J.M. Gorman (eds), *A Guide to Treatments that Work*. Oxford: Oxford University Press.

Williams, F. (2001) 'In and beyond New Labour: towards a new political ethics of care', *Critical Social Policy*, 21, 4, 467–493.

Wilson, D.B. and Chipungu, S.S. (1996) 'Introduction' to Special edition: Kinship Care, *Child Welfare*, 75, 5, 387.

Wilson, D.B. and MacKenzie, D.L. (2006) 'Boot camps', in B.C. Welsh and D.P. Farrington (eds), *Preventing Crime: What Works for Children, Offenders, Victims, and Places*. Dordrecht: Springer.

Wilson, D., Sharp, C. and Patterson, A. (2006) *Young People and Crime: Findings from the 2005 Offending, Crime and Justice Survey*. London: Home Office.

Wilson, E.O. (1998) *Consilience: The Unity of Knowledge*. London: Little, Brown & Co.

Wilson, T. and Fairburn, C. (1998) 'Treatments for eating disorders', in P. Nathan and J. Gorman (eds) *A Guide to Treatments that Work*. New York: Oxford University Press.

Winokur, M., Holtan, A. and Valentine, D. (2007) 'Kinship care for the safety, permanency, and well-being of children removed from the home for maltreatment. (Protocol)', *Cochrane Database of Systematic Reviews* 2007, Issue 2. Art. No.: CD006546. DOI: 10.1002/14651858.CD006546. Review in press.

Wodarski, J.S., Howing, P.T., Kurthz, P.D. and Gaudin, J.M. (1990) 'Maltreatment and the school-age child: major academic, socio-emotional and adaptive outcomes', *Social Work*, 35, 506–513.

Wolfe, D.A. and Sandler, J. (1981) 'Training abusive parents in effective child management', *Behavior Modification*, 5, 320–335.

Wolfe, D., Kaufman, K., Aragona, J. and Sandler, J. (1981) *The Child Management Program for Abusive Parents: Procedures for Developing a Child Abuse Intervention Program.* Winter Park, FL: Anna Publishing.

Wolfe, D.A., St Lawrence, J.S., Graves, K., Brehony, K., Bradlyn, A.S. and Kelly, J.A. (1982) 'Intensive behavioral parent training for a child abusive mother', *Behavior Therapy*, 13, 438–451.

Wolfe, D.A., Wekerle, C., Reitzel-Jaffe, D., Grasley, C., Pittman, A. and MacEachran, A. (1997) 'Interrupting the cycle of violence: empowering youth to promote healthy relationships', in D.A. Wolfe, R.J. McMahon and R. De V. Peters (eds) *Child Abuse: New Directions in Prevention and Treatment across the Lifespan.* Thousand Oaks, CA: Sage.

Wolpert, L. (1999) *Malignant Sadness: The Anatomy of Depression.* London: Faber & Faber.

Woodcock, A. and Davis, M. (1978) *Catastrophe Theory.* Harmondsworth: Penguin.

Woodroofe, K. (1966) *From Charity to Social Work.* London: Rowntree.

Woods, B., Spector, A., Jones, C., Orrell, M. and Davies, S. (2005) 'Reminiscence therapy for dementia', *Cochrane Database of Systematic Reviews* 2005, Issue 2. Art. No.: CD001120. DOI: 10.1002/14651858.CD001120.pub2.

Woods, R.T. (1997) 'Why should family caregivers feel guilty?', in M. Marshall (ed.) *State of the Art in Dementia Care.* London: Centre for Policy on Ageing.

Woolfenden, S.R., Williams, K. and Peat, J. (2001) Family and parenting interventions in children and adolescents with conduct disorder and delinquency aged 10–17. *Cochrane Database of Systematic Reviews* 2001, Issue 2. Art. No.: CD003015. DOI: 10.1002/14651858.CD003015.

Wright Mills, C. (1943) 'The professional ideology of social pathologists', *American Journal of Sociology*, 49, 165–180.

Wright, J. and Ruebain, D. (2002) *Taking Action! Your Child's Right to Special Education* (3rd edition). Birmingham: Questions Publishing Company.

Wurtele, S.K., Kast, L.C., Miller-Perin, C.L. and Kondrick, P.A. (1989) 'Comparison of programs for teaching personal safety to preschoolers', *Journal of Consulting and Clinical Psychology*, 57, 505–511.

Young, J. (1996) 'Rehabilitation and older people', *British Medical Journal*, 3213: 677–681.

Younghusband, E. (1951) *Social Work in Britain.* Edinburgh: Carnegie Trust.

Youth Justice Board (2002) *Intensive Supervision and Surveillance Programme (ISSP): A New Option for Dealing with Prolific and Serious Young Offenders.* London: Youth Justice Board Leaflet.

Youth Justice Board (2003) *Substance Misuse: Key Elements of Effective Practice.* London: Youth Justice Board Leaflet.

Youth Justice Board (2004) *Cognitive Behaviour Projects.* London: Youth Justice Board.

Youth Justice Board (2007) *Groups, Gangs and Weapons.* London: Youth Justice Board.

Zarit, S. and Edwards, A. (1999) 'Family caregiving: research and clinical intervention', in R.T. Woods (ed.) *Psychological Problems of Ageing: Assessment, Treatment and Care.* Chichester: John Wiley & Sons.

Zerbin-Rudin, E. (1967) 'Endogene Psychosen'. In *Humangenetik: em kurzes Handbuch.* V/2 ed Becker, P. E. Stuttgart.

Zimbardo, P.G. (2000) *Psychology and Life* (13th edn). New York: HarperCollins.

Zwi, K.J., Woolfenden, S.R., Wheeler, D.M., O'Brien, T.A., Tait, P. and Williams, K.W. (2007) 'School-based education programmes for the prevention of child sexual abuse', *Cochrane Database of Systematic Reviews* 2007, Issue 3. Art. No.: CD004380. DOI: 10.1002/14651858.CD004380.pub2.

Index